50% OFF

Online CHPN® Prep Course!

Dear Customer,

Thank you for your purchase of this CHPN Study Guide. Included with your purchase is **discounted access to our online CHPN Prep Course**. Many CHPN courses are needlessly expensive and don't deliver enough value. Our course provides the best CHPN prep material, and with discounted access, **you only pay half price**.

We have structured our online course to perfectly complement your printed study guide. The CHPN Prep Course contains **in-depth lessons** that cover all the most important topics, **600 practice questions** to ensure you feel prepared, and more than **350 digital flashcards**, so you can study while you're on the go.

Online CHPN Prep Course

Topics Included:

- Patient Care
  - Pain Management
  - Symptom Management
- Support, Education, Advocacy
  - Advance Care Planning
  - Therapeutic Communication
- Practice Issues
  - Standards of Practice
  - Strategies for Self-Care and Stress Management

Course Features:

- CHPN Study Guide
  - Get content that complements our best-selling study guide.
- 4 Full-Length Practice Tests
  - With 600 practice questions, you can test yourself again and again.
- Mobile Friendly
  - If you need to study on the go, the course is easily accessible from your mobile device.
- CHPN Flashcards
  - Our course includes a flashcard mode with over 350 content cards to help you study.

To lock in your discounted access, visit mometrix.com/university/chpn or simply scan this QR code with your smartphone. At the checkout page, enter the discount code: **CHPN50off**

If you have any questions or concerns, please contact us at support@mometrix.com.

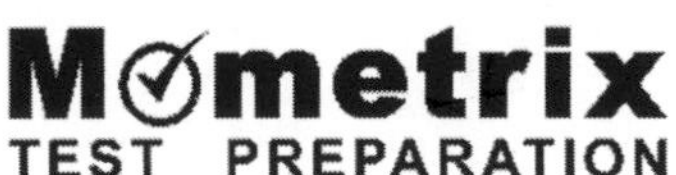

ACCESS YOUR ONLINE RESOURCES

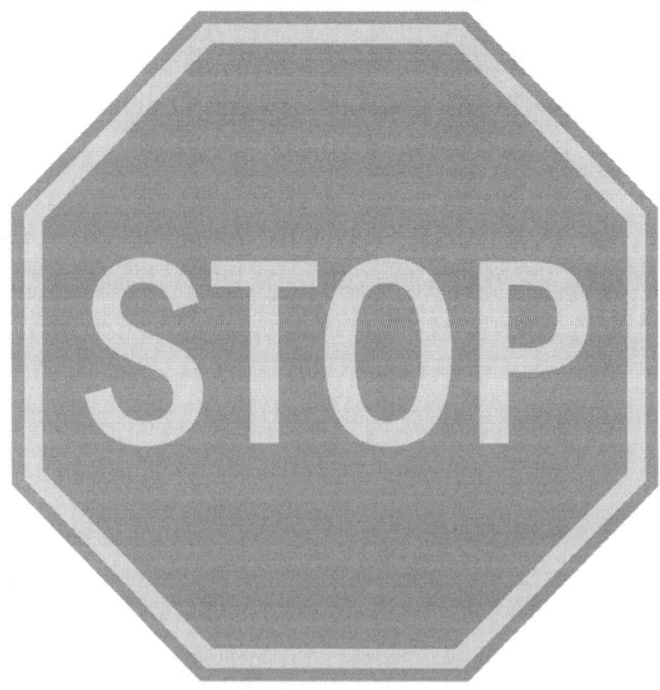

DON'T MISS OUT ON THE ONLINE RESOURCES INCLUDED WITH YOUR PURCHASE!

Your purchase of this product unlocks access to our Online Resources page. Elevate your study experience with our **interactive practice test interface**, along with all of the additional resources that we couldn't include in this book.

Flip to the Online Resources section at the end of this book to find the link and a QR code to get started!

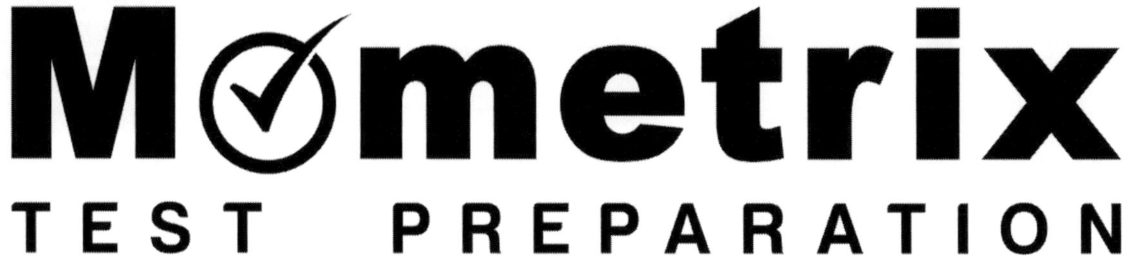

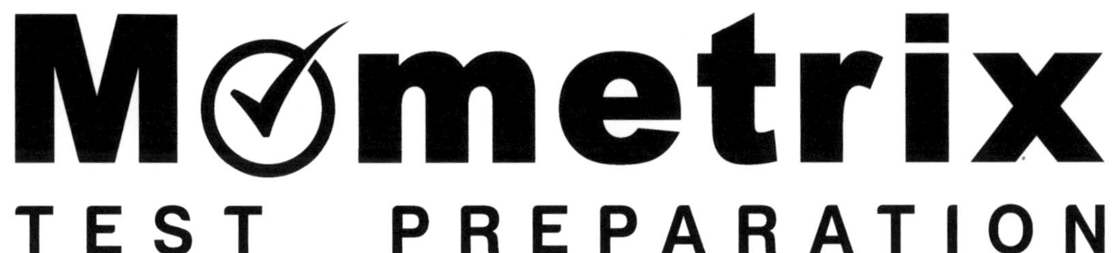

CHPN®

Exam Secrets Study Guide

2 Full-Length Practice Tests

Unofficial Exam Review and CHPN® Practice Test for the Certified Hospice and Palliative Nurse Test

Written and edited by Mometrix Test Prep

Printed in the United States of America

This paper meets the requirements of ANSI/NISO Z39.48-1992 (Permanence of Paper).

Paperback
ISBN 13: 978-1-5167-1900-6
ISBN 10: 1-5167-1900-X

DEAR FUTURE EXAM SUCCESS STORY

First of all, **THANK YOU** for purchasing Mometrix study materials!

Second, congratulations! You are one of the few determined test-takers who are committed to doing whatever it takes to excel on your exam. **You have come to the right place.** We developed these study materials with one goal in mind: to deliver you the information you need in a format that's concise and easy to use.

In addition to optimizing your guide for the content of the test, we've outlined our recommended steps for breaking down the preparation process into small, attainable goals so you can make sure you stay on track.

We've also analyzed the entire test-taking process, identifying the most common pitfalls and showing how you can overcome them and be ready for any curveball the test throws you.

Standardized testing is one of the biggest obstacles on your road to success, which only increases the importance of doing well in the high-pressure, high-stakes environment of test day. Your results on this test could have a significant impact on your future, and this guide provides the information and practical advice to help you achieve your full potential on test day.

Your success is our success

We would love to hear from you! If you would like to share the story of your exam success or if you have any questions or comments in regard to our products, please contact us at **800-673-8175** or **support@mometrix.com**.

Thanks again for your business and we wish you continued success!

Sincerely,
The Mometrix Test Preparation Team

Need more help? Check out our flashcards at:
http://mometrixflashcards.com/NBCHPN

Table of Contents

Introduction 1

Secret Key #1 – Plan Big, Study Small 2

Secret Key #2 – Make Your Studying Count 3

Secret Key #3 – Practice the Right Way 4

Secret Key #4 – Pace Yourself 6

Secret Key #5 – Have a Plan for Guessing 7

Test-Taking Strategies 10

Five-Week CHPN Study Plan 14
- Week 1: Patient Care: Assessment and Planning 14
- Week 2: Patient Care: Pain Management 15
- Week 3: Patient Care: Symptom Management 15
- Week 4: Support, Education, and Advocacy; Practice Issues 16
- Week 5: Practice Tests 17

Patient Care: Assessment and Planning 19
- Goals of Care and Shared Decision Making 19
- Interdisciplinary Care Planning and Ongoing Evaluation 28
- Life-Limiting Disease Progression, Complications, and Treatment 32
- Indicators of Imminent Death 50

Patient Care: Pain Management 57
- Etiology of Pain, Types of Pain, and Pain Syndromes 57
- Pain Scales 61
- Factors that Influence the Pain Experience 65
- Pharmacologic Pain Management 68
- Non-Pharmacologic Interventions 75
- Complementary and Alternative Therapies 78

Patient Care: Symptom Management 83
- Systems Review 83
- System-Specific End Stage Disease Progression 85
- Nutrition Assessment 101
- Psychosocial, Emotional, and Spiritual 102
- Hospice and Palliative Care Emergencies 109

Support, Education, and Advocacy 111
- Advance Care Planning 111
- Hospice and Palliative Care Benefits 113
- Patient Needs and Patient Safety 119
- Psychosocial, Spiritual, and Cultural Needs 123
- Life Completion and Search for Meaning 125
- Caregiver/Family Self-Care Activities 128
- Principles of Hospice and Palliative Education 131

Therapeutic Communication 137
Grief and Loss Support/Bereavement Services 140
Postmortem Care and Services 143
Ethical Issues Related to End of Life 146
Practice Issues 149
Standards of Practice 149
Strategies for Self-Care and Stress Management 151
Quality Improvement in Hospice and Palliative Care 153
CHPN Practice Test #1 155
Answer Key and Explanations for Test #1 179
CHPN Practice Test #2 205
Answer Key and Explanations for Test #2 228
How to Overcome Test Anxiety 248
Online Resources 254

Introduction

Thank you for purchasing this resource! You have made the choice to prepare yourself for a test that could have a huge impact on your future, and this guide is designed to help you be fully ready for test day. Obviously, it's important to have a solid understanding of the test material, but you also need to be prepared for the unique environment and stressors of the test, so that you can perform to the best of your abilities.

For this purpose, the first section that appears in this guide is the **Secret Keys**. We've devoted countless hours to meticulously researching what works and what doesn't, and we've boiled down our findings to the five most impactful steps you can take to improve your performance on the test. We start at the beginning with study planning and move through the preparation process, all the way to the testing strategies that will help you get the most out of what you know when you're finally sitting in front of the test.

We recommend that you start preparing for your test as far in advance as possible. However, if you've bought this guide as a last-minute study resource and only have a few days before your test, we recommend that you skip over the first two Secret Keys since they address a long-term study plan.

If you struggle with **test anxiety**, we strongly encourage you to check out our recommendations for how you can overcome it. Test anxiety is a formidable foe, but it can be beaten, and we want to make sure you have the tools you need to defeat it.

Secret Key #1 – Plan Big, Study Small

There's a lot riding on your performance. If you want to ace this test, you're going to need to keep your skills sharp and the material fresh in your mind. You need a plan that lets you review everything you need to know while still fitting in your schedule. We'll break this strategy down into three categories.

Information Organization

Start with the information you already have: the official test outline. From this, you can make a complete list of all the concepts you need to cover before the test. Organize these concepts into groups that can be studied together, and create a list of any related vocabulary you need to learn so you can brush up on any difficult terms. You'll want to keep this vocabulary list handy once you actually start studying since you may need to add to it along the way.

Time Management

Once you have your set of study concepts, decide how to spread them out over the time you have left before the test. Break your study plan into small, clear goals so you have a manageable task for each day and know exactly what you're doing. Then just focus on one small step at a time. When you manage your time this way, you don't need to spend hours at a time studying. Studying a small block of content for a short period each day helps you retain information better and avoid stressing over how much you have left to do. You can relax knowing that you have a plan to cover everything in time. In order for this strategy to be effective though, you have to start studying early and stick to your schedule. Avoid the exhaustion and futility that comes from last-minute cramming!

Study Environment

The environment you study in has a big impact on your learning. Studying in a coffee shop, while probably more enjoyable, is not likely to be as fruitful as studying in a quiet room. It's important to keep distractions to a minimum. You're only planning to study for a short block of time, so make the most of it. Don't pause to check your phone or get up to find a snack. It's also important to **avoid multitasking**. Research has consistently shown that multitasking will make your studying dramatically less effective. Your study area should also be comfortable and well-lit so you don't have the distraction of straining your eyes or sitting on an uncomfortable chair.

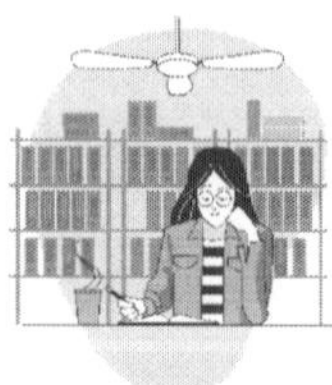

The time of day you study is also important. You want to be rested and alert. Don't wait until just before bedtime. Study when you'll be most likely to comprehend and remember. Even better, if you know what time of day your test will be, set that time aside for study. That way your brain will be used to working on that subject at that specific time and you'll have a better chance of recalling information.

Finally, it can be helpful to team up with others who are studying for the same test. Your actual studying should be done in as isolated an environment as possible, but the work of organizing the information and setting up the study plan can be divided up. In between study sessions, you can discuss with your teammates the concepts that you're all studying and quiz each other on the details. Just be sure that your teammates are as serious about the test as you are. If you find that your study time is being replaced with social time, you might need to find a new team.

Secret Key #2 – Make Your Studying Count

You're devoting a lot of time and effort to preparing for this test, so you want to be absolutely certain it will pay off. This means doing more than just reading the content and hoping you can remember it on test day. It's important to make every minute of study count. There are two main areas you can focus on to make your studying count.

Retention

It doesn't matter how much time you study if you can't remember the material. You need to make sure you are retaining the concepts. To check your retention of the information you're learning, try recalling it at later times with minimal prompting. Try carrying around flashcards and glance at one or two from time to time or ask a friend who's also studying for the test to quiz you.

To enhance your retention, look for ways to put the information into practice so that you can apply it rather than simply recalling it. If you're using the information in practical ways, it will be much easier to remember. Similarly, it helps to solidify a concept in your mind if you're not only reading it to yourself but also explaining it to someone else. Ask a friend to let you teach them about a concept you're a little shaky on (or speak aloud to an imaginary audience if necessary). As you try to summarize, define, give examples, and answer your friend's questions, you'll understand the concepts better and they will stay with you longer. Finally, step back for a big picture view and ask yourself how each piece of information fits with the whole subject. When you link the different concepts together and see them working together as a whole, it's easier to remember the individual components.

Finally, practice showing your work on any multi-step problems, even if you're just studying. Writing out each step you take to solve a problem will help solidify the process in your mind, and you'll be more likely to remember it during the test.

Modality

Modality simply refers to the means or method by which you study. Choosing a study modality that fits your own individual learning style is crucial. No two people learn best in exactly the same way, so it's important to know your strengths and use them to your advantage.

For example, if you learn best by visualization, focus on visualizing a concept in your mind and draw an image or a diagram. Try color-coding your notes, illustrating them, or creating symbols that will trigger your mind to recall a learned concept. If you learn best by hearing or discussing information, find a study partner who learns the same way or read aloud to yourself. Think about how to put the information in your own words. Imagine that you are giving a lecture on the topic and record yourself so you can listen to it later.

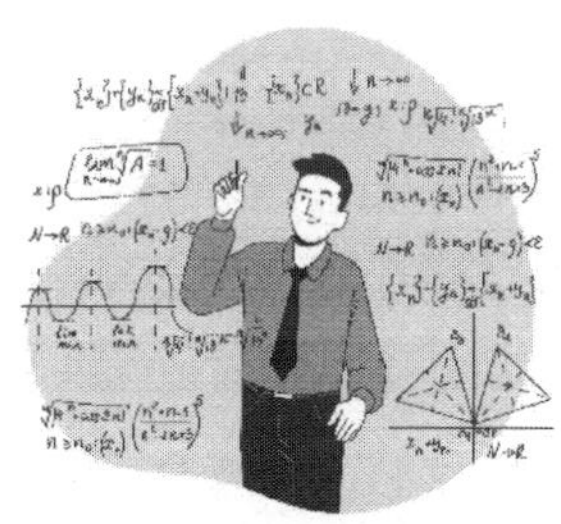

For any learning style, flashcards can be helpful. Organize the information so you can take advantage of spare moments to review. Underline key words or phrases. Use different colors for different categories. Mnemonic devices (such as creating a short list in which every item starts with the same letter) can also help with retention. Find what works best for you and use it to store the information in your mind most effectively and easily.

Secret Key #3 – Practice the Right Way

Your success on test day depends not only on how many hours you put into preparing, but also on whether you prepared the right way. It's good to check along the way to see if your studying is paying off. One of the most effective ways to do this is by taking practice tests to evaluate your progress. Practice tests are useful because they show exactly where you need to improve. Every time you take a practice test, pay special attention to these three groups of questions:

- The questions you got wrong
- The questions you had to guess on, even if you guessed right
- The questions you found difficult or slow to work through

This will show you exactly what your weak areas are, and where you need to devote more study time. Ask yourself why each of these questions gave you trouble. Was it because you didn't understand the material? Was it because you didn't remember the vocabulary? Do you need more repetitions on this type of question to build speed and confidence? Dig into those questions and figure out how you can strengthen your weak areas as you go back to review the material.

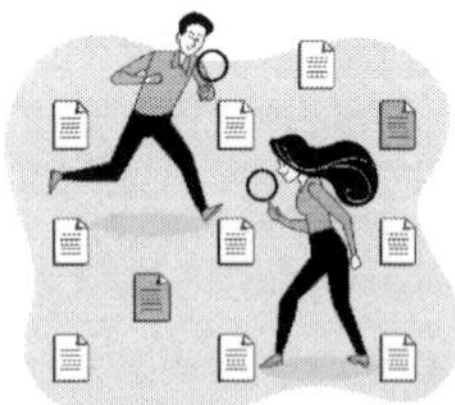

Additionally, many practice tests have a section explaining the answer choices. It can be tempting to read the explanation and think that you now have a good understanding of the concept. However, an explanation likely only covers part of the question's broader context. Even if the explanation makes perfect sense, **go back and investigate** every concept related to the question until you're positive you have a thorough understanding.

As you go along, keep in mind that the practice test is just that: practice. Memorizing these questions and answers will not be very helpful on the actual test because it is unlikely to have any of the same exact questions. If you only know the right answers to the sample questions, you won't be prepared for the real thing. **Study the concepts** until you understand them fully, and then you'll be able to answer any question that shows up on the test.

It's important to wait on the practice tests until you're ready. If you take a test on your first day of study, you may be overwhelmed by the amount of material covered and how much you need to learn. Work up to it gradually.

On test day, you'll need to be prepared for answering questions, managing your time, and using the test-taking strategies you've learned. It's a lot to balance, like a mental marathon that will have a big impact on your future. Like training for a marathon, you'll need to start slowly and work your way up. When test day arrives, you'll be ready.

Start with the strategies you've read in the first two Secret Keys—plan your course and study in the way that works best for you. If you have time, consider using multiple study resources to get different approaches to the same concepts. It can be helpful to see difficult concepts from more than one angle. Then find a good source for practice tests. Many times, the test website will suggest potential study resources or provide sample tests.

Practice Test Strategy

If you're able to find at least three practice tests, we recommend this strategy:

UNTIMED AND OPEN-BOOK PRACTICE

Take the first test with no time constraints and with your notes and study guide handy. Take your time and focus on applying the strategies you've learned.

TIMED AND OPEN-BOOK PRACTICE

Take the second practice test open-book as well, but set a timer and practice pacing yourself to finish in time.

TIMED AND CLOSED-BOOK PRACTICE

Take any other practice tests as if it were test day. Set a timer and put away your study materials. Sit at a table or desk in a quiet room, imagine yourself at the testing center, and answer questions as quickly and accurately as possible.

Keep repeating timed and closed-book tests on a regular basis until you run out of practice tests or it's time for the actual test. Your mind will be ready for the schedule and stress of test day, and you'll be able to focus on recalling the material you've learned.

Secret Key #4 – Pace Yourself

Once you're fully prepared for the material on the test, your biggest challenge on test day will be managing your time. Just knowing that the clock is ticking can make you panic even if you have plenty of time left. Work on pacing yourself so you can build confidence against the time constraints of the exam. Pacing is a difficult skill to master, especially in a high-pressure environment, so **practice is vital**.

Set time expectations for your pace based on how much time is available. For example, if a section has 60 questions and the time limit is 30 minutes, you know you have to average 30 seconds or less per question in order to answer them all. Although 30 seconds is the hard limit, set 25 seconds per question as your goal, so you reserve extra time to spend on harder questions. When you budget extra time for the harder questions, you no longer have any reason to stress when those questions take longer to answer.

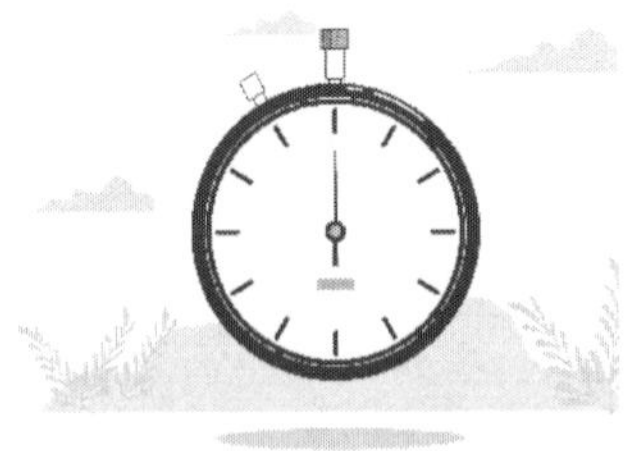

Don't let this time expectation distract you from working through the test at a calm, steady pace, but keep it in mind so you don't spend too much time on any one question. Recognize that taking extra time on one question you don't understand may keep you from answering two that you do understand later in the test. If your time limit for a question is up and you're still not sure of the answer, mark it and move on, and come back to it later if the time and the test format allow. If the testing format doesn't allow you to return to earlier questions, just make an educated guess; then put it out of your mind and move on.

On the easier questions, be careful not to rush. It may seem wise to hurry through them so you have more time for the challenging ones, but it's not worth missing one if you know the concept and just didn't take the time to read the question fully. Work efficiently but make sure you understand the question and have looked at all of the answer choices, since more than one may seem right at first.

Even if you're paying attention to the time, you may find yourself a little behind at some point. You should speed up to get back on track, but do so wisely. Don't panic; just take a few seconds less on each question until you're caught up. Don't guess without thinking, but do look through the answer choices and eliminate any you know are wrong. If you can get down to two choices, it is often worthwhile to guess from those. Once you've chosen an answer, move on and don't dwell on any that you skipped or had to hurry through. If a question was taking too long, chances are it was one of the harder ones, so you weren't as likely to get it right anyway.

On the other hand, if you find yourself getting ahead of schedule, it may be beneficial to slow down a little. The more quickly you work, the more likely you are to make a careless mistake that will affect your score. You've budgeted time for each question, so don't be afraid to spend that time. Practice an efficient but careful pace to get the most out of the time you have.

Secret Key #5 – Have a Plan for Guessing

When you're taking the test, you may find yourself stuck on a question. Some of the answer choices seem better than others, but you don't see the one answer choice that is obviously correct. What do you do?

The scenario described above is very common, yet most test takers have not effectively prepared for it. Developing and practicing a plan for guessing may be one of the single most effective uses of your time as you get ready for the exam.

In developing your plan for guessing, there are three questions to address:

- When should you start the guessing process?
- How should you narrow down the choices?
- Which answer should you choose?

When to Start the Guessing Process

Unless your plan for guessing is to select C every time (which, despite its merits, is not what we recommend), you need to leave yourself enough time to apply your answer elimination strategies. Since you have a limited amount of time for each question, that means that if you're going to give yourself the best shot at guessing correctly, you have to decide quickly whether or not you will guess.

Of course, the best-case scenario is that you don't have to guess at all, so first, see if you can answer the question based on your knowledge of the subject and basic reasoning skills. Focus on the key words in the question and try to jog your memory of related topics. Give yourself a chance to bring the knowledge to mind, but once you realize that you don't have (or you can't access) the knowledge you need to answer the question, it's time to start the guessing process.

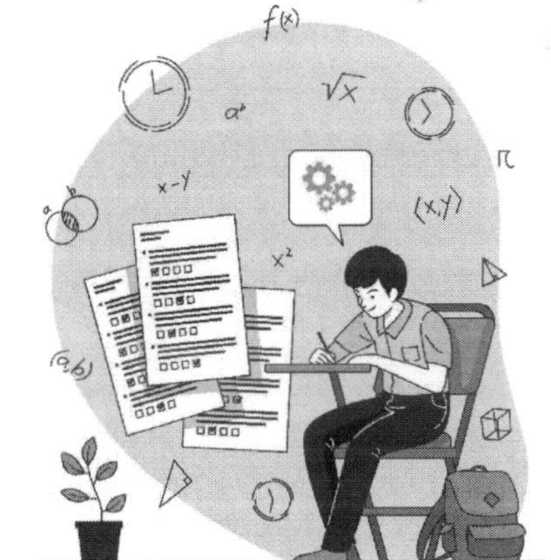

It's almost always better to start the guessing process too early than too late. It only takes a few seconds to remember something and answer the question from knowledge. Carefully eliminating wrong answer choices takes longer. Plus, going through the process of eliminating answer choices can actually help jog your memory.

Summary: Start the guessing process as soon as you decide that you can't answer the question based on your knowledge.

How to Narrow Down the Choices

The next chapter in this book (**Test-Taking Strategies**) includes a wide range of strategies for how to approach questions and how to look for answer choices to eliminate. You will definitely want to read those carefully, practice them, and figure out which ones work best for you. Here though, we're going to address a mindset rather than a particular strategy.

Your odds of guessing an answer correctly depend on how many options you are choosing from.

Number of options left	5	4	3	2	1
Odds of guessing correctly	20%	25%	33%	50%	100%

You can see from this chart just how valuable it is to be able to eliminate incorrect answers and make an educated guess, but there are two things that many test takers do that cause them to miss out on the benefits of guessing:

- Accidentally eliminating the correct answer
- Selecting an answer based on an impression

We'll look at the first one here, and the second one in the next section.

To avoid accidentally eliminating the correct answer, we recommend a thought exercise called **the $5 challenge**. In this challenge, you only eliminate an answer choice from contention if you are willing to bet $5 on it being wrong. Why $5? Five dollars is a small but not insignificant amount of money. It's an amount you could afford to lose but wouldn't want to throw away. And while losing $5 once might not hurt too much, doing it twenty times will set you back $100. In the same way, each small decision you make—eliminating a choice here, guessing on a question there—won't by itself impact your score very much, but when you put them all together, they can make a big difference. By holding each answer choice elimination decision to a higher standard, you can reduce the risk of accidentally eliminating the correct answer.

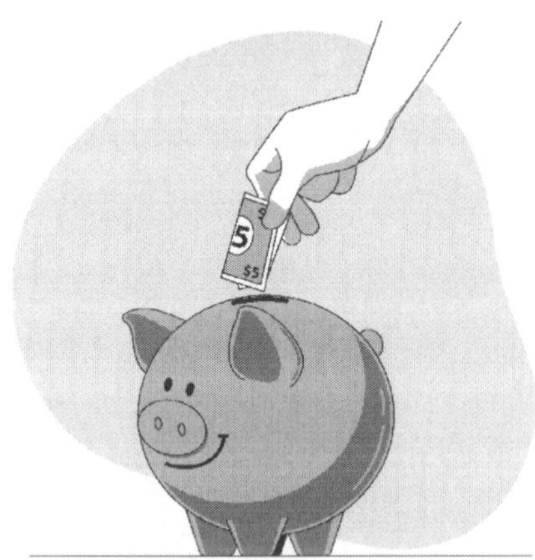

The $5 challenge can also be applied in a positive sense: If you are willing to bet $5 that an answer choice *is* correct, go ahead and mark it as correct.

Summary: Only eliminate an answer choice if you are willing to bet $5 that it is wrong.

Which Answer to Choose

You're taking the test. You've run into a hard question and decided you'll have to guess. You've eliminated all the answer choices you're willing to bet $5 on. Now you have to pick an answer. Why do we even need to talk about this? Why can't you just pick whichever one you feel like when the time comes?

The answer to these questions is that if you don't come into the test with a plan, you'll rely on your impression to select an answer choice, and if you do that, you risk falling into a trap. The test writers know that everyone who takes their test will be guessing on some of the questions, so they intentionally write wrong answer choices to seem plausible. You still have to pick an answer though, and if the wrong answer choices are designed to look right, how can you ever be sure that you're not falling for their trap? The best solution we've found to this dilemma is to take the decision out of your hands entirely. Here is the process we recommend:

Once you've eliminated any choices that you are confident (willing to bet $5) are wrong, select the first remaining choice as your answer.

Whether you choose to select the first remaining choice, the second, or the last, the important thing is that you use some preselected standard. Using this approach guarantees that you will not be enticed into selecting an answer choice that looks right, because you are not basing your decision on how the answer choices look.

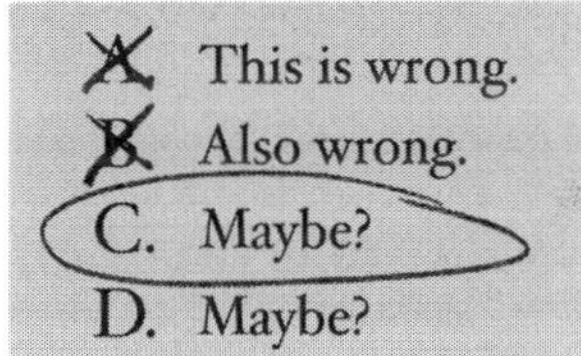

This is not meant to make you question your knowledge. Instead, it is to help you recognize the difference between your knowledge and your impressions. There's a huge difference between thinking an answer is right because of what you know, and thinking an answer is right because it looks or sounds like it should be right.

Summary: To ensure that your selection is appropriately random, make a predetermined selection from among all answer choices you have not eliminated.

Test-Taking Strategies

This section contains a list of test-taking strategies that you may find helpful as you work through the test. By taking what you know and applying logical thought, you can maximize your chances of answering any question correctly!

It is very important to realize that every question is different and every person is different: no single strategy will work on every question, and no single strategy will work for every person. That's why we've included all of them here, so you can try them out and determine which ones work best for different types of questions and which ones work best for you.

Question Strategies

✓ Read Carefully

Read the question and the answer choices carefully. Don't miss the question because you misread the terms. You have plenty of time to read each question thoroughly and make sure you understand what is being asked. Yet a happy medium must be attained, so don't waste too much time. You must read carefully and efficiently.

✓ Contextual Clues

Look for contextual clues. If the question includes a word you are not familiar with, look at the immediate context for some indication of what the word might mean. Contextual clues can often give you all the information you need to decipher the meaning of an unfamiliar word. Even if you can't determine the meaning, you may be able to narrow down the possibilities enough to make a solid guess at the answer to the question.

✓ Prefixes

If you're having trouble with a word in the question or answer choices, try dissecting it. Take advantage of every clue that the word might include. Prefixes can be a huge help. Usually, they allow you to determine a basic meaning. *Pre-* means before, *post-* means after, *pro-* is positive, *de-* is negative. From prefixes, you can get an idea of the general meaning of the word and try to put it into context.

✓ Hedge Words

Watch out for critical hedge words, such as *likely, may, can, often, almost, mostly, usually, generally, rarely*, and *sometimes*. Question writers insert these hedge phrases to cover every possibility. Often an answer choice will be wrong simply because it leaves no room for exception. Be on guard for answer choices that have definitive words such as *exactly* and *always*.

✓ Switchback Words

Stay alert for *switchbacks*. These are the words and phrases frequently used to alert you to shifts in thought. The most common switchback words are *but, although*, and *however*. Others include *nevertheless, on the other hand, even though, while, in spite of, despite*, and *regardless of*. Switchback words are important to catch because they can change the direction of the question or an answer choice.

✓ FACE VALUE

When in doubt, use common sense. Accept the situation in the problem at face value. Don't read too much into it. These problems will not require you to make wild assumptions. If you have to go beyond creativity and warp time or space in order to have an answer choice fit the question, then you should move on and consider the other answer choices. These are normal problems rooted in reality. The applicable relationship or explanation may not be readily apparent, but it is there for you to figure out. Use your common sense to interpret anything that isn't clear.

Answer Choice Strategies

✓ ANSWER SELECTION

The most thorough way to pick an answer choice is to identify and eliminate wrong answers until only one is left, then confirm it is the correct answer. Sometimes an answer choice may immediately seem right, but be careful. The test writers will usually put more than one reasonable answer choice on each question, so take a second to read all of them and make sure that the other choices are not equally obvious. As long as you have time left, it is better to read every answer choice than to pick the first one that looks right without checking the others.

✓ ANSWER CHOICE FAMILIES

An answer choice family consists of two (in rare cases, three) answer choices that are very similar in construction and cannot all be true at the same time. If you see two answer choices that are direct opposites or parallels, one of them is usually the correct answer. For instance, if one answer choice says that quantity *x* increases and another either says that quantity *x* decreases (opposite) or says that quantity *y* increases (parallel), then those answer choices would fall into the same family. An answer choice that doesn't match the construction of the answer choice family is more likely to be incorrect. Most questions will not have answer choice families, but when they do appear, you should be prepared to recognize them.

✓ ELIMINATE ANSWERS

Eliminate answer choices as soon as you realize they are wrong, but make sure you consider all possibilities. If you are eliminating answer choices and realize that the last one you are left with is also wrong, don't panic. Start over and consider each choice again. There may be something you missed the first time that you will realize on the second pass.

✓ AVOID FACT TRAPS

Don't be distracted by an answer choice that is factually true but doesn't answer the question. You are looking for the choice that answers the question. Stay focused on what the question is asking for so you don't accidentally pick an answer that is true but incorrect. Always go back to the question and make sure the answer choice you've selected actually answers the question and is not merely a true statement.

✓ EXTREME STATEMENTS

In general, you should avoid answers that put forth extreme actions as standard practice or proclaim controversial ideas as established fact. An answer choice that states the "process should be used in certain situations, if..." is much more likely to be correct than one that states the "process should be discontinued completely." The first is a calm rational statement and doesn't even make a definitive, uncompromising stance, using a hedge word *if* to provide wiggle room, whereas the second choice is far more extreme.

⊘ Benchmark

As you read through the answer choices and you come across one that seems to answer the question well, mentally select that answer choice. This is not your final answer, but it's the one that will help you evaluate the other answer choices. The one that you selected is your benchmark or standard for judging each of the other answer choices. Every other answer choice must be compared to your benchmark. That choice is correct until proven otherwise by another answer choice beating it. If you find a better answer, then that one becomes your new benchmark. Once you've decided that no other choice answers the question as well as your benchmark, you have your final answer.

⊘ Predict the Answer

Before you even start looking at the answer choices, it is often best to try to predict the answer. When you come up with the answer on your own, it is easier to avoid distractions and traps because you will know exactly what to look for. The right answer choice is unlikely to be word-for-word what you came up with, but it should be a close match. Even if you are confident that you have the right answer, you should still take the time to read each option before moving on.

General Strategies

⊘ Tough Questions

If you are stumped on a problem or it appears too hard or too difficult, don't waste time. Move on! Remember though, if you can quickly check for obviously incorrect answer choices, your chances of guessing correctly are greatly improved. Before you completely give up, at least try to knock out a couple of possible answers. Eliminate what you can and then guess at the remaining answer choices before moving on.

⊘ Check Your Work

Since you will probably not know every term listed and the answer to every question, it is important that you get credit for the ones that you do know. Don't miss any questions through careless mistakes. If at all possible, try to take a second to look back over your answer selection and make sure you've selected the correct answer choice and haven't made a costly careless mistake (such as marking an answer choice that you didn't mean to mark). This quick double check should more than pay for itself in caught mistakes for the time it costs.

⊘ Pace Yourself

It's easy to be overwhelmed when you're looking at a page full of questions; your mind is confused and full of random thoughts, and the clock is ticking down faster than you would like. Calm down and maintain the pace that you have set for yourself. Especially as you get down to the last few minutes of the test, don't let the small numbers on the clock make you panic. As long as you are on track by monitoring your pace, you are guaranteed to have time for each question.

⊘ Don't Rush

It is very easy to make errors when you are in a hurry. Maintaining a fast pace in answering questions is pointless if it makes you miss questions that you would have gotten right otherwise. Test writers like to include distracting information and wrong answers that seem right. Taking a little extra time to avoid careless mistakes can make all the difference in your test score. Find a pace that allows you to be confident in the answers that you select.

✓ Keep Moving

Panicking will not help you pass the test, so do your best to stay calm and keep moving. Taking deep breaths and going through the answer elimination steps you practiced can help to break through a stress barrier and keep your pace.

Final Notes

The combination of a solid foundation of content knowledge and the confidence that comes from practicing your plan for applying that knowledge is the key to maximizing your performance on test day. As your foundation of content knowledge is built up and strengthened, you'll find that the strategies included in this chapter become more and more effective in helping you quickly sift through the distractions and traps of the test to isolate the correct answer.

Now that you're preparing to move forward into the test content chapters of this book, be sure to keep your goal in mind. As you read, think about how you will be able to apply this information on the test. If you've already seen sample questions for the test and you have an idea of the question format and style, try to come up with questions of your own that you can answer based on what you're reading. This will give you valuable practice applying your knowledge in the same ways you can expect to on test day.

Good luck and good studying!

Five-Week CHPN Study Plan

On the next few pages, we've provided an optional study plan to help you use this study guide to its fullest potential over the course of 5 weeks. If you have 10 weeks available and want to spread it out more, spend two weeks on each section of the plan.

Below is a quick summary of the subjects covered in each week of the plan.

- Week 1: Patient Care: Assessment and Planning
- Week 2: Patient Care: Pain Management
- Week 3: Patient Care: Symptom Management
- Week 4: Support, Education, and Advocacy; Practice Issues
- Week 5: Practice Tests

Please note that not all subjects will take the same amount of time to work through.

Two full-length practice tests are included in this study guide. Take these practice tests without any reference materials a day or two before the real thing as practice runs to get yourself in the mode of answering questions at a good pace.

Week 1: Patient Care: Assessment and Planning

Instructional Content

First, read carefully through the **Patient Care: Assessment and Planning** chapter in this book, checking off your progress as you go:

❑ Goals of Care and Shared Decision Making
❑ Interdisciplinary Care Planning and Ongoing Evaluation
❑ Life-Limiting Disease Progression, Complications, and Treatment
❑ Indicators of Imminent Death

As you read, do the following:

- Highlight any sections, terms, or concepts you think are important
- Draw an asterisk (*) next to any areas you are struggling with
- Watch the review videos to gain more understanding of a particular topic
- Take notes in your notebook or in the margins of this book

After you've read through everything, go back and review any sections that you highlighted or that you drew an asterisk next to, referencing your notes along the way.

Week 2: Patient Care: Pain Management

Instructional Content

First, read carefully through the **Patient Care: Pain Management** chapter in this book, checking off your progress as you go:

❑ Etiology of Pain, Types of Pain, and Pain Syndromes
❑ Pain Scales
❑ Factors that Influence the Pain Experience
❑ Pharmacologic Pain Management
❑ Non-Pharmacologic Interventions
❑ Complementary and Alternative Therapies

As you read, do the following:

- Highlight any sections, terms, or concepts you think are important
- Draw an asterisk (*) next to any areas you are struggling with
- Watch the review videos to gain more understanding of a particular topic
- Take notes in your notebook or in the margins of this book

After you've read through everything, go back and review any sections that you highlighted or that you drew an asterisk next to, referencing your notes along the way.

Week 3: Patient Care: Symptom Management

Instructional Content

First, read carefully through the **Patient Care: Symptom Management** chapter in this book, checking off your progress as you go:

❑ Systems Review
❑ System-Specific End Stage Disease Progression
❑ Nutrition Assessment
❑ Psychosocial, Emotional, and Spiritual
❑ Hospice and Palliative Care Emergencies

As you read, do the following:

- Highlight any sections, terms, or concepts you think are important
- Draw an asterisk (*) next to any areas you are struggling with
- Watch the review videos to gain more understanding of a particular topic
- Take notes in your notebook or in the margins of this book

After you've read through everything, go back and review any sections that you highlighted or that you drew an asterisk next to, referencing your notes along the way.

Week 4: Support, Education, and Advocacy; Practice Issues

Instructional Content

First, read carefully through the **Support, Education, and Advocacy** and **Practice Issues** chapters in this book, checking off your progress as you go:

❑ Advance Care Planning
❑ Hospice and Palliative Care Benefits
❑ Patient Needs and Patient Safety
❑ Psychosocial, Spiritual, and Cultural Needs
❑ Life Completion and Search for Meaning
❑ Caregiver/Family Self-Care Activities
❑ Principles of Hospice and Palliative Education
❑ Therapeutic Communication
❑ Grief and Loss Support/Bereavement Services
❑ Postmortem Care and Services
❑ Ethical Issues Related to End of Life
❑ Standards of Practice
❑ Strategies for Self-Care and Stress Management
❑ Quality Improvement in Hospice and Palliative Care

As you read, do the following:

- Highlight any sections, terms, or concepts you think are important
- Draw an asterisk (*) next to any areas you are struggling with
- Watch the review videos to gain more understanding of a particular topic
- Take notes in your notebook or in the margins of this book

After you've read through everything, go back and review any sections that you highlighted or that you drew an asterisk next to, referencing your notes along the way.

Week 5: Practice Tests

Your success on test day depends not only on how many hours you put into preparing, but also on whether you prepared the right way. It's good to check to see if your studying is paying off. One of the most effective ways to do this is by taking practice tests to evaluate your progress. Practice tests are useful because they show exactly where you need to improve. Every time you take a practice test, pay special attention to these three groups of questions:

- The questions you got wrong
- The questions you had to guess on, even if you guessed right
- The questions you found difficult or slow to work through

This will show you exactly what your weak areas are, and where you need to devote more study time. Ask yourself why each of these questions gave you trouble. Was it because you didn't understand the material? Was it because you didn't remember the vocabulary? Do you need more repetitions on this type of question to build speed and confidence? Dig into those questions and figure out how you can strengthen your weak areas as you go back to review the material.

As you go along, keep in mind that the practice tests are just that: practice. Memorizing these questions and answers will not be very helpful on the actual test because it is unlikely to have any of the same exact questions. If you only know the right answers to the sample questions, you won't be prepared for the real thing. **Study the concepts** until you understand them fully, and then you'll be able to answer any question that shows up on the test.

Practice Test #1

Now that you've read over the instructional content, it's time to take a practice test. Complete Practice Test #1. Take this test with **no time constraints**, and feel free to reference the applicable sections of this guide as you go. Once you've finished, check your answers against the provided answer key. For any questions you answered incorrectly, review the answer rationale, and then **go back and review** the applicable sections of the book. The goal in this stage is to understand why you answered the question incorrectly, and make sure that the next time you see a similar question, you will get it right.

Practice Test #2

Next, complete Practice Test #2. This time, give yourself **3 hours** to complete all of the questions. You should again feel free to reference the guide and your notes, but be mindful of the clock. If you run out of time before you finish all of the questions, mark where you were when time expired, but go ahead and finish taking the practice test. Once you've finished, check your answers against the provided answer key, and as before, review the answer rationale for any that you answered incorrectly and then go back and review the associated instructional content. Your goal is still to increase understanding of the content but also to get used to the time constraints you will face on the test.

Patient Care: Assessment and Planning

Goals of Care and Shared Decision Making

Identifying Past and Present Goals and Expectations

When collaborating with the patient and family, the nurse should begin by educating the patient and family about patient rights and asking what **goals and expectations** they have. In order to develop the plan of care, the nurse must know what the patient and family desire, keeping in mind that goals may change. For example, if a patient's goal is to remain mentally alert until death, this may affect the plan for managing pain. If a desired outcome is that the patient die in the home, then the plan of care must include the resources needed to facilitate this. The nurse should ask that the patient and caregiver or other family members list the goals and outcomes that are most important to them and then should compare and discuss the items as they may not always be in agreement. Some negotiation and discussion may be required. While a patient may want to remain at home, for example, the caregiver may prefer that the patient be hospitalized.

Health Beliefs and Traditions Regarding Death

Individual beliefs and traditions regarding death vary widely, and these can affect how the patient and family deal with the end of life. The nurse should discuss these issues with the patient and/or family in order to ensure their needs are met. Those with strong spiritual beliefs may want spiritual advisors (priests, shamans, ministers, monks) present to provide support or perform rituals. People who have no belief in an afterlife may face death with resolution or may be frightened at the thought of the total end of their existence. Those who believe in reincarnation may find comfort in the thought of their rebirth but may also fear karma for the mistakes they made in this life. Some may feel that they will be in a loving place after death while others fear they will suffer torment for their sins. The nurse should remain supportive and allow patients and families to express their feelings, fears, and concerns.

Elements of Patient History

In addition to the physical assessment and review of systems, a patient history should include the following elements:

- **Biographical information**: Name, age, gender, ethnicity, marital status, occupation/profession
- **Family history/relationships**: Information about genetic diseases, genogram, health status of family members, family members' causes of death and ages at death, support systems, family system, and communication patterns
- **Physical environment**: Living arrangements, type of housing, homeless status, and environmental hazards
- **Cultural environment**: Attitudes and beliefs about wellness, sickness, death, complementary therapies, language spoken in the home, and customs
- **Spiritual environment**: Religious and/or spiritual beliefs, religious practices, belief system
- **Lifestyle**: Sexual preferences (straight, gay, bisexual, etc.), sexual habits (masturbation, multiple partners, high-risk behaviors), personal habits (sleeping, eating, exercising), and substance abuse (alcohol, drugs, nicotine)

- **Social environment**: Friends, relationships, clubs, social media, sports participation
- **Disability**: Physical disabilities (hearing, vision, smell), mobility disorders and need for assistive devices (walkers, canes, wheelchairs) and mental disabilities (cognitive impairment, psychiatric/psychological disorders)

Special History-Taking Challenges

Special history-taking challenges exist when dealing with special populations. The following considerations should be taken:

- **Silent patient**: Be patient, sensitive, and alert for nonverbal clues.
- **Talkative patient**: Allow the patient to speak freely for a few minutes and then periodically summarize.
- **Anxious patient**: Be patient, provide reassurance, explain all procedures.
- **Patient with multiple complaints**: Ask the patient to help prioritize issues.
- **Hostile/angry patient**: Remain calm, respond as appropriate.
- **Intoxicated patient**: Avoid cornering, belittling, or challenging the patient or asking the patient to lower voice or stop swearing. Remain calm and treat the patient with respect.
- **Depressed, crying patient**: Assess the severity of depression, listen, and remain supportive and non-judgmental.
- **Patient with language barrier**: Use a translator, utilize hand gestures, show equipment before using and point to the part of the body where the equipment will be used.
- **Patient with visual impairment**: Announce presence, explain all procedures verbally, tell the patient before touching them.
- **Patient with hearing impairment**: Determine if the patient has a hearing aid and obtain it if possible. Speak slowly and clearly facing patient for hearing deficit. If the patient has complete hearing loss, use writing use hand gestures and demonstrations to communicate.

Previous/Current Therapies

The patient history should include information about previous and current therapies:

- **Medications**: Note any previous and current prescribed medications, including dosages, frequency, and duration as well as the reason for the drug.
- **Allergies**: Make note of any drug allergies or reactions, history of anaphylaxis, other allergies (dust, foods, latex, animals, plants, pollens).
- **Vitamins, minerals, and herbal preparations**: Be aware of types, dosages, frequency, and duration. If using herbal preparations or those not readily identified, determine where they were obtained as some from overseas may include substances banned in the US or dangerous to the health.
- **Complementary therapies**: Complementary therapies include relaxation, visualization, homeopathy, acupuncture, music therapy, aromatherapy, Ayurveda, biofeedback, chiropractic medicine, hypnosis, meditation, massage, traditional Chinese medicine, yoga, naturopathy, reflexology, acupuncture, and Tai Chi.
- **Cultural therapies**: Cultural therapies include the use of healers, shamans, coining, cupping, pricking (with a needle).
- **Fasting and cleanses**: Note the specific program, duration, and substances utilized for cleanses (oral, rectal).

Assessment of Functional Abilities

ADL and IADL

Functional impairment may affect the ability to prepare and receive adequate fluids and nutrition. Functional assessment may include:

- **Activities of daily living (ADL)**: This assesses the ability to care for oneself, including dressing, bathing, and preparing food. Inability to carry out ADL may relate to physical impairment (paralysis, paresis, frailty), or cognitive impairment (dementia, confusion).
- **Instrumental activities of daily living (IADL)**: This assesses managing affairs (including finances), arranging transportation, using prosthetic devices, shopping, and telephoning. Inability to carry out IADL may relate to cognitive impairment, poverty, or inaccessibility and can prevent people from shopping for or ordering food.

Gait Speed, TUG, and POMA

Gait assessments include:

- **Gait speed** in 5 meters with slow gait (<0.6 m/second) predictive of limitations.
- **Timed up and go (TUG)**: Patient stands from chair with armrests, walks 3 meters, turns, and sits back down. Those requiring ≥14 seconds are at risk for falls (Normal: 7-10 seconds).
- **Performance-oriented mobility assessment (POMA)** tests mobility and gait under different conditions.

Index of Independence of Activities of Daily Living and Palliative Performance Scale

The **Index of Independence of Activities of Daily Living (Katz Index)** tool is a check list that does not use scores but rather evaluates the individual in 6 areas (bathing, dressing, toileting, transfer, continence, and feeding) to provide an assessment of the person's need for assistance and progression of disease and/or disability.

The **Palliative Performance Scale** assesses the functional ability of older adults receiving palliative care. Categories are assessed by percentage of ability from 0% (death) to 100% with lower percentages indicative of functional impairment. The scores are used as a guide to determine probable life expectancy with 60-100% at 108 days, 30-50% at 41 days, and 10-20% at 6 days although survival rates have been primarily correlated with cancer rather than other terminal illness. Categories include:

- Ability to ambulate
- Activity level and evidence of disease
- Self-care
- Intake
- Level of consciousness

Assessing the Quality of Life

QOLS

The Quality-of-Life Scale (QOLS) is a self-administered test often used with adults, including the chronically ill, to assess the patient's perception of their quality of life. The tool has 7 categories with a total of 16 elements that are assessed with a 1-7 scale that ranges from satisfaction to dissatisfaction. The possible scores range from 16-112 with an average normal finding of about 90. The higher the score, the higher the perceived quality of life. Categories include:

- **Material/physical wellbeing**: Includes material wellbeing/financial security as well as health and personal safety
- **Interpersonal relationships**: Includes family members, spouse, children, and friends
- **Activities (social, community, civic)**: Includes those activities that involve assisting others and those related to local/national government
- **Personal development/fulfillment**: Includes intellectual development, personal understanding, creative expression, and role in occupation
- **Recreation**: Hobbies and leisure activities
- **Independence**: The ability to live and manage independently

Psychosocial Assessment

A psychosocial assessment should provide additional information to the physical assessment to guide the patient's plan of care and should include:

- **Previous hospitalizations and experience with healthcare**
- **Psychiatric history**: suicidal ideation, psychiatric disorders, family psychiatric history, history of violence and/or self-mutilation
- **Chief complaint**: patient's perception
- **Complementary therapies**: acupuncture, visualization, and meditation
- **Occupational and educational background**: employment, retirement, and special skills.
- **Social patterns**: family and friends, living situation, typical activities, support system.
- **Sexual patterns**: orientation, problems, and sex practices
- **Interests/abilities**: hobbies and sports
- **Current or past substance abuse**: type, frequency, drinking pattern, use of recreational drugs, and overuse of prescription drugs
- **Ability to cope**: stress reduction techniques
- **Physical, sexual, emotional, and financial abuse**: whether the individual feels safe at home or where they live
- **Spiritual/cultural assessment**: religious/spiritual importance, practices, restrictions (such as blood products or foods), and impact on health/health decisions

Assessment of Patient/Family Knowledge of and Response to Advanced Illness

Assessment of patient/family knowledge of and response to advanced illness begins with a determination of how much they actually know about the illness and how much they want to know through direct interview and questioning. This includes questions like, "What do you understand about your disease?" and "What do you want to know about your disease?" Open-ended questions (as opposed to those answered with "yes" or "no") are most effective in eliciting information. Questioning can help evaluate the patient's/family's general health literacy and cognitive abilities as well as readiness to learn (related to physical, emotional, experiential, and knowledge readiness). Issues that should be covered during the **assessment include patient/family understanding** of:

- Disease and disease process
- Medications or treatments
- Adverse effects
- Signs and symptoms, including progression over time
- Prognosis
- End-of-life options for care
- Personal preferences

During the assessment, it's important to note both the patient's verbal and nonverbal communication and to remain supportive and non-judgmental.

Assessment of Patient/Family Support Systems

Patient/family **support systems** may vary widely and can include those that provide physical and/or emotional support:

- **Family members**: Family members (parents, spouse, siblings, children, grandparents) remain the primary support system for many patients and family, especially if they live nearby and can provide assistance, though even distant communication can provide emotional support.
- **Friends**: Close friends may provide support in lieu or in addition to family members and may, in some cases, be more aware of emotional needs because of longstanding close association.
- **Co-workers**: Co-workers may donate sick time, ease workload, and provide support in various manners.
- **Organizations**: Community organizations may help in provision of meals, transportation, visitors, and other types of support.
- **Religion/Spirituality**: Some religions/spiritual organizations provide not only emotional support but also nursing care and financial assistance.
- **Online support groups/message boards**: Internet support systems, such as message boards for specific types of cancer, can provide emotional support as well as useful information on treatment and coping.

Substance Abusers

Assessment of substance abusers (drugs, alcohol) can be met with resistance because of the patient's unwillingness to admit to substance abuse, so the nurse should begin by discussing the importance of the information for diagnosis and treatment. When possible, the nurse should use standardized assessment tools, such as the Addiction Severity Index (ASI), the CAGE tool, and/or the Drinker Inventory of Consequences in order to quantify the presence of abuse. The nurse must remain nonjudgmental and supportive throughout the assessment and should ensure privacy and confidentiality to the fullest extent possible. For example, a patient may not want family members to know about substance abuse. Patients with substance abuse should also be assessed for psychiatric conditions for which they may be self-medicating, homelessness, malnutrition, financial difficulties, and substance-specific illnesses, such as liver disease (alcohol), heart and kidney disease (methamphetamine), lung disease (nicotine), and tachycardia and Parkinson's disease (cocaine). Patients who inject drugs should be assessed for HIV and hepatitis B.

Indications of Substance Abuse

Many people with substance abuse (alcohol or drugs) are reluctant to disclose this information. Common agents include **cannabis** (marijuana), **hallucinogens** (LSD), **stimulants** (cocaine, methamphetamine), **barbiturates** (secobarbital [Seconal], amobarbital [Amytal]), **sedatives** (zolpidem [Ambien], eszopiclone [Lunesta]), **hypnotics/benzodiazepines** (alprazolam [Xanax], diazepam [Valium], lorazepam [Ativan]), and **opiates** (heroin, morphine, fentanyl, oxycodone, hydrocodone). A number of indicators are suggestive of substance abuse:

Physical signs

- Needle tracks on arms or legs
- Burns on fingers or lips
- Pupils abnormally dilated or constricted, eyes watery
- Slurring of speech, slow speech
- Lack of coordination, instability of gait
- Tremors
- Sniffing repeatedly, nasal irritation
- Persistent cough
- Weight loss
- Dysrhythmias (abnormal pulse)
- Pallor, puffiness of face

Other signs

- Odor of alcohol/marijuana on clothing or breath
- Labile emotions, including mood swings, agitation, and anger
- Inappropriate, impulsive, and/or risky behavior.
- Lying
- Missing appointments
- Difficulty concentrating/short term memory loss, disoriented/confused
- Blackouts
- Insomnia or excessive sleeping
- Lack of personal hygiene

CAGE Assessment Tool

The CAGE tool is used as a quick assessment tool to determine if people are drinking excessively or are problem drinkers. Moderate drinking (1 drink a day for older adults), unless contraindicated by health concerns, is usually not harmful, but drinking more than that can lead to serious physical and psychosocial problems. One drink is defined as 12 oz beer, 5 oz wine, or 1.5 oz liquor.

C	Cutting down	Do you think about trying to cut down on drinking?
A	Annoyed at criticism	Are people starting to criticize your drinking?
G	Guilty feeling	Do you feel guilty or try to hide your drinking?
E	Eye opener	Do you increasingly need a drink earlier in the day?

A "Yes" on one question suggests the possibility of a drinking problem while a "yes" on at least two indicates a drinking problem, in which case, the patient should be provided with information about reducing drinking and appropriate referrals made.

Homeless Population

The homeless population has disproportionate rates of mental illness, estimated at 40-45%, many with serious illnesses, such as schizophrenia and bipolar disorder, complicated by substance abuse, so assessment must be multi-faceted, including assessment of substance abuse, nutritional status, functional status, and cognitive status. The need for adequate housing is an ongoing problem with homeless patients. Once released from inpatient care services, the homeless often return directly to the streets or to shelters. They often resist treatment (sometimes not believing themselves to be ill), fail to keep appointments, and lack transportation or money for transportation. They may be victims of violence, have no money for medications, and may not qualify for assistance or may be reluctant to deal with government agencies in order to gain assistance, so referral to social service is often critical.

COGNITIVELY IMPAIRED

Patients with evidence of **cognitive impairment**, often associated with Alzheimer's disease, should have cognition assessed. The Mini-mental state exam (MMSE) or the Mini-cog test is commonly used. Both require the patient to carry out specified tasks:

- MMSE
    - Remembering and later repeating the names of 3 common objects
    - Counting backward from 100 by 7s or spelling "world" backward
    - Naming items as the examiner points to them
    - Providing the location of the examiner's office, including city, state, and street address.
    - Repeating common phrases
    - Copying a picture of interlocking shapes
    - Following simple 3-part instructions, such as picking up a piece of paper, folding it in half, and placing it on the floor
- Mini-cog
    - Remembering and later repeating the names of 3 common objects.
    - Drawing the face of a clock with all 12 numbers and the hands indicating the time specified by the examiner.

ELDERLY ASSESSMENTS

FALL RISKS

The American Geriatrics Society **Guidelines for the Prevention of Falls in Older Persons**:

- All geriatric patients should be asked if they have had falls in the past year.
- If no falls, no intervention is needed.
- If one fall, the patient should be assessed for gait and balance, including the get-up-and-go test in which the patient stands up from a chair without using arms to assist, walks across the room, and returns. If the patient is steady, no further assessment is needed. If the patient demonstrates unsteadiness, further assessment to determine the cause is necessary.
- If multiple falls, a full assessment should be completed: history, vision, neurological status, muscle strength, joint function, mental status, reflexes, cardiovascular status, including rate and rhythm), postural pulse and blood pressure. Referral to a geriatric specialist may be appropriate.

RISK FOR PRESSURE SORES

The Braden scale for predicting **risk of developing pressure sores** scores 6 different areas with 1-4 points. The first 4 areas include sensory perception, moisture, activity, and mobility. The last 2 areas include:

Usual nutrition pattern	Very poor (eats < half of meals; inadequate protein, intake, and hydration) Inadequate (eats about 1/2 of food with 3 protein servings or not enough liquid or tube feeding) Adequate (eats more than half of meals and 4 protein servings) Excellent
Friction and sheer	*(3 parameters only)* Problem moving (skin frequently slides down sheets, needs help to move) Potential problem (moves weakly or needs some assistance, skin slides somewhat during moves) No apparent problem

The scores for all six items are totaled, and a risk is assigned according to the number:

- 23 (best): Prognosis is excellent, very minimal risk.
- ≤16: Breakpoint for risk of pressure ulcer (will vary somewhat for different populations).
- 6 (worst): Prognosis is very poor, strong likelihood of developing pressure ulcers.

Geriatric Depression Scale

The Geriatric Depression Scale is a self-assessment tool to identify older adults with depression. The test can be used for those with normal cognition and those with mild to moderate impairment. The test poses 15 questions to which patients answer "yes" or "no." A score of more than 5 "yes" answers is indicative of depression:

1. Are you basically satisfied with your life?
2. Have you dropped many of your activities and interests?
3. Do you feel your life is empty?
4. Do you often get bored?
5. Are you in good spirits most of the time?
6. Are you afraid that something bad is going to happen to you?
7. Do you feel happy most of the time?
8. Do you often feel helpless?
9. Do you prefer to stay at home rather than going out and doing new things?
10. Do you feel you have more problems with memory than most?
11. Do you think it is wonderful to be alive now?
12. Do you feel pretty worthless the way you are now?
13. Do you feel full of energy?
14. Do you feel that your situation is hopeless?
15. Do you think that most people are better off than you are?

Pharmacological Concerns

There are a number of issues that can affect **gerontological pharmacology** and should be assessed:

- Antidepressants are associated with excess sedation, so typical doses are only 16-33% of a younger adult's dose. SSRIs are safest, but Prozac may cause anorexia, anxiety, and insomnia, so it should be avoided.
- Older antipsychotics, such as haloperidol, have high incidence of side effects. Atypical antipsychotics appear to be safer with risperidone (<2 mg daily) having the fewest adverse effects. The lowest possible doses should be tried first with careful monitoring of any antipsychotic.
- Adverse effects of drugs are 2-3 times more common in older adults than younger, often related to polypharmacy.
- Drug and nutrient interactions may impact nutrition by impairing appetite. Interactions may also alter the pharmacokinetics of nutrients or drugs, interfering with absorption, distribution, metabolism, and elimination.

VETERANS

Assessment of veterans must include not only the standard assessments appropriate for the patient's age and gender but also assessment of combat-associated injuries and illnesses:

- Shrapnel and/or gunshot injuries: Associated physical limitations, pain
- Amputations: Mobility and prosthesis issues
- PTSD: Extent, frequency of attacks, limiting factors, triggers
- Depression, suicidal ideation
- Substance abuse: Type and extent
- Agent orange-associated illnesses: Multiple types of cancer (including Hodgkin's disease, prostate cancer, lung cancer, and leukemia), Parkinson's disease, diabetes mellitus (type 2), chloracne, and heart disease

Because a large number of veterans are among the homeless population, the veteran's living arrangements should be explored and appropriate referrals made if the patient is in need of housing. Veterans may be unaware of programs offered through the US Department of Veterans Affairs and should be provided information about these programs as appropriate for the patient's needs.

Interdisciplinary Care Planning and Ongoing Evaluation

Developing Plan of Care

The patient's plan of care is based on different types of **goals**:

- **Patient/family goals for care and outcomes** are a primary concern, especially for hospice and palliative care patients, whose care focuses on comfort and emotional support. These goals may relate to goals of life closure. Families, including young children, often want to be involved in developing the plan of care because participation increases feelings of self-worth and respect for healthcare providers.
- **Clinical needs/obligations** are aimed at preventing complications, treating disorders, and promoting comfort. The plan should focus on the problem list identified as part of the history and physical examination. Each item in the problem list must be addressed in the plan of care, including interventions, nursing goals (immediate, intermediate, and long-term), and expected outcomes and utilization of appropriate clinical pathways that are realistic for the patient's condition.

Review Video: Plan of Care
Visit mometrix.com/academy and enter code: 300570

Prioritizing Nursing Diagnoses and Problems

One method of prioritizing nursing and/or differential diagnoses is to consider consequences (high, medium, low) if treatment is delayed:

- **High** (Life threatening): Acute myocardial infarction, suicidal ideation
- **Medium** (Delay may cause problems): Malnutrition, manic episodes
- **Low** (Treatment can be delayed safely): Osteoarthritis, mild anxiety

Needs can also be prioritized according to **Maslow's Hierarchy of Needs**. American psychologist Abraham Maslow defined human motivation in terms of needs and wants. His hierarchy of needs is classically portrayed as a pyramid sitting on its base divided into horizontal layers. He theorized that, as humans fulfill the needs of one layer, their motivation turns to the layer above.

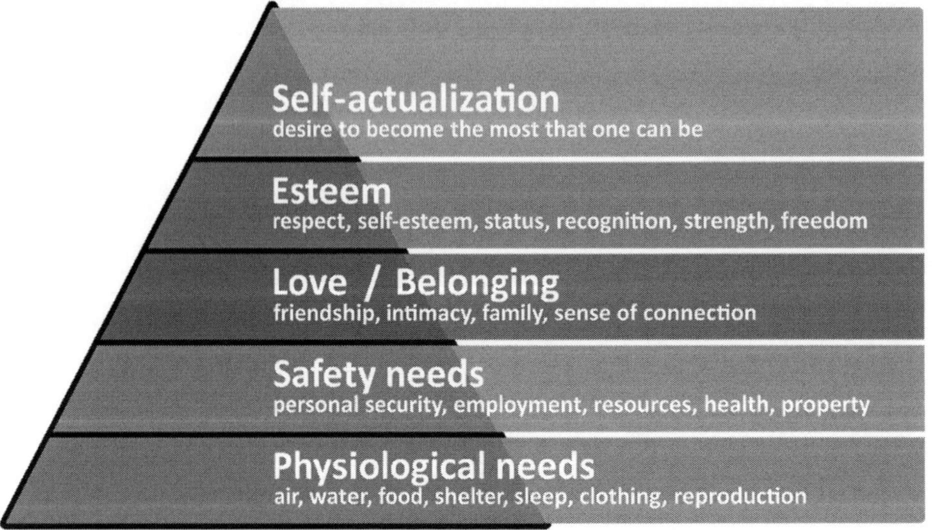

Level	Need	Description
Physiological	Basic needs to sustain life—oxygen, food, fluids, sleep	These basic needs take precedence over all other needs and must be dealt with first before individuals can focus on other needs.
Safety and security	Freedom from physiological and psychological threats	Once basic needs are met, individuals become concerned about safety, including freedom from fear, job security, war, and disasters. Children respond more intensely to threats than adults.
Love/Belonging	Support, caring, intimacy	Individuals tend to avoid isolation and loneliness and have a need for family, intimacy, or membership in a group where they feel they belong.
Self-esteem	Sense of worth, respect, independence	To have confidence, individuals need to develop self-esteem and receive the respect of others.
Self-actualization	Meeting one's own sense of potential and finding fulfillment	Individuals choose a path in life that leads to fulfillment and contentment.

Review Video: Maslow's Hierarchy of Needs
Visit mometrix.com/academy and enter code: 461825

Assisting Patient/Family in Evaluating Resources

The steps in assisting patient/family in evaluating appropriate and available resources includes:

- Develop a problem list and plan of care in collaboration with patient and family.
- Identify needs associated with plan of care, including those associated with hospitalization and home care.
- Categorize needs as follows:
    - **General care**: Hospital bed, bedpan, wheelchair, walker, assistive devices, meal preparation (home, Meals-on-Wheels)
    - **Treatment**: Medications, dressings, IVs, catheters, nutritional supplements
    - **Transportation**: Availability and requirements (car, ambulance, bus, taxi)
    - **Financial**: Insurance/Medicare coverage, co-pay, income, savings
    - **Caregiver**: Who will provide care, how often, where, when, and how, including the need to hire caregivers; need for respite care and/or homemaking services
    - **Consultation/Therapy**: Speech therapy, physical therapy, occupational therapy, etc.
    - **Psychological care**: Counseling, support programs
- Review categories and determine where additional resources are needed to ensure needs are met and what the patient/family can afford or attend to without further assistance.
- Provide lists of resources and/or referrals for deficits where additional resources are needed.

Unique Needs of Special Population

Certain populations require special considerations when developing their plan of care:

- **Substance abusers**: May need referral for drug/alcohol rehabilitation or drug maintenance (such as methadone) program. May require referrals for dental care and treatment of infections. Interventions may include dealing with drug-seeking behaviors and ongoing substance abuse.
- **Homeless**: May need treatment for lice and malnutrition. May need referral for psychiatric care and/or substance abuse (as above). Discharge planning may require assistance from social services and housing authorities.
- **Cognitively impaired**: Special interventions may be needed for safety, such as movement alarms, keeping side rails down, or attendants. Interventions may include alternative communication devices/approaches and dysphagia precautions. Consultation may be needed regarding effective management.
- **Elderly**: Fall and dysphagia precautions are often needed as well as functional assessment to ensure the patient receives adequate assistance with ADLS. This population may need nutritional supplementation and monitoring of intake and output and bowel movements.
- **Veterans**: Any of the needs/interventions above may apply. Interventions to deal with PTSD include determining triggers and maintaining a quiet environment when possible.

Patient Goals/Outcomes

The plan of care is developed from information gained from patient interviews, history and physical exam, and medical records. Once a problem list is generated, the nurse must review and prioritize the list and determine **patient goals/outcomes**, depending on the type of problem. Goals should be specifically related to the problem, measurable by some method, and attainable:

- Some problems (such as cardiac arrhythmias) can improve with treatment, so goals will aim toward resolution: "Pulse rate will not exceed 90 at rest."
- Other problems (such as chronic conditions) probably won't resolve, so the goals will aim toward preventing deterioration or further complications: "Patient will maintain current weight."
- Some problems (terminal cancer) cannot be resolved and deterioration of condition is inevitable, so the goal will aim toward palliation and ensuring the patient's comfort and support: "Patient will not experience breakthrough pain."

Outcomes Evaluation

Outcomes evaluation is an important component of evidence-based practice, which involves both internal and external research, and is important when modifying the plan of care. All treatments are subjected to review to determine if they produce positive outcomes, and policies and protocols for outcomes evaluation should be in place. **Outcomes evaluation** includes the following:

- Monitoring over the course of treatment involves careful observation and record keeping that notes progress, with supporting laboratory and radiographic evidence as indicated by condition and treatment.
- Evaluating results includes reviewing records as well as current research to determine if outcomes are within acceptable parameters.
- Sustaining involves continuing treatment, but continuing to monitor and evaluate.
- Improving means to continue the treatment but with additions or modifications in order to improve outcomes.
- Replacing the treatment with a different treatment must be done if outcomes evaluation indicates that current treatment is ineffective.

Change in Level of Care

Advocating for the hospice and palliative care patient to have a **change in the level of care** includes discussing care needs and options with the patient and family to ascertain their feelings and wishes. It also involves discussing changes in the patient's condition and the patient's wishes with the physician. For a patient on palliative care, the change in level of care may involve:

- **Lesser form of care**: This change is indicated because the patient is responding well to treatment, such as may occur following palliative radiotherapy.
- **Hospice care**: If the patient's condition has deteriorated and death is expected within 6 months, then hospice care provides more benefits than palliative care. Patients and family are often unaware of these benefits, so providing information can help them make a decision. Hospice care is appropriate when no further curative treatment is available or when a patient opts to discontinue curative treatments in favor of comfort care.

Life-Limiting Disease Progression, Complications, and Treatment

Autoimmune Disorders

HIV/AIDS

HIV (human immunodeficiency virus) is the retrovirus that causes AIDS (acquired immune deficiency syndrome). Diagnosis is determined by the CD4+ T-cell count with AIDS currently diagnosed with a CD4+ count of <200 cells per mm^3. HIV is transmitted in bodily fluids (blood, semen, vaginal secretions, breast milk) that contain free virions and infected CD4+ T-cells. Categories of HIV include:

- **Category A**: (CD4+ count <500). Asymptomatic or lymphadenopathy, sore throat, fatigue.
- **Category B**: (CD4+ count 200-499). Conditions include candidiasis, pelvic inflammatory disease, bacillary angiomatosis, fever, diarrhea, herpes zoster, low platelet count, weight loss, and peripheral neuropathy.
- **Category C (AIDS)**: (CD4+ count <200). Late-stage illness. Invasive diseases are common.

Risk factors include unprotected sex, especially males having sex with other males, and needle sharing. Patients often need support in dealing with anxiety, coping with increasing symptoms, adhering to medical protocols, and finding meaning and value in their lives.

Effects on Cells

The **AIDS virus** attaches itself to the **CD4 cell surface protein** of T-4 lymphocytes with a viral envelope of glycoprotein (gp120). This protein binds to CD4 receptors and coreceptors (CXCR4 and CCR5). HIV is a **retrovirus** that quickly infects circulating immune cells or finds safe harbors in body reservoirs that are inaccessible to drug therapy. The retrovirus uses an enzyme called **reverse transcriptase** to convert the HIV viral RNA to a viral DNA. This conversion allows the viral DNA to take over the host cell DNA of lymphocytes, macrophages, and other immune system cells. When the viral DNA has taken over, it produces viral proteins that assemble into **virions** using viral enzyme protease. Each reproductive cycle of HIV can produce up to 100 billion virions with minor protective mutations.

Common Associated Infections and Malignancies

The AIDS patient is highly **susceptible** to many bacterial, viral, fungal, and parasitic infections as well as certain types of cancers, such as Kaposi sarcoma, Hodgkin's lymphoma, and non-Hodgkin's lymphoma.

- **Bacterial infections** include *Streptococcus pneumoniae, Mycobacterium intracellulare* (MAI) and Mycobacterium avium complex (MAC), tuberculosis (TB), salmonellosis, syphilis, and Bacillary angiomatosis.
- **Viral infections** include cytomegalovirus (CMV), viral hepatitis, herpes simplex virus (HSV), human papillomavirus (HPV), and progressive multifocal leukoencephalopathy (PML).
- **Fungal infections** include Candida albicans, Histoplasma capsulatum, and cryptococcal meningitis.
- **Parasitic infections** include toxoplasmosis and cryptosporidium.

The rates of infection with these types of infections in AIDS patients far exceed the rates found within the general population.

AIDS Dementia Complex

The exact cause of **AIDS dementia** is unknown, but it is a primary result of the disease process of AIDS itself. Current theories suggest that the HIV infection stimulates an invasion of **macrophages** in the brain (microglia). These release **cytokines** that directly damage the nervous tissue by disrupting the neurotransmitter functions and cause encephalopathy. This condition affects as many as 15% of all AIDS patients. Prognosis is poor, and the disease is not reversible. However, **retrovirals** can delay its onset. Central nervous system HIV infection in children tends to have a more dramatic and pronounced effect than that in adults. AIDS dementia is characterized by gradual memory loss, decreased concentration, and cognition and mood disorders. The patient may also experience physical symptoms of ataxia, incontinence, and seizures.

Systemic Lupus Erythematosus

Systemic lupus erythematosus is a systemic reaction to collagen or connective tissue in the body, believed to be triggered by an antibody-antigen immune response to an environmental agent, resulting in widespread damage of vessels and organs, primarily in females. Onset is usually age 9-15 and is more common in African American, Hispanic, and Asian females than Caucasian.

Symptoms (vary widely)	Treatment (varies with severity)
• Butterfly rash (scaly erythematous maculopapular patches) on face, chest, and arms. • Arthritic-type pain, stiffness, and swelling of joints. • CNS involvement with seizures, headache, and psychosis. • Heart/vessels (pericarditis, vasculitis) and lung (pleurisy) inflammation. • Kidney failure. • Anemia (erythrocytopenia and pancytopenia, hemolytic). • Spleen, liver, and lymph nodes enlarged. • GI symptoms: Nausea, vomiting, pain, and hepatitis.	• NSAIDs for pain and inflammation. • Steroids for organ inflammation and hemolytic anemia. • Antimalarial drugs for skin involvement. • Immunosuppressant agents if steroids not adequate. • Patients may need support dealing with fatigue (rest, energy-conservation methods), pain, decreased mobility, nutrition, and anxiety/depression.

Rheumatoid Arthritis

Rheumatoid arthritis is a chronic systemic autoimmune inflammatory disorder of the connective tissue of synovial joints, resulting in loss of cartilage and joint deformity. RA has onset at 25 to 50 years, usually beginning with pain and stiffness in the hands, wrists, and feet. Joint inflammation and deformity increases over time. Symptoms include pain, stiffness, swelling, erythema, nodules, and lack of function in affected joints, and generalized weakness, fatigue, weight loss, and fever. Involvement is systemic, bilateral, and symmetric. Treatment includes light exercise to prevent contractures and pharmacologic treatment: salicylates (ASA), NSAIDs, COX-2 inhibitors (Celebrex), disease-modifying antirheumatic drugs (gold-containing compounds, methotrexate, azathioprine, adalimumab), immunomodulator (abatacept), interleukin-1 receptor inhibitors (anakinra), and glucocorticoids (prednisone) and topical analgesics. RA may be classified according to joint damage and/or functional status. Those in class 4 (functional) generally have limitations in ability to carry out all activities and require assistance in all ADLs. Patients often experience severe fatigue because of joint pain and disturbed sleep, so patients may especially need support in managing pain and conserving energy.

Oncologic Disorders

End-Stage Disease Progression of Oncologic Disorders

End-stage progression of oncologic disorders may vary depending on the type of cancer and the areas of metastasis but often includes the following:

- **Pain**: This is the most common complication and may be localized or generalized. Opioids are the treatment of choice, usually on a continuous round-the-clock schedule with additional doses for breakthrough pain at end-stage to provide as much comfort as possible.
- **Nausea/vomiting**: Anti-emetics and/or medical marijuana may help to reduce nausea and vomiting. The patient's diet should be altered to include those foods the patient can best tolerate, often soft, bland, or liquid foods.
- **Dyspnea**: Dyspnea is common, and supplementary oxygen may help to provide some relief.
- **Confusion**: Supportive care and reorienting the patient may help to reduce confusion, but confusion often persists, especially with high doses of opioids.
- **Bowel/bladder dysfunction**: This is common because of dehydration and opioid use. Stool softeners, laxatives and encouraging fluid intake may help. If the patient is still able to eat, adding yogurt, fiber, and prune juice to the diet may be helpful.

Advanced Renal Cancer

Renal cancers generally occur **asymptomatically** in the early stages. Symptoms begin to appear as the condition worsens. Gross hematuria, dull, aching pain, and palpable abdominal mass are generally the first signs. When all three of these are evidenced in the patient, it is generally a well-advanced cancer. **Hematuria** is the most common symptom but may not be noticed until it has reached the gross stage where it is visible to the naked eye. Other late signs and symptoms can include fever, anemia, weight loss, night sweats, elevated erythrocyte sedimentation rate, dyspnea, hypertension, hypercalcemia, and polycythemia. **Polycythemia** may cause headaches, dizziness, vein inflammation, itchiness, and a general feeling of bloating. **Hypercalcemia** causes tiredness, decreased appetite, frequent urination, thirst, nausea, vomiting, confusion, difficulty concentrating, and constipation.

Renal Failure

When the kidneys become unable to function, either short or long-term, it is referred to as renal failure. Causes for kidney failure range from toxins (including some medications that may become nephrotoxic), tumors, infections, diabetes, and hypertension to collagen vascular diseases such as lupus. When there is hope of restoring normal kidney function, peritoneal dialysis or hemodialysis as well as diuretics and the treatment of underlying causes such as hypertension may be used. Dietary treatments typically focus on a low sodium, low protein, and low potassium regimen. Dialysis, and its supplementary treatments, is the treatment of choice for chronic kidney failure. When there is no hope of return to normal kidney function, the patient faces the difficult decision of whether or not to start, continue, or even stop dialysis. This decision will either prolong the patient's life or bring death within just a few days. As the disease progresses it brings more pronounced complications in fluid and electrolyte balances, anemia, and uremia. At this point, the patient's treatment may turn to a focus on comfort and palliative medications rather than on prolonging life by the use of dialysis.

LEUKEMIA

Leukemia is an acute or chronic condition in which proliferating white blood cells compete with normal cells for nutrition. Leukemia affects all cells because the abnormal cells in the bone marrow depress the formation of all elements, resulting in the following consequences, regardless of the type of leukemia:

- Decrease in production of erythrocytes (RBCs), resulting in anemia.
- Decrease in neutrophils, resulting in increased risk of infection.
- Decrease in platelets, with subsequent decrease in clotting factors and increased bleeding or hemorrhage with pallor petechiae, purpura, and bleeding mucous membranes. Patients may need guidance regarding dental care.
- Increased risk of physiological fractures because of invasion of bone marrow that weakens the periosteum.
- Infiltration of liver, spleen, and lymph glands, resulting in enlargement and fibrosis.
- Infiltration of the CNS, resulting in increased intracranial pressure, ventricular dilation, and meningeal irritation with headaches, vomiting, papilledema, nuchal rigidity, and coma progressing to death.
- Hypermetabolism that deprives cells of nutrients, resulting in anorexia, weight loss, muscle atrophy, and fatigue. Patients often need support regarding nutrition and fatigue.

COLORECTAL CANCERS

Colorectal cancers are the third most common cancer, and adenocarcinomas account for up to 95% of all colorectal cancers. There are two additional subtypes of adenocarcinomas that are less common:

- **Signet ring** is a very aggressive form that is harder to treat but accounts for only 0.1% of adenocarcinomas.
- **Mucinous** is also an aggressive form that is composed of about 60% mucous, allowing the cells to spread faster and making it hard to treat. This form accounts for 10-15% of adenocarcinomas.

Because symptoms often do not appear before the disease is advanced, many patients will undergo colectomy with re-anastomosis or with formation of a colostomy, which requires ongoing care. Patients with advanced disease may be unable to care for a colostomy independently, and the psychological impact of the stoma may be profound. Patients need not only physical support for pain and colostomy care but also often emotional support to deal with changing body image and depression.

LUNG CANCER

Lung cancer is the most common cause of cancer-related deaths. Symptoms vary with type of tumor but are often not evident until metastasis has occurred. The most common symptom is cough that changes in character. Later symptoms include hemoptysis, dyspnea, weight loss, fatigue, nausea and vomiting, hoarseness, dysphagia, and unilateral diaphragmatic paralysis. Lung cancers may be primary, arising within the tissue of the lung, or secondary, spreading from a distant tumor. Secondary tumors can be identified by the type of tumor cells, as the cells are the same as those of the primary tumor site. Most primary lung cancers arise from the lining of the bronchi or bronchioles. Treatment may include surgical excision, radiotherapy, and/or chemotherapy, depending on the type and stage of the tumor. Most forms of lung cancer are associated with cigarette smoking or exposure to second-hand smoke. Even after treatment, dyspnea is common, and the nurse must be alert for signs of metastasis (most commonly to adrenals, bone, brain, liver, or other lung sites).

Breast Cancer

The most common type (75%) of breast cancer is infiltrating ductal carcinoma. This cancer progresses from ductal carcinoma in situ and originates in ductal cells but spreads to adjacent tissue and often metastasizes to axillary nodes. Treatment includes lumpectomy with radiation or mastectomy. If lymph nodes are positive, chemotherapy may be administered. Follow-up treatment depends on whether the cancer is hormone receptive and may include trastuzumab (Herceptin), tamoxifen, or aromatase inhibitor (Femara). Patients must deal with pain, fear of metastasis (most commonly to bone, brain, liver, or lung), and altered self-image, especially after mastectomy. About 15% develop cancer in the other breast. The nurse must be aware of the psychological impact of the disease and provide relief of symptoms but also encourage the patient to express feelings and help the patient to develop coping strategies. Anxiety and depression are common. Patients may benefit from peer support groups.

Prostate Cancer

Cancer of the prostate primarily occurs in older adults, average age 72. Many tumors are non-lethal or progress so slowly that they pose little threat to the person, but increased screening with PSA, ultrasound, and digital rectal exam in asymptomatic males has resulted in earlier diagnosis and more aggressive treatment. Both benign prostatic hypertrophy and prostatic carcinoma are frequently treated with transurethral resection of the prostate (TURP), especially if the volume of the gland reaches only 40-50 mL. Prostate cancer tends to be more aggressive with earlier onset.

Signs and symptoms	Treatment
• Dysuria—difficulty initiating flow • Frequency, urgency • Hematuria • Bloody semen • Difficulty achieving erection • Lower back pain • Pain in hips and proximal thighs	Note: Treatment varies depending on age of onset, size of lesion, stage, and symptoms and may include one or more of the following: • Monitoring (watch and wait) • Surgical excision • Hormone therapy • Chemotherapy • Radiation • Supportive care to help the patient cope with pain, erectile dysfunction, impotence, and metastasis (most commonly to adrenals, bone, liver, and lungs)

Primary Hepatocellular Carcinoma

Primary hepatocellular carcinoma, the most common liver cancer, is usually associated with a history of cirrhosis (especially from chronic hepatitis) but can result from hemochromatosis or alcoholism. Even with removal, many cancers recur, especially if the tumor is >5 cm. Diagnostic findings include ultrasound, liver function tests, elevation of serum alpha fetoprotein (occurs in 70% in Western countries), elevation of serum des-gamma-carboxyl prothrombin (in 90%), abdominal CT, liver scan, and liver biopsy. Metastasis is commonly to the lungs and regional lymph nodes.

Signs and symptoms	Treatment
• Cachexia and loss of weight • Bruising • Fever • Splenomegaly • Hepatic bruit or friction rub • Lethargy • RUQ discomfort, sometimes radiating to right shoulder • Jaundice • Ascites (fluid may be bloody)	• Surgical removal or transplantation for small tumors <3 cm • Chemotherapy/radiation may shrink large masses prior to surgery, but response is usually poor. Transcatheter arterial chemoembolization (TACE) or chemoinfusion (TACI) into hepatic arteries may provide palliation. • Multikinase inhibitor (tumor blocking medication): Sorafenib (Nexavar) orally • Support care with analgesia (opioids)

Secondary Hepatic Cancer

Secondary hepatic cancer occurs more frequently than primary hepatic cancer because cancer cells in the blood filter through the liver from primary tumors throughout the body, such as pulmonary, colon, prostatic, gastric, renal, and breast cancers. Secondary hepatic cancer has characteristics of the primary tumor and may, in fact, be diagnosed first when symptoms indicate hepatic abnormality. Prognosis is poor because metastasis has already occurred. Diagnostic tests include ultrasound, liver function tests, and extreme drug resistance testing to determine the most effective chemotherapeutic agent, PET, and MRI. In some cases, liver biopsy may be needed, especially if the primary tumor has not been identified.

Signs and symptoms	Treatment
• Anorexia and loss of weight • Bruising • Fever • Splenomegaly • Lethargy • RUQ discomfort, sometimes radiating to right shoulder • Jaundice • Ascites	• Chemotherapy appropriate for the primary tumor may include TACE and/or TACI • Surgical removal/radiofrequency ablation of small lesions to reduce obstruction and spread • Cryosurgery • Supportive and/or palliative care, emotional support

Bladder Cancer

Bladder cancer and most other urinary cancers begin in the inside lining of the urinary organs (urothelium) and then invade the deeper layers.

Symptoms	Treatment
• **Gross hematuria**: Frank bright red blood may be evident. Sometimes urine is brown or rust-colored. This is usually the first sign of bladder cancer. Blood in urine may appear, disappear, and reappear, usually without pain. • **Microscopic hematuria**: Blood may be present but only visible under microscope examination. • **Dysuria**: Patient may have burning on urination or pain, the feeling that the bladder does not completely empty on urination, and frequency.	**Options include**: • Transurethral resection with fulguration • Radical or segmental cystectomy • Urinary diversion **Post-surgical options include**: • Chemotherapy • Radiation • Biologic therapy • Clinical trials • Supportive care

Brain Tumors

Brain tumors may be primary or secondary, resulting from metastasis from other organs. The most common primary neoplastic brain tumors in adults are astrocytoma and oligodendroglioma; and, in pediatric patients, medulloblastomas, astrocytoma, brain stem glioma, and ependymoma. Symptoms may vary widely but often include deficits in vision or hearing, ataxia, changes in mental status, nausea and vomiting, headaches, dizziness, paresthesias, and seizures. Diagnosis is usually through neurological exam and MRI. Treatment most often involves surgical excision of all or part of the tumor, radiotherapy, and/or chemotherapy. Patients may need to maintain head elevation after surgery to reduce cerebral edema and pressure, so they may need positioning assistance. Patients often need medications to control nausea and vomiting as well as pain. Some patients may exhibit personality changes (especially if the frontal lobe was involved), and family may need support in dealing with the changes.

Neurologic Disorders

Amyotrophic Lateral Sclerosis (ALS)

ALS is a rapidly progressing **degenerative neuromuscular disease** with an unknown origin. The main area of involvement is the **motor neurons** of the brain and spinal cord. Approximately half of those patients presenting with ALS will have difficulty swallowing as their first symptom. Other patients will experience distal weakness. As the disease progresses, weakness affects both the upper and lower neurons. Death generally results from **respiratory failure** due to weakness in the diaphragm along with decreased laryngeal and lingual functionality. Swallowing and oral nourishment are of high concern for these patients. Loss of motility in the tongue and hypopharynx result in the loss of ability to manipulate food as well as creating speech and communication barriers.

Review Video: Amyotrophic Lateral Sclerosis (ALS)
Visit mometrix.com/academy and enter code: 178603

CEREBROVASCULAR ACCIDENTS

Cerebrovascular accidents most commonly occur in the right or left hemisphere, but the exact location and the extent of brain damage affects the type of presenting symptoms. If the frontal area of either side is involved, there tends to be memory and learning deficits. Some **symptoms** are common to specific areas and help to identify the area involved:

- **Right hemisphere**: This results in left paralysis or paresis and a left visual field deficit that may cause spatial and perceptual disturbances so that people may have difficulty judging distance. Fine motor skills may be impacted, resulting in trouble dressing or handling tools. People may become impulsive and exhibit poor judgment, often denying impairment. Left-sided neglect (lack of perception of things on the left side) may occur. Difficulty following directions, short-term memory loss, and depression are also common. Language skills usually remain intact.
- **Left hemisphere**: This results in right paralysis or paresis and a right visual field defect. Depression is common and people often exhibit slow, cautious behavior, requiring repeated instruction and reinforcement for simple tasks. Short-term memory loss and difficulty learning new material or understanding generalizations is common. Difficulty with mathematics, reading, writing, and reasoning may occur. Aphasia (expressive, receptive, or global) is common.
- **Brain stem**: Because the brain stem controls respiration and cardiac function, a brain attack (stroke) frequently causes death, but those who survive may have a number of problems, including respiratory and cardiac abnormalities. Strokes may involve motor or sensory impairment or both.
- **Cerebellum**: This area controls balance and coordination. Strokes in the cerebellum are rare but may result in ataxia, nausea and vomiting, and headaches and dizziness or vertigo.

DEMENTIAS

End-stage progression of **dementia** results in patients becoming increasingly confused and unable to care for themselves. They may eventually lose the ability to speak, walk, or carry out any ADLs and become bedridden and non-responsive. Patients with dementia are at increased **risk** for falls, dysphagia, pressure sores, aspiration, delirium, and seizures. Some patients may become aggressive or violent, especially if frightened or severely confused. In advanced stages, medications (such as cholinesterase inhibitors, which are used for mild to moderate dementia and NMDA antagonists, used to treat moderate to severe dementia) to **control behavior** or **improve cognition** may be of limited value. SSRIs, such as citalopram, sertraline, and duloxetine are sometimes used to treat associated depression or aggressive behavior when other strategies have been unsuccessful. Anticonvulsants, such as carbamazepine and sodium valproate, may help to control aggressive behavior, but antipsychotic drugs are generally avoided because of increased risk of death. The CHPN should maintain a calm, quiet environment and use a friendly tone of voice to speak to the patient, even if the patient cannot respond.

Alzheimer's Disease

In Alzheimer's disease, there is disruption in both the electrical activity and the neurotransmitters in the brain. The cerebral cortex begins to atrophy, especially in the area of the hippocampus, which controls storage of new memories, resulting in characteristic short-term memory loss. Seven stages of disease progression (Reisberg) include:

- **Stage 1**: Preclinical with no evident impairment
- **Stage 2**: Mild cognitive decline, misplaces items, forgets words
- **Stage 3**: Mild, early-stage, problems with reading, retention, planning, handling money, organizing
- **Stage 4**: Moderate cognitive decline, difficulty with complex tasks, social withdrawal, can manage most ADLs
- **Stage 5**: Moderately severe cognitive decline, obvious confusion and disorientation, difficulty using language and managing ADLs, dress inappropriately, forget to eat, forget address, telephone number
- **Stage 6**: Moderately severe cognitive decline, profoundly confused and unable to care for self, may wander, develop sundowner's syndrome and obsessive behavior
- **Stage 7**: Very severe, wheelchair/bedbound, lose ability to speak, incontinent, muscles weak and rigid, dysphagia occurs

Non-Alzheimer's Dementias

Dementia can result from various non-Alzheimer's related conditions, including the following:

- **Creutzfeldt-Jakob disease**: CJD causes rapidly progressive dementia with impaired memory, behavioral changes, and incoordination.
- **Dementia with Lewy Bodies**: Cognitive and physical decline is similar to Alzheimer's, but symptoms may fluctuate frequently. This form of dementia may include visual hallucinations, muscle rigidity, and tremors.
- **Fronto-temporal dementia**: This may cause marked changes in personality and behavior and is characterized by difficulty using and understanding language.
- **Mixed dementia**: Dementia mirrors Alzheimer's and another type because of two different causes of dementia.
- **Normal pressure hydrocephalus**: This is characterized by ataxia, memory loss, and urinary incontinence.
- **Parkinson's dementia**: This form of dementia may involve impaired decision making and difficulty concentrating, learning new material, understanding complex language, sequencing, inflexibility, and short or long-term memory loss.
- **Vascular dementia**: Memory loss may be less pronounced than that common to Alzheimer's, but symptoms are similar.

CARDIAC DISORDERS

HEART FAILURE

Heart failure (HF) is a cardiac disease that includes disorders of contractions (systolic dysfunction) or filling (diastolic dysfunction) or both. It may include pulmonary, peripheral, or systemic edema. Congestive heart failure occurs in end-stage HF in which edema is pronounced. Left ventricular dysfunction usually precedes right. Common causes include coronary artery disease, systemic or pulmonary hypertension, cardiomyopathy, and valvular disorders. The incidence of chronic heart failure correlates with age. There are two main types of HF: systolic and diastolic. The **New York Heart Association classification** is based on function:

- **Class I**: The patient is essentially asymptomatic during normal activities with no pulmonary congestion or peripheral hypotension. There is no restriction on activities, and prognosis is good.
- **Class II**: Symptoms appear with physical exertion but are usually absent at rest, resulting in some limitations of ADL. Slight pulmonary edema may be evident by basilar rales. Prognosis is good.
- **Class III**: Obvious limitations of ADL and discomfort on any exertion. Prognosis is fair.
- **Class IV**: Symptoms at rest. Prognosis is poor.

PERICARDIAL EFFUSION

Pericardial effusion is defined as an accumulation of fluid within the pericardial cavity. Effusions (whether pleural or pericardial) will affect nearly 20% of patients with lung cancer during the advanced stages of the disease. They are also associated with breast cancer, leukemia, and lymphoma. This condition carries a poor prognosis for these patients. Pericardial effusion can be caused by the presence of cancerous cells or by the treatments used in defense of these malignancies, as well as potentially having other nonmalignant causes. Other possible causes include pericarditis, congestive heart failure, uremia, myocardial infarction, autoimmune diseases, infections, hypothyroidism, and renal and hepatic failure. Clinical signs and symptoms are dependent on the amount of fluid, how quickly it accumulates, and the general health of the cardiac tissue. Dyspnea is the most common presenting symptom, and the patient may be unable to speak more than one word with each breath. There may also be complaints of chest heaviness, dry cough, and generalized weakness. Physically, tachycardia is present as the body tries to compensate for the reduced cardiac output.

Pulmonary Disorders

COPD

Functional dyspnea, body mass index (BMI), and spirometry are used to assess the stages of **COPD**. Spirometry measures used are the ratio of forced expiratory volume in the 1st second of expiration (FEV_1) after full inhalation to total forced vital capacity (FVC). Normal lung function decreases after age 35; so, normal values are adjusted for height, weight, gender, and age:

- **Stage I (mild)**: Minimal dyspnea with or without cough and sputum. FEV_1 is ≥80% of predicted rate and FEV_1: FVC <70%.
- **Stage 2 (moderate)**: Moderate to severe chronic exertional dyspnea with/without cough and sputum. FEV_1 is 50-80% of predicted rate and FEV_1: FVC <70%.
- **Stage 3 (severe)**: Same as stage 2 but repeated episodes with increased exertional dyspnea and condition impacting quality of life. FEV_1 is 30-50% of predicted rate and FEV_1: FVC <70%.
- **Stage 4 (very severe)**: Severe dyspnea and life-threatening episodes that severely impact quality of life. FEV_1 is 30% of predicted rate or <50% with chronic respiratory failure and FEV_1: FVC <70%.

Management of End-Stage COPD

End-stage COPD is characterized by severe dyspnea. Some patients may be confused from lack of oxygen, and tachycardia is common. **Management** includes:

- Bronchodilators, such as albuterol (Ventolin) and salmeterol (Serevent), may help relieve bronchospasm and airway obstruction.
- Corticosteroids, both inhaled (Pulmicort, Vanceril) and oral (prednisone) may improve symptoms but are used most for associated asthma. High doses may result in numerous adverse effects.
- Oxygen therapy may be long term continuous or used during exertion.
- Patients should be placed in a position of comfort, usually with the head elevated.
- Eating and drinking may exhaust patient, so small frequent feedings are best.
- Skin tears and bruising are common with steroid therapy, so patients must have frequent skin care and use appropriate pressure-reducing surfaces, especially for those who insist on sitting upright and move little.
- Remain patient and supportive because patients are often irritable because of poor oxygenation and general discomfort.

Pleural Effusion

A pleural effusion occurs when fluid accumulates in the pleural space. Secretion rates are increased and/or fluid absorption becomes restricted causing excessive fluid to collect. The onset of a pleural effusion can be slow or rapid. The patient will most often present with dyspnea. Dyspnea generally results from the collapse of a lung due to increased pleural fluid pressure. The inability to expand the lung leads to the complaint of dyspnea. As the affected area increases, dyspneic distress also increases along with orthopnea and tachypnea, anorexia, malaise, and fatigue. The patient may also complain of a dry, nonproductive cough and an aching, heaviness, or dull pain in the chest. Treatment of a cancer-induced pleural effusion is palliative and symptomatic in nature, and is dependent on the surrounding circumstances, the overall patient condition, and proximity to death.

Review Video: Pleural Effusions
Visit mometrix.com/academy and enter code: 145719

Chronic Renal Failure

Chronic renal failure (resulting in end-stage renal disease) occurs when the kidneys are unable to filter and excrete wastes, concentrate urine, and maintain electrolyte balance because of hypoxic conditions, kidney disease, or obstruction in the urinary tract. It results first in azotemia (increase in nitrogenous waste in the blood) and then in uremia (nitrogenous wastes cause toxic symptoms). When >50% of the functional renal capacity is destroyed, the kidneys can no longer carry out necessary functions, and progressive deterioration takes place over months or years. Symptoms are often non-specific in the beginning with loss of appetite and energy.

Symptoms and complications	Treatment
• Weight loss • Headaches, muscle cramping, general malaise • Increased bruising and dry or itching skin • Increased BUN and creatinine • Sodium and fluid retention with edema • Hyperkalemia • Metabolic acidosis • Calcium and phosphorus depletion, resulting in altered bone metabolism, pain, and restricted growth • Anemia with decreased production on RBCs • Increased risk of infection • Uremic syndrome	• Supportive/symptomatic therapy • Dialysis and transplantation • Diet control: Low protein, salt, potassium, and phosphorus • Fluid limitations • Calcium and vitamin supplementation • Phosphate binders

Gastrointestinal Disorders

Cirrhosis and Liver Failure

Cirrhosis is a chronic hepatic disease in which normal liver tissue is replaced by fibrotic tissue that impairs liver function. Decompensated cirrhosis occurs when the liver can no longer adequately synthesize proteins, clotting factors, and other substances so that portal hypertension and liver failure occur.

Signs and symptoms	Treatment
• Hepatomegaly • Chronic elevated temperature • Clubbing of fingers • Purpura resulting from thrombocytopenia, with bruising and epistaxis • Portal obstruction resulting in jaundice and ascites • Bacterial peritonitis with ascites • Esophageal varices • Edema of extremities and presacral area resulting from reduced albumin in the plasma • Vitamin deficiency from interference with formation, use, and storage of vitamins, such as A, C, and K • Anemia from chronic gastritis and reduced intake • Hepatic encephalopathy with alterations in mentation • Hypotension • Atrophy of gonads	• Treatment varies according to the symptoms and is supportive rather than curative as the fibrotic changes in the liver cannot be reversed: • Dietary supplements and vitamins • Diuretics (potassium sparing), such as Aldactone and Dyrenium, to decrease ascites • Colchicine to reduce fibrotic changes • Liver transplant (the definitive treatment) • Paracentesis may be done for palliative relief

Ascites

Ascites involves the accumulation of serous fluid in the abdominal cavity. There are three **types of ascites**:

- **Central ascites** results from compression of the portal venous or lymphatic system from tumor invasion. With this process, there may also be a decrease in plasma oncotic pressure favoring the development of ascites, as a result of reduced dietary protein intake and cancer-induced catabolism.
- **Peripheral ascites** results from deposits of tumor cells on the parietal or visceral peritoneum, functionally interfering with normal lymph and venous drainage. The presence of macrophages also increases capillary permeability and thereby contributes to increasing fluid retention within the peritoneal cavity.
- **Mixed-type ascites** is a combination of both peripheral and central ascites.

Chylous malignant ascites occurs when cancer cells invade the retroperitoneal space causing lymph flow obstruction through the lymph nodes or pancreas. Malignant ascites generally has a poor prognosis. Tumor cells make it difficult to reduce fluid accumulation. Cancers most often associated with ascites include ovarian, endometrial, breast, colon, gastric, and pancreatic cancer. Less common sources include mesothelioma, non-Hodgkin's lymphoma, and prostate cancer.

Bowel Obstruction

Bowel obstruction is a mechanical obstruction of the passage of intestinal contents because of constriction or occlusion of the lumen or lack of muscular contractions (paralytic ileus). In pediatric hematologic/oncologic patients, bowel obstruction is most often associated with non-Hodgkin's lymphomas because tumors may form in the small and/or large intestine (most common), especially Burkitt lymphoma. Bowel obstruction may also occur with hematological malignancies, such as leukemia, and intraabdominal tumors. Symptoms include abdominal pain and distention, vomiting, dehydration, diminished or absent bowel sounds, severe constipation, respiratory distress, shock, and sepsis. Sudden and frequent nausea and vomiting in large volumes, often immediately after intake, usually indicates a bowel obstruction in the small intestines while obstructions of the colon usually result in more delayed vomiting, with fecal emesis. If obstruction is partial or inoperable, dexamethasone may relieve some of the symptoms because it reduces inflammation and swelling and provides relief of nausea. With paralytic ileus, an NG tube may be inserted for decompression. Surgical intervention is used for complete obstruction.

Constipation

Constipation may be caused by primary or metastasized cancers, diabetes, hypothyroidism, hemorrhoids, diverticular disease, neurological diseases, dehydration, changes in toileting, and hypercalcemia. Medications that can cause constipation include opioids, anticholinergics, tricyclic antidepressants, antiparkinsonian drugs, iron, antihypertensives, antihistamines, antacids, and diuretics. Vinca alkaloid chemotherapy also causes constipation by damaging the myenteric plexus of the colon, causing increased contractions without increased movement. Stool laxative/softeners should be taken daily to prevent/treat constipation, especially if associated with opioid use. If patients cannot tolerate oral medications, then methylnaltrexone subcutaneously may relieve constipation. For opioid-induced constipation, reducing the dose of opioid may increase the patient's pain, so treating the adverse effect is more important than removing the cause. Bulking agents should be avoided as they can increase constipation and impaction if the patient is not able to drink adequate fluids, as is common with debilitated patients. While adequate fluid intake is preferred, forcing fluids may increase a patient's discomfort and cause nausea.

DIARRHEA

Diarrhea may be acute or chronic and is often associated with treatment (chemotherapy, radiotherapy) or disease (HIV/AIDS, GVHD). Diarrhea may be osmotic (hyperosmolar preparations/enteric feedings), secretory (chemotherapy and radiotherapy), hypermotile (partial bowel obstruction), or exudative (abdominal radiotherapy). The **National Cancer Institute Scale of Severity of Diarrhea:**

- **Grade 0**: Normal stools
- **Grade 1**: Two to three stools daily but essentially no other symptoms
- **Grade 2**: Four to six stools daily with stools at night and/or moderate abdominal cramping
- **Grade 3**: Seven to nine stools daily with fecal incontinence and/or severe abdominal cramping
- **Grade 4**: >10 stools daily with stools grossly blood and/or fluid depletion results in need for parenteral support

Management may include oral/IV fluids and electrolytes, loperamide 2-4 mg 1-2 times daily, diphenoxylate 1-2 tablets up to 8 times daily, codeine, tincture of opium (decreases peristalsis), octreotide (secretory diarrhea), bismuth salicylate, and clonidine (watery diarrhea associated with bronchogenic cancer). Pectin and methylcellulose may improve stool consistency. Milk products and foods that are high fiber, gas producing, sugary, or spicy should be avoided.

DIABETES

End-stage progression of diabetes may include:

- **Nephropathy and renal failure**: Patients may have recurrent urinary infections, difficulty urinating because of impaired sensation, and progressing to kidney failure and uremia. Some patients may be maintained on hemodialysis or peritoneal dialysis. Others may require catheterization.
- **Retinopathy and vision impairment**: Patients may need orientation to objects about them and vision aids.
- **Peripheral neuropathy**: Lack of sensation increases risks of ulcerations and infections, and some patients may develop severe pain in the feet and legs, requiring pain medications. Patients should be turned frequently with limbs supported and cushioned, and skin assessed.
- **Diabetic ulcers**: Various treatments, including dressings, debridement, and hyperbaric oxygen treatments may be utilized to prevent worsening and promote healing.
- **Gastroparesis**: Patients may have frequent heartburn and feeling of fullness and discomfort. Sitting upright for 1-2 hours after eating and taking metoclopramide may help promote gastric emptying.
- **Hypoglycemia/Hyperglycemia**: Management of glucose levels may become more difficult, especially if the patient is unable to eat adequately, so glucose levels must be monitored frequently, especially to avoid ketoacidosis and hypoglycemia.

Diabetic Neuropathy

Up to 70% of patients with diabetes mellitus develop diabetic neuropathy. **Types of neuropathy** include:

- **Sensory (peripheral)**: Usually bilateral and affecting hands and feet ("stocking-glove neuropathy"). Patients have sensory loss, paresthesias (tingling, itching), and pain (burning, cramping, tearing). Pain usually worsens at night. Foot injuries and ulcerations may occur because of loss of sensation. Some experience hyperesthesia and cannot tolerate any pressure on skin. Patients have increased risk of ulceration and amputation because of loss of protective sensation (LOPS) and peripheral arterial disease (a common finding). Feet should be examined daily, and the patient should not go barefoot. Patients may develop foot deformity (Charcot's foot).
- **Autonomic**: Can affect all body systems, leading to fecal incontinence, diarrhea, hypoglycemic unawareness, neurogenic bladder, gastroparesis, postural hypotension, tachycardia, erectile dysfunction, decreased libido, and vaginitis. Some patients may develop urinary retention and may require intermittent catheterization.

Hematologic Disorders

Neutropenia

Neutropenia refers to an abnormally low blood count of neutrophil granulocytes—the main form of white blood cells and the body's primary defense against infection. It is sometimes also called "leucopenia" in reference to the lack of white blood cells. **Neutropenia** is diagnosed as a polymorphonuclear neutrophil count equal or less than 500/mL. Chronic neutropenia is a sustained condition of minimal neutrophils lasting 3 or more months. Neutropenia may occur from a decreased production of white blood cells following chemotherapy or radiation therapy. It may also occur from a loss of white blood cells due to an autoimmune disease. Neutropenia is silent but dangerous. It leaves essentially no neutrophils to fight any threat of infection. Neutrophils make up as much as 70% of the white blood cells circulating in the blood. Neutropenia can ultimately result in a severe septic situation which can be life threatening. Up to 70% of patients experiencing a fever while in a neutropenic state will die within 48 hours if not treated aggressively.

DIC

The onset of symptoms of **disseminated intravascular coagulation** (DIC) may be very rapid or a slower chronic progression from a disease. Those who develop the chronic manifestation of the disease usually have fewer acute symptoms and may slowly develop ecchymosis or bleeding wounds.

Signs and symptoms	Treatment
• Bleeding from surgical or venous puncture sites • Evidence of GI bleeding with distention, bloody diarrhea • Hypotension and acute symptoms of shock • Petechiae and purpura with extensive bleeding into the tissues • Laboratory abnormalities: • Prolonged prothrombin and partial prothrombin times • Decreased platelet counts and fragmented RBCs • Decreased fibrinogen	• Identifying and treating underlying cause • Replacement blood products, such as platelets and fresh frozen plasma • Anticoagulation therapy (heparin) to increase clotting time • Cryoprecipitate to increase fibrinogen levels • Coagulation inhibitors and coagulation factors

Burn Injuries

Burn injuries may be chemical, electrical, or thermal and are assessed by the area, percentage of the body burned, and depth:

- **First-degree burns** are superficial and affect the epidermis, causing erythema and pain. Treatment: Soothing lotion, cool compresses, analgesia.
- **Second-degree burns** extend through the dermis (partial thickness), resulting in blistering and sloughing of epidermis with severe pain. Treatment: Silver sulfadiazine, non-adherent dressings, and analgesia.
- **Third-degree burns** affect underlying tissue, including vasculature, muscles, and nerves (full thickness), with no pain because of nerve damage. Treatment: Varies but may include debridement, skin grafts, oxygen, IV fluids/electrolytes, antibiotics, high protein diet, and analgesia.

American Burn Association Criteria	
Minor	<10% body surface area (BSA) 2% BSA with 3rd degree without serious risk to face, hands, feet, or perineum
Moderate	10-20% BSA combined 2nd and 3rd degree burns ≤10% full thickness without serious risk to face, hands, feet, or perineum
Major	20% BSA; ≥10% 3rd degree burns All burns to face, hands, feet, or perineum that will result in functional/cosmetic defect Burns with inhalation or other major trauma

Head Trauma

Concussions and Contusions/Lacerations

A variety of different injuries can occur as a result of **head trauma**:

- **Concussions** are the most common injury and are usually relatively transient, causing no permanent neurological damage. When the concussion is severe, or multiple concussion occur, however, permanent damage can occur. Concussions may result in confusion, disorientation, and mild amnesia, which last only minutes or hours.
- **Contusions/lacerations** are bruising and tears of cerebral tissue. There may be petechial areas at the impact site (coup) or larger bruising. Contrecoup injuries are less common in children than in adults. Areas most impacted by contusions and lacerations are the occipital, frontal, and temporal lobes. The degree of injury relates to the amount of vascular damage, but initial symptoms are similar to a concussion; however, symptoms persist and may progress, depending upon the degree of injury. Lacerations are often caused by fractures.

Glasgow Coma Scale

The Glasgow coma scale (GCS) measures the depth and duration of coma or impaired level of consciousness and is used for postoperative assessment. The GCS measures three parameters (best eye response, best verbal response, and best motor response) with a total possible score that ranges from 3 to 15. The same scale is used with slight modifications for infants.

Eye opening	4: Spontaneous 3: To verbal stimuli 2: To pain (not of face) 1: No response
Verbal	5: Oriented (Infant: Smiles, exhibits appropriate interactions) 4: Conversation confused, but can answer questions (Infant: crying but consolable) 3: Uses inappropriate words (Infant: Moaning, sometimes inconsolable) 2: Speech incomprehensible (Infant: Inconsolable, agitated) 1: No response
Motor	6: Moves on command (Infant: Moves spontaneously or with purpose) 5: Moves purposefully to respond to pain 4: Withdraws in response to pain 3: Decorticate posturing (flexion) in response to pain 2: Decerebrate posturing (extension) in response to pain 1: No response

Review Video: Glasgow Coma Scale
Visit mometrix.com/academy and enter code: 133399

Classifications of Acute Traumatic Brain Injuries

Traumatic brain injuries may range from mild to severe and may result from impact (falls, motor-vehicle accidents, assaults, or penetration (gunshot and stabbing injuries)). Injuries may be primary with direct assault on the brain or secondary, resulting from hypoxia or hypotension, so initial treatment focuses on maintaining adequate blood pressure and preventing increased intracranial pressure that interferes with oxygenation. TBIs are classified according to symptoms and Glasgow coma score:

- **Mild (GCS 13-15)**: Brief loss of consciousness (LOC), headache, and mild confusion. Recovery is good although some may have persistent symptoms.
- **Moderate (GCS 9-12)**: LOC, confused, focal neurologic defects may be present. Prognosis is usually good, but 12% progress to severe TBI.
- **Severe (GCS ≤8)**: Comatose, severe symptoms, increased intracranial pressure, 20% mortality rate with survivors usually having significant neurological deficits. With severe injuries, patients may require intubation and mechanical ventilation. If injuries are inconsistent with life, patients may become organ donors.

Management of Complications from Acute Traumatic Head Injuries

Head injuries that occur at the time of trauma include fractures, contusions, hematomas, and diffuse cerebral and vascular injury. These injuries may result in hypoxia, increased intracranial pressure, and cerebral edema. Open injuries may result in infection. Patients often suffer initial hypertension, which increases intracranial pressure, decreasing perfusion. Often the primary problem with head trauma is a significant increase in swelling, which also interferes with perfusion, causing hypoxia and hypercapnia, which trigger increased blood flow. This increased volume at a time when injury impairs auto-regulation increases cerebral edema, which, in turn, increases intracranial pressure and results in a further decrease in perfusion with resultant ischemia. If pressure continues to rise, the brain may herniate. Concomitant hypotension may result in hypoventilation, further complicating treatment. Treatments include:

- Monitoring ICP and CCP
- Providing oxygen
- Elevating head of bed and maintaining proper body alignment
- Giving medications: Analgesics, anticonvulsants, and anesthetics
- Providing blood/fluids to stabilize hemodynamics
- Managing airway, providing mechanical ventilation if needed
- Providing osmotic agents, such as mannitol and hypertonic saline solution, to reduce cerebral edema

SPINAL CORD INJURIES

Spinal cord injuries may result from blunt trauma, falls from a height, various types of sports injuries (especially contact sports, gymnastic, diving), and penetrating trauma. Damage results from mechanical injury and secondary responses resulting from hemorrhage, edema, and ischemia. The type of symptoms relates to the area and degree of injury.

Anterior cord	The posterior column functions remain so there is sensation of touch, vibration, and position remaining below injury but with complete paralysis and loss of sensations of pain and temperature. Injury to the anterior portion of the spinal cord usually results from herniated disks, hyperflexion injuries, or damage to the anterior spinal artery. Prognosis is poor.
Brown-Séquard /Lateral cord	The cord is hemisected resulting in spastic paresis, loss of sense of position and vibration on the injured side and loss of pain and thermal sensation on the other side below level of injury. Prognosis is good. Injury to the right or left half of spinal cord usually occurs from transverse hemisection by knife injury or fracture dislocations.
Cauda equina	Damage is below L-1 with variable loss of motor ability and sensation and bowel and bladder dysfunction. Injury is to peripheral nerves, which can regenerate so prognosis is better than for other lesions of the spinal cord.
Central cord	Results from hyperextension and ischemia or stenosis of cervical spine, causing quadriparesis (more severe in upper extremities) with some loss of sensations of pain and temperature). Prognosis is good, but fine motor skills are often impaired in upper extremities. The trunk area may suffer incomplete loss of sensation and control, and bowel and bladder control may remain intact.
Conus medullaris	Injury to lower spine (lower lumbar and sacral nerves) causes lumbar pain, loss of sensation in medial thighs, numbness and weakness in legs and feet, unstable ambulation, impotence, and lack of bladder control.
Posterior cord	Motor function is preserved but without sensation.
Spinal shock	Injury at T6 or above, results in flaccid paralysis below lesion with loss of sensations and rectal tone, bradycardia, and hypotension.

Indicators of Imminent Death

Nurse's Role in the Final Hours of Life

The nurse and nursing assistant are important members of the healthcare team throughout the process leading to death, and often develop significant bonds with the patient and family. Many patients and families prefer the presence of a nurse in the final hours of a patient's life, rather than a doctor, because of the close, consistent care-giving relationship. Some patients and families prefer to share those last moments privately. Accept whatever the patient and family choose. The presence of the nurse can be beneficial, as it provides the patient and family with immediate access to a member of the healthcare team who can answer questions regarding the actual process of death. The nurse ensures that everybody has a seat, points out where washroom, telephone, and cafeteria facilities are located, and offers to remain with the patient when family members need a break. If asked to be present, the nurse intervenes only as necessary, out of respect for the family's need for time with their loved one.

The interdisciplinary healthcare team prepares patients and their families for the **imminent death** of the patient. Nevertheless, the actual event is a time of great emotion. *If specific rituals cannot be conducted in a facility because they are against regulations, ensure that the family understands the limitations prior to the death.* Ensure that the patient and family are treated with dignity and respect prior to and after death occurs. Check the patient's vital signs. Record the time vital signs are absent in the patient's chart. If death occurred in a hospice, the nurse pronounces death. If death occurred at home, the CNA or nurse notifies the doctor, who comes to legally pronounce death and complete the death certificate. Do not begin postmortem care until after death is officially pronounced. Offer family caregivers the opportunity to assist in preparing the body if their cultural and religious traditions require participation in postmortem care. The body must be prepared before 2 hours elapse, when decomposition and rigor mortis start.

If it appears death will occur while the nurse is present, alert the family. Assist with contacting family members who are not present, and gathering those that are together. Be cognizant of visitors that are tiring the patient. Close the curtain around the patient for privacy. The patient is the top priority. Encourage family members to enter behind the curtain and speak to the patient singly or in pairs, if this is allowed under the family's customs and they wish to be present. Respect the family's specific religious or cultural observances surrounding the moment of death. If family members choose to remain outside the room, relay information to them as necessary.

Nearing Death Awareness

Nearing death awareness (**NDA**) is a common phenomenon among patients who are dying. When NDA occurs, the patient seems to be aware that death is imminent and may exhibit a sudden change in **mental status**, which may be dismissed as simple confusion. Patients may, for example, begin to talk about going on a journey or taking a trip. Others may say directly that they are going to die, or state a time ("I'm doing to die tomorrow"). Many patients begin to talk about seeing or speaking to someone close to them who has died ("Mother is there waiting for me") or may report seeing angels, Jesus, Buddha, or heaven, depending on their religious beliefs. Some may report a bright light, report a feeling of peace, or report their mind is separate from their body. Others may stare into space and appear to be seeing or listening to something or someone although they can return to awareness if spoken to, so in this sense the experience is different from usual hallucinations. The **Greyson NDE scale** assesses this state with questions in 4 areas: cognitive, affective, paranormal, and transcendental.

ACTIVELY DYING

Active dying, or imminent death, is defined by physical signs and symptoms that indicate likely demise within hours or days. Typically, the patient shows signs of profound weakness, appears gaunt and pale, and the extremities are cool and mottled. He or she lacks interest in food or drink and has difficulty swallowing, which significantly decreases oral intake. Changes in breathing patterns are also common, including shallow respirations with decreased oxygen concentration, dyspnea, Cheyne-Stokes or other irregular patterns, and gurgling or gravelly sounds in the back of the throat from excess secretions. There may be transient improvements in comfort, pain sensation and mental status, but the overall state is one of varying agitation, restlessness, delirium and confusion, increased pain, profound sleepiness, reduced awareness, difficulty concentrating and disorientation to time and place. A semi-comatose or fully comatose state may emerge.

The patient may also experience incontinence of both bowel and bladder. Third-space fluids may gradually be reabsorbed, decreasing the amount of swelling present. The pupils may become fixed and dilated.

FEEDING

A dying patient is not taking in **adequate nutrition**, so his or her metabolism changes and energy declines. When this happens, the patient will have less awake time, which can cause the family concern. Food is often associated with comfort. The family's inability to provide this comfort for their loved one can be a source of distress. The CNA or nurse can assist the family by educating them to the problems a patient may experience by consuming more than desired at this point. The dying patient's altered metabolism means his or her body is unable to handle nutrients in a normal way. Excess food and fluid will cause an increase in respiratory and gastric secretions that can result in dyspnea, abdominal distention, pain, and peripheral edema. All of these conditions put the patient at risk for infection, skin breakdown, and pain.

PROVIDING FLUIDS

Most actively dying patients are **dehydrated** because they are no longer consuming adequate food and fluids, but there is little discomfort associated with this. Dehydration helps reduce nausea, vomiting, and edema for end-stage patients. The most common complaint is dry lips, nasal membranes, and mouth. Oral and nasal drying often results from increased mouth breathing, medication side effects (e.g., antihistamines), and supplementary oxygen delivered by mask or nasal cannula. The family may wish to provide the patient with fluids to drink as a way to relieve suffering and offer comfort. However, the result could be to increase the patient's distress by increasing respiratory and gastrointestinal secretions. Increased secretions lead to dyspnea, abdominal pain and distention, and peripheral edema. A bloated patient is at risk for skin breakdown, infection, and pain. Cleanse the patient's mouth and lips frequently with cool water or protective gel that help them retain moisture, to ease the discomfort without creating more problems.

EDUCATING THE FAMILY

It is often difficult for family members to cope with the physical changes associated with the dying patient. One of the most alarming is significant weight loss and muscle wasting, called **cachexia**. Food is associated with comfort and caring. When asking the family to withhold food, it can leave them feeling frustrated and unable to do anything to help. Reaching this point with the patient may force family members to accept that death is imminent. Educate the family about the physiological changes that take place in the dying patient to help them understand that the withholding of food is actually beneficial. The change in metabolism that results from decreased nutrition causes the body to produce and release endorphins, which are peptide hormones for natural pain control.

Dehydration reduces the production and accumulation of secretions in the respiratory and gastrointestinal tract and reduces edema. It may also decrease pain caused by the pressure tumors exert on surrounding tissues, all of which make the patient more comfortable.

Changes in Bowel Habits

As patients approach death, it is almost universal that their intake of food and fluids decreases. Decreased input means **decreased output of urine and feces**. Monitor the intake and output of patients and be aware of the signs and symptoms of constipation and urinary retention. Constipation, abdominal distention, nausea, and vomiting can indicate bowel obstruction or volvulus (twisted intestine). Urinary retention can indicate kidney failure or a blockage from a stone or tumor. Diarrhea creates significant fluid loss and unbalances electrolytes, which can result in heart attack. Constipated patients are uncomfortable and more difficult to manage. Follow instructions in the care plan for the treatment of constipation.

Congestion

Patients experience **increased respiratory secretions** as they approach death, and are unable to clear them independently. Many experience a drowning sensation. Frequent episodes of coughing leave patients fatigued. Assist the patient with dyspnea to clear the airway by repositioning, and encourage deep breathing and coughing exercises. Use caution, because patients with osteoporosis may fracture ribs if they cough hard. Note the quality of the patient's cough—dry and non-productive, or wet and productive. The RN may suction the airway and ask the doctor to prescribe antihistamines and decongestants. If the patient has a productive cough, the doctor may order the nurse or CNA to assist the patient to collect a sputum sample. The best time of collection is when the patient awakes in the morning, because fluid collects overnight. Wear gloves. Label the jar in ink. Open the sterile jar and ask the patient to expel lung fluid into it, *not saliva*. Cap the jar, place it in a biohazard bag, and refrigerate until pick-up by the lab.

Increased Sleepiness

During the last four weeks of life, end-stage patients experience a marked increase in **sleepiness** due to decreased intake of calories, dehydration, hypoxia, psychological withdrawal, organ failure, and vital exhaustion. As caloric intake decreases, the body conserves energy and shunts blood flow from the periphery to the core to preserve the vital organs (brain, heart, lungs, and kidneys). Rerouting the blood supply triggers the brain to decrease the amount of time a patient is awake. Depending on the underlying disease process, the amount of awake time a patient experiences may be related to a significant decrease in oxygen availability. A low blood oxygen level (hypoxia) will result in sleepiness. For those patients receiving opiates, an increase in sleepiness occurs as a side effect of the medication. Azotemia (also called uremia) causes sleepiness as the kidneys fail. Azotemia causes death 8-12 days after a patient decides to stop dialysis.

Agitation or Restlessness

Patients experience **acute agitation** from urinary retention, constipation, dyspnea, medication side effects, and pain over the course of their diseases. When death is imminent in one or two days, many patients experience another final flare of agitation, which is difficult for families and caregivers to watch. It is the responsibility of the hospice team to monitor the patient for signs of agitation and be prepared with appropriate interventions. The most common cause of agitation in the dying patient is pain. If the patient is nonverbal, rely on physical symptoms to determine when the patient is experiencing pain. Reposition the patient. Monitor for signs that the patient needs pain medication. Divert the patient's attention through music or reading. If the patient approaches death with fear or spiritual unrest, it may express itself as agitation. Ask if he or she wants to speak to a chaplain. Chaplains have contacts among many religions and can arrange visits from the appropriate spiritual leader.

When Death Is Imminent

It is important for the nurse and nursing assistant to understand the cultural and religious beliefs of the patient and his or her family, because these two aspects are highlighted when death is approaching. It is the responsibility of the hospice/palliative care team to support the patient and family and to respect the wishes of the patient. The patient must be monitored for physiological signs that indicate death is imminent, even if the patient does not complain of symptoms. Most patients, within the last four weeks of life, will experience significant fatigue and weakness and require additional assistance. Pain may increase in the dying patient, or the patient's requirement for pain control medication may decrease as the body releases endorphins. Endorphins are polypeptide hormones produced by the pituitary gland and hypothalamus in the brain that act as natural pain suppressants. Most patients experience difficulty breathing (dyspnea) and this is most distressing for families. Careful positioning of the patient and improving air circulation facilitates breathing.

Use of Air Circulation

One of the most common symptoms at the end of life is difficulty breathing (dyspnea). While this can be related to the underlying disease process, most patients near death experience dyspnea as a result of:

- Increased respiratory secretions
- Increased breathing muscle weakness
- Decreased ability to clear respiratory secretions
- Metabolic changes that alter the effectiveness of gas exchange in the lungs

Dyspnea is often the most distressing of symptoms, as the patient fears the sensation of suffocating, and the family is concerned because they are unable to provide relief and comfort to their loved one. The easiest and least invasive way for the nurse and nursing assistant to relieve dyspnea is to use fans to increase the **circulation of air** in the patient's room. Many patients report a decrease in dyspnea when they feel air moving across their faces. If fans are ineffective, inform the respiratory therapist or doctor that supplemental oxygen seems indicated.

Patients' Belief System

Often, patients approaching death feel they have lost control of their lives, which can be as distressing as their physical symptoms. The hospice/palliative care team must understand the cultural, gender, and religious beliefs of patients and their families. **Belief systems** play a vital role in the expectations of the patient and family members. It is also important that nurses and nursing assistants recognize their own personal beliefs surrounding death, and do not impose their own belief systems on the patient and family. Most patients find familiar family and/or religious objects comforting. Treat religious and family artifacts with the utmost respect. Regardless of where the patient is receiving hospice care, he or she deserves to spend time in an environment tailored to his or her preferences. A home-like environment provides comfort and security. Allow the patient to reach the end of life in peace, which will look different for each individual.

The nurse and nursing assistant must accept how the **cultural and religious beliefs** of the patient and family require environmental changes as death nears. They may be required to place particular objects of sentimental value or religious significance around the sick room. The schedule may change to allow for religious rites. They may be asked to assist with ritual washing and dressing.

Some patients prefer quiet and few visitors. If the patient prefers to be surrounded by family and friends, the nurse must rearrange the sick room to ensure the patient's privacy when performing personal care. Support the patient's choice of environment, whether hospice and palliative care is being given in a facility or the patient's home. Develop strategies so that the patient's choices do not interfere with those of other dying patients, such as encouraging the use of headphones. Examine one's own belief systems surrounding death and do not impose personal beliefs or preferences on the patient's environment. Respect the wishes of the patient and attempt to provide the environment the patient desires.

Cultural Influences on Nutrition and Hydration at End of Life

Most cultures attach significant importance to the **role of consuming meals together**. As patients experience the progression of disease and approach death, the goals of nutrition and hydration change. Changing feeding routines often proves distressing for patients and their families. It is the responsibility of the nurse/nursing assistant to understand the changes and help support the patient and their family as the need for food decreases. As death approaches, the goal of eating and drinking is no longer to meet the nutritional needs of the patient. In fact, introducing food and/or fluids as the patient's organs shut down can cause or increase discomfort for the patient. End-stage patients produce increased mucous in the respiratory tract, which leads to dyspnea and the death rattle. If fluids are introduced, the body uses it to increase secretions, which causes increased respiratory difficulty. A more appropriate use of fluid is to moisten the patient's mouth for speaking.

Most cultures attach significant social importance to eating meals together and the hospice/palliative care team must understand the cultural background and the significance of sharing meals in that culture. As a patient approaches death, the goal of eating and drinking becomes social, rather than meeting the diminished nutritional needs of the patient. Anorexia in the patient signals that the dying process has begun. Families often exhibit distress because they perceive that the patient is starving. It is important that the nurse/nursing assistant understands the metabolic changes occurring in the patient's body, and educates and supports the patient and family. Patients who continue to consume food after metabolic changes have started organ shutdown will experience increased edema and discomfort. End-stage patients are unable to process food comfortably, as the intestinal tract slows significantly or stops functioning altogether.

Providing Comfort Measures and Dignity at Time of Death

The nurse should prepare family and friends for the changes they will see as the patient nears death and provide guidance in **comfort measures** for the dying patient:

- Ensuring pain is managed adequately, including medications, such as analgesics and muscle relaxants (if the patient is having muscle spasms), and complementary therapies, such as massage, Reiki, and music therapy
- Providing mouth care with premoistened swabs
- Gently washing and moisturizing the patient's kin with a warm cloth if the patient is cold and cool cloth if feverish
- Talking softly to the patient even if the patient appears to be in a coma and non-responsive
- Accepting and not challenging if the patient appears to be seeing or communicating with deceased loved-ones
- Using FaceTime or Skype to allow family/friends who are not present to participate

After the patient has died, some people will want to spend time sitting with the body and may want to participate in washing and dressing the body, and the nurse should respect their wishes.

Discontinuing Life Support

Discontinuation or withholding of life support often occurs when a patient is dying and unlikely to benefit from treatment. Patients (and surrogates if the patient is unable to make decisions) have the right to refuse life-supporting/life-prolonging therapy. Before withdrawing life-support, a DNR order should be documented as well as the reason and rationale for discontinuation of treatment. Most commonly, life-supporting therapies are withdrawn in the following sequence:

1. Blood products, such as packed red blood cells
2. Hemodialysis
3. Vasopressors
4. Mechanical ventilation
5. Total parenteral nutrition
6. Antibiotics (allowing infection to take its course)
7. Intravenous fluids
8. Tube feedings

Bedside monitors should be shut off during the withdrawal procedures. The family should be included in decision-making and apprised of the steps taken to discontinue life support and to provide for the patient's comfort. The time to death after discontinuation of treatment varies depending on a number of factors, but discontinuation of ventilation usually results in death within a few minutes or hours while discontinuation of hemodialysis usually results in death in 2-3 days.

Removal of Mechanical Ventilation

Steps for the removal of mechanical ventilation include:

1. Decrease provided analgesia (opioid) and decrease intermittent mandatory ventilation to <10, then discontinue neuromuscular blockade so that the level of discomfort can be more accurately assessed.
2. Turn off alarms and monitors.
3. Position patient at 30° or higher and suction mouth if secretions are copious.
4. Set PEEP to 0.
5. Gradually reduce the fractional oxygen content (FiO_2).
6. Reduce or stop mandatory inspirations.
7. Reduce level of pressure support.
8. Place T-piece to flow-by.
9. Extubate.
10. Administer humidified oxygen.
11. Administer opioid (morphine, fentanyl, or midazolam) and/or diazepam if the patient exhibits signs of distress.

The time period from beginning of the weaning process to extubation usually takes 15-60 minutes.

Discontinuing Nutrition and Hydration

Artificial nutrition and hydration (per TPN, tube feedings, IV fluids) are medical treatments and can be withdrawn along with other treatments for patients who are nearing death or in a permanent vegetative state. As the patient's systems begin to shut down, continuing artificial nutrition and hydration can increase edema, secretions, and heart failure, resulting in increased discomfort. Additionally, TPN and tube feedings may lead to a number of different complications. As patients near death, they typically do not experience hunger or thirst. Some healthcare providers feel that providing fluids to dying patients may be a comfort measure, but most adverse effects (dry mouth, cracked lips) can be alleviated effectively with good medical and nursing care. Often the decision regarding artificial hydration rests with the patient or family, but if hydration is continued, a minimal volume should be used to avoid fluid overload.

Turning Off LVAD and ICD

Ventricular assist devices (VAD) can provide support to the left (most common; LVAD) or right ventricle or both. With most devices, blood drains from the base of the left ventricle into the pump through an inflow cannula and back into the aorta through an outflow cannula. The LVAD pump is placed preperitoneally in the abdomen with electrical cables and air vent tunneled through a percutaneous line to the external controller and battery pack. The **implantable cardioverter defibrillator (ICD)** is usually placed in the upper chest with electrodes into the right atrium. It paces the heart and delivers a shock when necessary. Before the devices are discontinued, the patient is usually sedated to reduce the perception of dyspnea associated with abrupt reduction in cardiac output, especially with the LVAD. In most cases, patients will die within minutes of the LVAD being shut off, but if the patient has some residual cardiac function, death may be delayed for a few days. Death after removal of the ICD may vary depending on residual cardiac function.

Withholding or Withdrawing Medications from Dying Patients

Withholding or withdrawing medications of dying patients must include the following considerations:

- Antihypertensives and other drugs (diuretics, antibiotics, hormones, antidysrhythmics, hypoglycemic agents, and laxatives) that do not directly contribute to patient comfort are usually discontinued in the final days.
- Abrupt discontinuation of corticosteroids can cause severe effects, so discontinuation should be tapered. If used to reduce cerebral edema and intracranial pressure in order to control pain and seizures, as the corticosteroid dose is tapered, the dosage of anticonvulsant should be increased.
- Medications that are usually continued as long as possible include sedatives and analgesics and medications to control symptoms, such as antipyretics, antiemetics, anticholinergics, and anticonvulsants.
- Oral medications can be continued as long as a patient can swallow, often in liquid form rather than pills or capsules. Other medications may be administered parenterally.
- Patients should be medicated prior to extubation, and additional medications should be available to control symptoms. The medications that are most indicated to relieve a sense of breathlessness are opioids. Benzodiazepines are also usually administered to relieve anxiety. Oxygen is usually continued at about 21%.

Patient Care: Pain Management

Etiology of Pain, Types of Pain, and Pain Syndromes

Pathophysiology of Pain

Nociceptors

Nociceptors are the primary neurons, or **sensory receptors**, responding to stimuli in the skin, muscle, and joints, as well as the stomach, bladder, and uterus. These neurons have specialized responses for mechanical, thermal, or chemical stimuli. The **neuron stimulation** is a direct result of tissue injury and follows four stages: **transduction** where a change occurs, **transmission** where the impulse is transferred along the neural path, **modulation** or translation of the signal, and **perception** by the patient. When injury occurs, the nociceptors initiate the process that begins **depolarization of the peripheral nerve**. Nociceptors may consist of either A-fiber axons or C-fiber axons. The message travels along the neural pathway and creates a perception of pain. A-fiber axons carry these pain messages at a much faster rate than C-fiber axons.

Nociceptive Pain

Nociceptive pain is an umbrella term for pain caused by **stimulation of the neuroreceptor**. This stimulation is a direct result of tissue injury. The severity of pain is proportionate to the extent of the injury. Nociceptive pain can be subdivided into two classifications: somatic and visceral pain. **Somatic pain** is located in the cutaneous tissues, bone joints, and muscle tissues. **Visceral pain** is specific to internal organs protected by a layer of viscera, such as the cardiovascular, respiratory, gastrointestinal, or genitourinary systems. Both types are treatable with opioids.

Visceral Pain

Visceral pain is associated with the internal organs. It can be very different depending on the affected organ. Not all internal organs are sensitive to pain (some lack **nociceptors**, such as the spleen, kidney, and pancreas), and may withstand a great deal of damage without causing pain. Other internal organs, such as the stomach, bladder, and ureters, can create significant pain from even the slightest damage. Visceral pain generally has a **poorly defined area**. It is also capable of referring pain to other remote locations away from the area of injury. It is described as a squeezing or cramping: a deep ache within the internal organs. The patient may complain of a generalized sick feeling or have nausea and vomiting. Visceral pain generally responds well to treatment with **opioids**.

Review Video: Visceral Pain
Visit mometrix.com/academy and enter code: 430402

Somatic Pain

Somatic pain refers to messages from pain receptors located in the **cutaneous or musculoskeletal tissues**. When the pain occurs within the musculoskeletal tissue, it is referred to as **deep somatic pain**. Metastasizing cancers commonly cause deep somatic pain. **Surface pain** refers to pain concentrated in the **dermis and cutaneous layers** such as that caused by a surgical incision. Deep somatic pain is generally described as a dull, throbbing ache that is well focused on the area of trauma. It responds well to **opioids**. Surface somatic pain is also directly focused on the injury. It is frequently described as sharper than deep somatic pain. It may also present as a burning or pricking sensation.

Review Video: Somatic Pain
Visit mometrix.com/academy and enter code: 982772

Review Video: Somatic Nervous System
Visit mometrix.com/academy and enter code: 100382

Neuropathic Pain

Neuropathic pain results from injury to the **nervous system**. This can result from cancer cells compressing the nerves or spinal cord, from actual cancerous invasion into the nerves or spinal cord, or from chemical damage to the nerves caused by chemotherapy and radiation. Other causes include diabetes- and alcohol-related damage, trauma, neuralgias, or other illnesses affecting the neural path either centrally or peripherally. When the nerves become damaged, they are unable to carry accurate information. This results in more severe, distinct **pain messages**. The nerves may also relay pain messages long after the original cause of the pain is resolved. It can be described as sharp, burning, shooting, shocking, tingling, or electrical in nature. It may travel the length of the nerve path from the spine to a distal body part such as a hand, or down the buttocks to a foot. NSAIDs and opioids are generally ineffective against neuropathic pain, though adjuvants may enhance the therapeutic effect of opioids. Nerve blocks may also be used.

Review Video: Neuropathic Pain
Visit mometrix.com/academy and enter code: 780523

Adverse Systemic Effects of Pain

Acute pain causes adverse systemic effects that can negatively affect many body systems.

- **Cardiovascular**: Tachycardia and increased blood pressure is a common response to pain, causing increased cardiac output and systemic vascular resistance. In those with pre-existing cardiovascular disease, such as compromised ventricular function, cardiac output may decrease. The increased myocardial need for oxygen may cause or worsen myocardial ischemia.
- **Respiratory**: Increased need for oxygen causes an increase in minute ventilation and splinting due to pain, which may compromise pulmonary function. If the chest wall movement is constrained, tidal volume falls, impairing the ability to cough and clear secretions. Bed rest further compromises ventilation.
- **Gastrointestinal**: Sphincter tone increases and motility decreases, sometimes resulting in ileus. There may be an increased secretion of gastric acids, which irritates the gastric lining and can cause ulcerations. Nausea, vomiting, and constipation may occur. Reflux may result in aspiration pneumonia. Abdominal distension may occur.
- **Urinary**: Increased sphincter tone and decreased motility result in urinary retention.
- **Endocrine**: Hormone levels are affected by pain. Catabolic hormones such as catecholamine, cortisol, and glucagon increase, and anabolic hormones such as insulin and testosterone decrease. Lipolysis increases along with carbohydrate intolerance. Sodium retention can occur because of increased ADH, aldosterone, angiotensin, and cortisol. This in turn causes fluid retention and a shift to extracellular space.
- **Hematologic**: There may be reduced fibrinolysis, increased adhesiveness of platelets, and increased coagulation.
- **Immune**: Leukocytosis and lymphopenia may occur, increasing risk of infection.

- **Emotional**: Patients may experience depression, anxiety, anger, decreased appetite, and sleep deprivation. This type of response is most common in those with chronic pain, who usually have different systemic responses from those with acute pain.

Core Principles of Pain Assessment and Management

According to the Joint Commission, assessing pain should be a priority in patient care, and organizations must establish **policies** for assessment and treatment of pain and must educate staff members about these policies. The Joint Commission considers a **plan of care** regarding pain control an essential patient right. Hospitals should be consistent in the use of the same assessment tools throughout the organization, specific to different patient populations (for example, pediatrics and geriatrics). The latest standards (2018) of evidence-based practice include the following:

- Organizations must establish a clinical leadership team to oversee pain management and safe prescription of opioids.
- Patients must be involved in planning and setting goals and should receive education regarding safe use of opioid and non-opioid medications.
- Patients should be screened for pain in all assessments, including visits to the emergency department.
- Patients at high risk for opioid misuse or adverse effects must be identified and monitored.
- Healthcare providers should have access to prescription drug monitoring safety databases, such as the prescription databases provided by most states.
- Organizations must provide performance improvement educational programs regarding pain assessment and management and must collect and analyze data on its pain assessment and management.

Areas Addressed When Assessing Pain

Information concerning a patient's pain can be gathered from a variety of sources, including observations, interviews with the patient and family, medical records, and observations of other health care providers. However, it is important to remember that each patient's pain is **subjective** and **personal**. Pain is defined as whatever the patient says it is. Having the patient give parameters of quality, location, duration, speed of onset, and intensity can all be beneficial in forming a treatment plan based on the patient's needs. Pain is also influenced by psychological, social, and spiritual factors. Behavioral, psychological, and subjective assessment information such as physical demeanor and vital signs can be helpful in further defining a patient's pain parameters.

Physical Signs of Pain

The best assessment of the patient's pain is **the patient's own report**. All other information is assessed as supporting this report. However, when this method is restricted or unavailable, **physical signs and symptoms** can help the nurse's assessment capabilities. It is important to be familiar with the patient's **baseline** or resting information to give a clear picture of the changes the body may go through when experiencing significant pain. Systolic blood pressure, heart rate, and respirations may all increase above the patient's normal parameters. Tightness or tension may be felt in major muscle groups. Posturing can also occur: the patient may guard areas of the body, curl themselves up into a fetal position, or hold only certain body portions rigid. Calling out, increased volume in speech, and moaning can also be indicators. Facial expressions, such as flat affect or grimacing, and distraction from their surroundings also indicate a significant increase in stressful stimuli.

Importance of Pain Assessments in Advanced Disease

As many as 90% of all **advanced disease patients** will experience some level of pain. The hospice and palliative care philosophy focuses on the relief of pain and provision for comfort measures for all patients who desire it to improve quality of life. Each patient has the right to accept or refuse treatment for their pain. This becomes difficult when the patient is unable to **communicate** their desires and pain level. It can be assumed that if a patient was experiencing pain when able to communicate, they will continue to experience pain when the ability to communicate has been compromised—pain will be present even in an unconscious state. Changes from previous behavioral, psychological, and subjective and objective assessment data provide the supporting information for continued pain assessments in a nonverbal patient.

Pain Scales

Pain Assessment Tools

ABCDE Mnemonic Approach to Pain Assessment

The Agency for Healthcare Policy and Research recommends use of the **ABCDE method** for assessing and managing pain:

- **Asking** the patient about the extent of pain and assessing systematically.
- **Believing** that the degree of pain the patient reports is accurate.
- **Choosing** the appropriate method of pain control for the patient and circumstances.
- **Delivering** pain interventions appropriately and in a timely, logical manner.
- **Empowering** patients and family by helping them to have control of the course of treatment.

The **5 key elements of pain assessment** include:

- **Quality**: Words are used to describe pain, such as *burning, stabbing, deep, shooting,* and *sharp.* Some may complain of pressure, squeezing, and discomfort rather than pain.
- **Intensity**: Use of a 0-10 scale or other appropriate scale to quantify the degree of pain.
- **Location**: Where does the patient indicate pain?
- **Duration**: Is it constant; does it come and go; is there breakthrough pain?
- **Aggravating/alleviating factors**: What increases the intensity of pain and what relieves the pain?

Unidimensional Tools for Pain Assessment

Unidimensional tools for pain assessment focus on one aspect only: the patient's level of pain. Tools include:

- **Visual analog/numeric rating scale**: A 1-10 rating scale presented visually or verbally from which the patient chooses a number to describe the degree of pain the patient is experiencing. Zero represents no pain, 1 very mild pain, and 10 the most severe pain the patient can imagine.
- **Descriptive**: Pain is described in simple terms that a patient can choose from: mild, moderate, or severe. This may be especially helpful for patients from other countries or cultures where the 1-10 scale is not generally used.
- **FACES**: A chart shows a facial expression scale of simple drawings showing faces with different emotions, such as happiness, fear, and pain. Used primarily for children over age 3 and for nonverbal adults, although both a child's and an adult's version are available. A revised version applies numeric values to expressions so that pain can be assessed according to a numeric rating scale as well.

Review Video: How to Accurately Assess Pain
Visit mometrix.com/academy and enter code: 693250

Review Video: Assessment Tools for Pain
Visit mometrix.com/academy and enter code: 634001

Multidimensional Tools for Pain Assessment

Multidimensional tools used for pain assessment include:

- **Multidimensional pain inventory**: The patient begins by identifying a significant other and then answering 20 questions (rating scale 0-6) about the current rate of pain, the degree of interference in daily life, the ability to work, satisfaction from social/recreational activities, support level of the significant other, mood, pain during the previous week, changes brought about by pain, concerns of the significant other, ability to deal with pain, irritability, and anxiety.
- **Brief pain inventory**: Patients are assessed on the severity of pain (on a 1-10 scale), location of pain, impact of pain on daily function, pain medication, and amount of pain relief in the past 24 hours or the past week. They are asked if the pain interferes with general activity, walking, normal work, mood, interpersonal relations, sleep, or enjoyment of life.
- **McGill pain questionnaire**: The patient marks areas of internal and external pain on body diagrams and selects appropriate adjectives for 20 different sections regarding sensory, affective, and evaluative perceptions. For example, the questionnaire allows the patient to indicate if the pain is "flickering, quivering, pulsing, throbbing, beating, or pounding." The patient also rates present pain intensity (PPI) from 0 (none) to 5 (excruciating).

Assessment Tools for Cognitively Impaired or Nonverbal Patients

The following are types of assessment tools available for use with cognitively impaired or nonverbal patients:

- **Discomfort Scale for Dementia of the Alzheimer Type (DS-DAT)**: For use with elderly persons experiencing dementia, decreased cognition, and decreased verbalization
- **Assessment of Discomfort in Dementia Protocol (ADD)**: Particularly designed for use with patients exhibiting difficult behaviors
- **Checklist of Nonverbal Pain Indicators (CNPI)**: Pain measurement with cognitive impairment
- **Noncommunicative Patient's Pain Assessment Instrument (NOPPAIN)**: Specifically for use by nursing assistants
- **Pain Assessment for the Dementing Elderly (PADE)**: Assessing physical pain behaviors
- **Pain Assessment Tool in Confused Older Adults (PATCOA)**: Focuses on the observation of nonverbal cues
- **Pain Assessment in Advanced Dementia (PAINAD)**: Adapted from the DS-DAT
- **Pain Assessment Checklist for Seniors with Limited Ability to Communicate (PACSLAC)**: To assess common and subtle symptoms
- **Abbey Pain Scale**: For late-stage dementia in nursing home environments

Neuropathic Pain Scale

The neuropathic pain scale (NPS) is the first tool designed specifically to assess the types of pain associated with neuropathy. The NPS comprises 10 sections with 9 assessed with a 0 to 10 (not unpleasant to intolerable) scale:

- Intensity of pain
- Sharpness of pain
- Heat of pain
- Dullness of pain
- Coldness of pain
- Skin sensitivity to touch, clothing
- Itchiness
- Overall unpleasantness of pain
- Intensity of deep and surface pain

The 10th section asks for narrative descriptions of the **time quality** of pain. The patient chooses from three options:

- Feeling background pain all of the time with occasional flare-ups
- Feeling a single type of pain all the time
- Feeling a single type of pain sometimes while having some pain-free periods. The patient then is asked to describe the pain experienced

Assessing Pain in Pediatric Patients

When assessing the pediatric patient, the nurse must take into consideration the **chronological and developmental age** of the child. These factors help determine which measure the child might use to express pain, as well as treatments that might prove most successful. Assessment parameters must also include the presence of and parameters surrounding chronic illness, as well as neurological impairment. The nurse must identify the underlying cause of the pain, what nonpharmacological measures have been tried for pain control, and what methods can be used to deliver pharmacological interventions. The weight of the child in kilograms determines the appropriate dosages of medications. If the child is able to speak, do the child and the parents speak the same language as the health care provider, and are there any other obvious barriers to communication or pain relief measures?

Preteen/Adolescent Pain Scale

Pain is subjective and may be influenced by the individual's pain sensation threshold (the smallest stimulus that produces the sensation of pain) and tolerance threshold (the maximum degree of pain that a person can tolerate). The most common current pain assessment tool for preteens and adolescents is the 1-10 pain scale:

- 0 = no pain
- 1-2 = mild pain
- 3-5 = moderate pain
- 6-7 = severe pain
- 8-9 = very severe pain
- 10 = excruciating pain

However, assessment also includes information about onset, duration, and intensity. Identifying pain triggers and what relieves the pain is essential when developing a pain management plan. Children may show very different behaviors when they are in pain. Some may cry and moan with minor pain, and others may seem indifferent even when they are truly suffering. Thus, judging pain by behavior alone can lead to the wrong conclusions.

Non-Communicating Children's Pain Checklist

The **Non-Communicating Children's Pain Checklist** (NCCPC) is designed for children ages 3-8 who are cognitively impaired, but a modified version may be used for children recovering from anesthesia. The checklist contains 7 categories with sub-listings that are each scored: 0 (not occurring), 1 (occurring occasionally), 2 (occurring fairly often), 3 (occurring frequently), and NA (not applicable).

- **Vocal**: Moaning, whining, crying, screaming, yelling, or using a specific word for pain
- **Social**: Uncooperative, unhappy, withdrawn, seeking closeness, or can't be distracted
- **Facial**: Furrowed brow, eye changes, not smiling, lips tight or quivering, or clenching or grinding teeth.
- **Activity**: Not moving and quiet or agitated and fidgety.
- **Body and limbs**: Floppy, tense, rigid, spastic, pointing to a part of body that hurts, guarding part of the body, flinching, or positioning body to show pain.
- **Physiological**: Shivering, pallor, increased perspiration, tears, gasping, or holding breath
- **Eating and sleeping**: Eating less or sleeping significantly more or less than usual

The child is usually observed for 2 hours and then scored. All scores are then added together, A score of ≥7 indicates pain.

QUESTT Pediatric Pain Assessment Tool

QUESTT is designed to focus on assessment, action, and consequent reassessment for results.

- **Question** both the child and parent about the pain experience.
- **Use** assessment tools and rating scales that are appropriate to the developmental stage and situation and understanding of the child.
- **Evaluate** the patient for both behavioral and physiological changes.
- **Secure** the parent's participation in all stages of the pain evaluation and treatment process.
- **Take the cause of the pain into consideration** during the evaluation and choice of treatment methods.
- **Take action** to treat the pain appropriately, and then evaluate the results on a regular basis.

Factors that Influence the Pain Experience

Barriers to Optimal Pain Assessments

Barriers to optimal pain assessments include:

- **Professional**: Health care providers may lack knowledge about pain assessment and management of different patient populations or may carry out assessments based on personal perceptions rather than validated pain assessment instruments. Some may be concerned about managing adverse effects or the patient's development of tolerance or addiction. In other cases, healthcare providers may lack empathy for patients' suffering. Lack of cultural awareness may affect interpretation of pain. For example, patients in cultures that encourage expression of pain may be assessed as having more pain than patients from cultures that value stoicism.
- **System**: The organization may lack clear policies regarding pain assessment and management, and may not have established clear guidelines for consistent use of pain assessment instruments. Additionally, supervision and accountability may be inadequate, and the organization may be concerned about costs and reimbursement for treatment.
- **Patient**: For personal or cultural reasons, patients may minimize or overstate the degree of pain, interfering with assessment. Some patients may be concerned about addiction or the effects of drugs on cognition (confusion, disorientation, lethargy) or other side effects (constipation, nausea, itching). Some may want to protect family from knowing the extent of pain.
- **Family**: Cultural biases may influence how the family responds to a patient's pain, and this can influence the patient's response as well. Families may lack understanding of the role of pain assessment and management. Some lack understanding about the difference between addiction and pain control at the end of life.
- **Society**: Concerns about drug abuse and addiction often permeate society and influence societal attitudes toward pain control and appropriate drugs to use. Laws and regulations may make access to certain drugs, such as those derived from marijuana, difficult or impossible to obtain.

Influential Factors in Pain Perception

Factors that can influence the perception of pain include:

- **Emotional state/Attitude**: Patients who are extremely upset or anxious may be so overwhelmed they don't feel the pain, or they may experience pain as more severe than those who are relaxed and calm. If patients expect to suffer from pain, they are also more likely to report severe pain than patients who expect that their pain will be controlled.
- **Cultural expectations**: Perception may vary according to cultural beliefs about pain. For example, if a patient believes that pain is punishment, the patient may agonize over past sins. If a patient believes that pain is fate and reflects karma, then the patient may feel that bearing pain is necessary.
- **Pain threshold**: Different patients simply perceive and experience pain to different degrees. What may be a minor pain to one individual may be severe to another.

Effects of Gender on Pain Experience

Gender can affect pain sensitivity, tolerance, distress, and exaggeration of pain, and the patient's willingness to report pain, as well as displayed nonverbal cues concerning the pain experience. Studies indicate that women generally have **lower pain thresholds** and **less tolerance** for noxious stimuli or pain factors that hinder them from doing things they enjoy. Women seek help for pain-related problems sooner than men and respond better to therapy. Women also experience more **visceral pain** than men. Men are more prone to experience **somatic pain** and show more stoicism regarding pain experiences than women. **Neuropathic pain** seems to be experienced equally between men and women. Nurses need to be careful that biases concerning gender experiences with pain do not skew their assessments of pain. However, they need to be aware that pain experiences are always individual and may differ between the sexes.

Cultural Considerations for Pain Management

The following are cultural considerations for pain management:

- **American Indian** and **Alaskan natives** may be unwilling to show pain or request medications. Pain is a difficulty that must be endured rather than treated.
- **Asian and Pacific Islanders** may not vocalize pain and may have an interest in pursuing nontraditional and nonpharmacological treatments to help relieve pain.
- **Black and African American** cultures may tend to openly express their pain but still believe that it is to be endured. They may avoid medication because of personal fears of addiction or cultural stigmatism.
- **Hispanic cultures** may value the ability to endure pain and suffering as a personal quality of strength. Expression of pain, especially for a male, may be considered a sign of weakness. They may feel that pain is a form of divine punishment or trial.

Psychological Factors in Experience of Pain

Psychological factors that may influence a patient's experience of pain include:

- **Fear**: The fear of pain and the anticipation of having pain are factors in how much pain a person feels, because the fear stimulates areas of the brain that focus attention on the body so that the patient experiences an increased sensation of pain. Fear also causes muscles to tense, blood pressure to increase, and the heart rate to increase, and all of these can exacerbate the perception of pain. While pain medications may be necessary, practicing relaxation and mindfulness exercises may help to reduce anxiety and have a positive effect.
- **Depression**: The same neurotransmitters that transmit sensations of pain are also those that transmit moods, so many people with depression present first with complaints of pain or discomfort, and this can result in chronic pain if the depression is not resolved. In some cases, pain may lead to depression, but then the depression worsens the pain so it becomes a cycle of worsening discomfort. Patients may benefit from cognitive behavioral therapy or medication such as SSRIs.

PAIN DOCUMENTATION IN MEDICAL RECORDS

Recommendations for **pain documentation** in the medical record include:

- Describe the time of onset, the location of pain, the character of the pain, and the degree of pain, using a validated pain assessment instrument (either a self-reporting instrument, such as the visual analog scale, or one based on observation, such as PAINAD).
- Document all interventions, both pharmacological (opioids, adjuvants) and nonpharmacological (positioning, massage, relaxation exercises), including the time, the dosage, and the method of administration.
- Assess and document the initial response to the medication based on the expected response time. For example, an IV medication should take effect almost immediately, but oral medications may take up to 20 minutes to take effect.
- Assess and document the duration of response based on the expected duration of the medication. For example, if a medication response is expected to last for 6 hours, the patient's pain level should be assessed at least every 2 hours and more frequently if the rate of pain increases.
- Describe any adverse effects, such as itching or nausea.

Review Video: Pain Assessment Documentation
Visit mometrix.com/academy and enter code: 248521

Pharmacologic Pain Management

WHO Pain Ladder

The WHO pain ladder was developed as an algorithm for treating pain through medications with progressively increasing potency. The approach can be used effectively with both adult and pediatric patients. Beginning with the least potent medication option, each step adds a stronger analgesic until optimum pain relief is reached.

The **WHO pain ladder** has three steps.

- **Step 1**: The patient is given a non-opioid medication which may be used alone or in conjunction with other adjuvant therapies.
- **Step 2**: If the patient reports no change in the pain level, mild- to moderate-level pain-relieving opioids are introduced along with adjuvants if they have not been previously introduced.
- **Step 3**: Uncontrolled pain is then treated with opioids for moderate to severe pain. Adjuvants may also be continued.

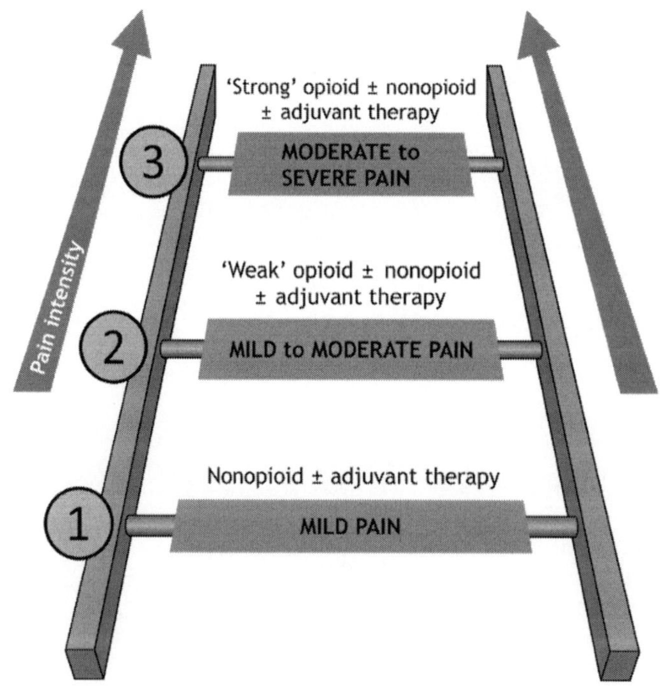

Scheduling of Pain Medications

For mild to moderate pain, patients may take **acetaminophen** alternating with an **NSAID** such as ibuprofen on a regularly scheduled basis or as needed (PRN) at the onset of pain or when pain is anticipated (such as before a dressing change). However, for severe chronic pain, long-acting **opioid pain medications**, such as time-released MS Contin, Duragesic, and OxyContin, should be given regularly around the clock, because these medications help not only control but also prevent pain. The patient should not skip a dose when free of pain, because this makes control more difficult when the pain recurs. In addition to **time-scheduled medications**, the patient may need **short-acting supplementary medications**, such as Percocet, to take on a PRN basis. When taking short-acting medications, the patient should take the medication at the onset of pain, before anticipated pain, or at the onset of increased pain, rather than waiting until the pain is severe, because the goal should always be to keep the pain under control.

Acetaminophen

Acetaminophen remains one of the safest analgesics for **long-term use**. It can be used to treat mild pain or as an adjuvant with other analgesics for more severe pain. Nonspecific musculoskeletal pain and osteoarthritis are particularly responsive to acetaminophen therapy. Acetaminophen also has a limited **anti-inflammatory nature**.

Acetaminophen should, however, be used cautiously in persons with altered liver or kidney function, as well as those with a history of significant alcohol use, regardless of liver function compromise. It should be dosed separately from any opioid analgesic, which should be given separately as well. This allows for individual titration of each drug to assess the individual needs and side effects separately.

NSAIDs

NSAIDs act by inhibiting the cyclooxygenase (COX) enzyme, which controls prostaglandin formation. COX-1 affects platelet clumping, gastric blood flow, and mucosal integrity. COX-2 affects pain, inflammation, and fever. COX-1 and 2 inhibitors include aspirin and ibuprofen. Ibuprofen has a lower occurrence of side effects, such as gastric bleeding, than aspirin does. A COX-2 inhibitor, such as Celebrex, must be used with caution due to increased cardiovascular risks when used for over 18 months. NSAIDs are useful for both arthritis and bone cancer pain and work well with opioids for relief of postoperative and other severe pain. NSAIDs may increase the effects of antiseizure drugs and warfarin. Smaller doses are needed if kidney function is impaired.

Review Video: NSAID Side Effects
Visit mometrix.com/academy and enter code: 569064

Local Anesthetic Pain Relief

Local anesthetics block neural conduction of pain through the application of the anesthetic directly to the nerve endings in the area of pain. It can be injected prior to minor surgery or suturing. It can be injected intercostally for thoracic or high abdominal surgeries. The addition of a vasoconstrictor prolongs effectiveness of the anesthetic. A cream containing local anesthetics (EMLA) can be rubbed on the skin to decrease pain from IV starts or lumbar punctures. It should be applied 60-90 minutes prior to the procedure. A lidocaine 5% patch is approved to relieve pain from postherpetic neuralgia. The patient applies up to 3 patches for 12 hours at a time. Local anesthetics can be applied via the use of an epidural catheter to provide pain control for surgery, childbirth, or postoperative pain control. Opioids can be infused along with the anesthetic agent. Patients using an epidural catheter for postoperative pain tend to ambulate sooner, suffer fewer complications as a result, and go home more quickly.

Opioids

Guidelines for Opioid Use

Opioid analgesic therapy is a widely used method of chronic pain control. By adhering to clinical guidelines, pain control can be safely optimized. **Intramuscular administration** should be used as a last resort except in the presence of a "pain emergency" when no other treatment is readily available. Such cases are rare since subcutaneous delivery is almost always an alternative. Noninvasive routes such as **transdermal** and **transmucosal**, which bypass the enteral route, are optimal for continuous pain control and are often effective in eliminating breakthrough pain as well. Changing from one opioid to another, or altering the delivery method, may become necessary under the assumption that incomplete cross-tolerance among opioids occurs. Changing analgesics or method of delivery may result in a decreased drug requirement. When altering opioid delivery regimens, use **morphine equivalents** as the common factor for all dose conversions. This method will help reduce medication errors. Side effects such as sedation, constipation, nausea, and myoclonus should be anticipated in every care plan, and require both prevention and treatment methods.

Side Effects of Opioid Analgesics

Examples of **opioid analgesics** are numerous and include morphine, hydromorphone, oxymorphone, methadone, meperidine, fentanyl, sufentanil, alfentanil, levorphanol, codeine, oxycodone, hydrocodone, propoxyphene, pentazocine, nalbuphine, and buprenorphine. Opioid analgesics have multiple effects on most of the organ systems of the body. Central nervous system (CNS) effects include respiratory depression, analgesia, euphoria, sedation, miosis, cough suppression, truncal rigidity, nausea, and vomiting. Cardiovascular effects are usually slight and include bradycardia, hypotension, reduced blood volume, and increased cerebral blood flow. Gastrointestinal effects can include constipation, decreased gastric motility, and decreased hydrochloric acid. Genitourinary effects are urinary retention and decreased renal function. Other effects are sweating, flushing, and histamine release with itching.

Opioid Use During Last Few Hours of Life

Assessment of pain continues in the **last hours of life**, and medication is adjusted according to assessment. Pain does not necessarily increase as death approaches. It can be assumed that if pain was present prior to loss of consciousness it will continue in the patient's unconscious state. It should be assessed for and treated accordingly. Research has confirmed that administering opioids at the end of life does not hasten nor prolong the dying process. The patient's **prior medication regimen** should be continued. However, adjustments may be made in consideration of reduced renal or hepatic clearance. The **route of administration** should also be assessed for appropriateness and adjusted as needed (e.g., loss of consciousness, inability to swallow).

Oral Transmucosal Fentanyl Citrate

Oral transmucosal fentanyl citrate consists of **fentanyl** on an oral applicator. The patient applies the dosage (starting at 200 mcg) to the **buccal mucosa** between the cheek and gum for rapid absorption and subsequent pain relief. This makes transmucosal fentanyl particularly useful for managing **breakthrough pain**. Pain relief generally begins within 5 minutes, but the patient should be instructed to wait 15 minutes after the previous dose has been completed before taking another dose. Swallowing even part of the dose rather than having it completely absorbed through the oral mucosa can affect the timing of pain relief onset. **Peak effect** occurs in 20-40 minutes with the total pain relief duration lasting 2-3 hours. Side effects can include somnolence, nausea, and dizziness. Consuming drinks such as coffee, tea, and juices that alter the oral secretion pH can also alter the absorption rate of transmucosal fentanyl.

Methadone

Methadone is useful for treating **severe or chronic pain** and may be particularly helpful in the presence of **neuropathic pain**. It has a long-acting pain relief factor for a lower cost than many comparable medications. However, the exact dosing ratios with morphine remain unclear within the available research. Metabolism of methadone can also be swayed (either increased or decreased) by many other medications normally taken by patients with chronic conditions. Methadone can also be used to treat opioid addiction. US law for the prescription of methadone for addiction in detoxification or maintenance programs requires a special license and patient enrollment. The words "for pain" need to be clearly stated in the prescription. Methadone can cause drowsiness, weakness, headache, nausea, vomiting, constipation, sweating, and flushing, as well as sedation, decreased respirations, or an irregular heart rate.

Oxycodone

Oxycodone, a synthetic formulation, is a long-acting opioid for **moderate to severe pain relief**. Side effects are similar to those of morphine. It has a similar pain relief ratio, with the possibility of less nausea and vomiting. Because of its extended-release nature, the medication cannot be cut or crushed for administration. Oxycodone does not carry any greater addiction risk than other types of opioids; however, public sensationalism related to this formulation may create hesitation for use among patients. Pharmacies may also limit the amount of this medication they will make available to an individual. Oxycodone should be used cautiously in patients with a history of hypothyroidism, Addison's disease, urethral stricture, prostatic hypertrophy, or lung or liver disease.

Hydromorphone

Hydromorphone is available as tablets, liquid, suppository, and parenteral formulations. It offers the advantage of being synthetic, allowing for its use in the presence of a true **morphine allergy**. It is also helpful when significant side effects have occurred in the past or pain has been inadequately controlled with other medications. It may also be useful for controlling cough. However, neurotoxicity may occur, particularly myoclonus, hyperalgesia, and seizures. It should also be used cautiously in the presence of kidney, liver, heart, and thyroid disease, seizure disorders, respiratory disease, prostatic hypertrophy, or urinary problems. Common *side effects* include dizziness, lightheadedness, drowsiness, upset stomach if taken without food, vomiting, and constipation.

Titration of Morphine for Pain Control

Morphine titration protocols vary according to the type of morphine used, the severity of pain, and the patient's tolerance:

Type	Peak	Duration (hours)
Short-acting	60 minutes	4-5
Long-acting	3-4 hours	8-24
IM	30-60 minutes	4-5
SQ	50-90 minutes	4-5
IV	20 minutes	4-5
Rectal	20-60 minutes	3-7

For example, **optimal dosage** is usually calculated by starting with short-acting oral morphine at 30 mg every 3-4 hours with doses increased by 25-50% for moderate pain or 50-100% for severe pain each time until the patient has at least 50% reduction in pain on a scale of 1-10 or a behavior scale. The dose may need to be reduced if excessive sedation occurs. Once the patient's pain is controlled on short-acting morphine and 24-hour dosage needs are calculated, the patient could be switched to extended-release. **Breakthrough pain** is usually treated with dosages that are 10% of the 24-hour dose. Dosages may be repeated or increased if there is inadequate relief of pain at the peak time. Increasing the dose prior to peak time will result in increased drowsiness.

Morphine Use for Chronic Cancer Pain

One advantage of morphine for chronic cancer pain is that it has no **ceiling dose**. As tolerance to the medication increases or the disease progresses in severity, the dose can be gradually increased to an infinite level. It is also available in many different forms for administration, including intravenous, intramuscular, immediate release, sustained release, long-acting, liquid oral preparations, and suppositories. Morphine is often used as the **equivalency standard** for other opioid analgesics. Common *side effects* of morphine include sedation, respiratory depression, itching, nausea, chronic spasms or twitching of muscle groups, and constipation. Constipation is experienced by all patients receiving opioids. This inevitability should be planned for and treated aggressively. Hallucinations are common when morphine is initiated. After the first few days, most patients will overcome the respiratory depression, nausea, itching, and extreme sedation as tolerance for the medication is developed.

Dosages for Morphine, Codeine, Hydromorphone, and Levorphanol

The dosages for both the enteral and parenteral routes of morphine, codeine, hydromorphone, and levorphanol are as follows:

- **Morphine**: Enteral dosage is 30 mg (available as continuous and sustained-release formulations to last 12-24 hours); parenteral dosage is 10 mg.
- **Codeine**: Enteral dosage is 200 mg (not generally recommended); parenteral dosage is 130 mg.
- **Hydromorphone**: Enteral dosage is 7.5 mg (available as a continuous-release formula lasting 24 hours); parenteral dosage is 1.5 mg.
- **Levorphanol**: In acute pain episodes, enteral dosage is 4 mg; parenteral dosage is 2 mg. For chronic pain, dosage is equivalent for both enteral and parenteral at 1 mg. Levorphanol has a long half-life, increasing the chances of dosage accumulation over time.

Adhering to the statement "If the gut works, use it," as much as 90 percent of all patients will at least start out able to use oral medications instead of other routes.

Calculation for Converting Medication Regimen Between Two Opioids

Calculate the current 24-hour drug dose, or the total amount given in a 24-hour period. Multiply the current 24-hour dose times the ratio of the 24-hour equivalent dose for the new drug over the 24-hour equivalent of the old drug. This calculation provides the **equivalent 24-hour dose** for the new drug. Divide the new dose amount by the number of doses to be provided during the day. This amount equals the new **target dosage**.

$$\text{current 24 hr dose} \times \frac{\text{new drug 24 hr equiv dose}}{\text{current drug 24 hr equiv dose}} = \text{new 24 hr dose}$$

$$\frac{\text{new 24 hr dose}}{\text{doses per day}} = \text{new target dosage}$$

Ketamine

Ketamine is a dissociative anesthetic that can provide pain relief as an alternate or complement to an opioid. The dissociative quality is an effective way to help the patient separate from the sensation of pain. Ketamine treatment begins with an initial bolus of 0.1 mg/kg IV. If there is no improvement, a second bolus with double the dosage is provided in 5 minutes. This can be repeated as needed. Boluses should be followed by a decrease in the patient's current opioid dose by 50% and an infusion of ketamine. **Infusion dosing** for ketamine is 0.015 mg/kg/min, or about 1 mg/min for a 70 kg person. If IV access cannot be attained, subcutaneous infusion is a possibility with dosing of 0.3-0.5 mg/kg. Consider concurrent treatment with a **benzodiazepine** to prevent hallucinations or frightful dreams and observe for increased secretions, as these are all possible side effects of ketamine. The secretions may be treated with glycopyrrolate, scopolamine, or atropine as needed.

Treating Breakthrough Pain

The three basic types of breakthrough pain, and their treatment measures are as follows:

- **Incident pain**: Pain that can be specifically tied to an activity or event, such as a dressing change or physical therapy. These events can be anticipated and treated with a rapid-onset, short-acting analgesic just prior to the painful event.
- **Spontaneous pain**: This type of pain is unpredictable and cannot be pinpointed to a relationship with any certain time or event. There is no way to anticipate spontaneous pain. In the presence of neuropathic pain, adjuvant therapy may be useful. Otherwise, a rapid-onset, short-acting analgesic is used.
- **End-of-dose failure**: Pain that specifically occurs at the end of a routine analgesic dosing cycle when medication blood levels begin to taper off. Careful evaluation of end-of-dose failure can help prevent it sooner. It may indicate an increased dose tolerance and the need for medication dose alterations.

Treating Neuropathic Pain

Treatment options for neuropathic pain are often different from the methods used to treat other types of pain. The three drug classes most commonly used and proven effective for treating neuropathic pain are **anticonvulsants**, **anesthetics**, and **antidepressants**. Some are given on an as-needed basis, but most require consistent dosing with **24-hour symptom control**. Examples of the most common medications include amitriptyline, nortriptyline, duloxetine, gabapentin, topical lidocaine, opioids, and pregabalin. Medication choice is dependent on factors such as the type and progression of the disorder and the associated physical and emotional problems, such as nerve injury, muscle weakness or spasms, anxiety, depression, or sleep disturbances.

Review Video: Neuropathic Pain
Visit mometrix.com/academy and enter code: 780523

Treating Bone Pain

Treatment options for bone pain may depend on the causative agent related to the pain, such as the primary cancer site, severely weakened bones, or fractures. **Systemic treatment choices** include chemotherapy, radiation, and hormone therapy. **Hormone therapy** is used in the presence of estrogen and androgen receptors within the cancer cells. **Bisphosphonates**, such as ibandronate, zoledronate, and alendronate, may help strengthen the bones, slow damage, and prevent fractures; they can also help reduce pain. However, side effects can include fatigue, fever, nausea, vomiting, and anemia. **Surgery** may also be considered to remove cancerous cells or reinforce weakened areas of bone. **Opioids** and **NSAIDs/COX-2 inhibitors** are most often used for pain relief and need to be provided on a consistent basis.

Morphine combined with ibuprofen provides the benefit of a centrally acting opioid with a peripherally acting NSAID. Ibuprofen also acts as an effective adjuvant analgesic agent to enhance the relief provided by the opioid without increasing opioid side effects.

Measures Taken During Pain Crisis

During a pain crisis, assess for a change in the mechanism or location of the pain and attempt to differentiate between **terminal anxiety** or agitation and the **physical causes** of pain. Begin with a rapid increase in **opioid treatment**. If the pain is unresponsive to opioid titration, switching to **benzodiazepines**, such as diazepam and lorazepam, may produce a more effective response. If terminal symptoms remain unresponsive, assess for **drug absorption**. While invasive routes of medication delivery are generally avoided unless necessary, the only guaranteed route of drug delivery is the IV route. If there is any question about absorption, it is appropriate to establish parenteral access. IM delivery should be considered as a last resort. When all accessible resources have been exhausted, seek a pain management consultation as quickly as possible. Alternative methods of terminal pain control include radiotherapy, anesthetic, or neuroablative procedures.

CONCERNS SURROUNDING USE OF PAIN MEDICATIONS WITH END-OF-LIFE PATIENTS

Common concerns surrounding the use of pain medications with end-of-life patients include:

- **Adequacy**: Patients are often concerned that medication may not be adequate to control pain and that chronic or breakthrough pain will occur. Patients may be concerned that if they take adequate pain medication, it will be less effective later when pain may be worse.
- **Sedation/addiction**: Some patients and family members are concerned about the risks of addiction, and others may be concerned about the effects of the medication on the patient's cognition, as some patients may become confused, disoriented, or sedated, depending on the medication or dosage.
- **Adverse effects**: Nausea and vomiting may be almost as debilitating to a patient as the pain it is intended to alleviate. Constipation, a common adverse effect, may be very uncomfortable for a patient. Some medications may result in itching and others may cause myoclonus, both of which are uncomfortable for the patient.

Non-Pharmacologic Interventions

PALLIATIVE SURGERY

Palliative surgery is sometimes carried out to reduce pain and symptoms although in most cases it does not appreciably prolong life. Palliative surgery may be **cancer-directed**, such as palliative nephrectomy with renal cell carcinoma, partial or total gastrectomy for gastric cancer, or endoscopic paranasal debulking for facial metastasis, and aimed at removing cancerous tissue. Decompression of the vertebra (in the case of bony metastases) and arthroplasty of the femur may be carried out to reduce pain and the risk of pathological fractures. Palliative surgery may also be **non-cancer-directed**, which includes procedures that do not remove cancerous tissue, such as palliative colonic splinting and nerve block procedures. Patients may undergo pleurodesis, thoracentesis, thoracotomy, paracentesis, and pericardiocentesis to relieve discomfort. The risks and pain associated with surgical procedures must be balanced against improvement in the quality of life with consideration of the expected length of survival.

PALLIATIVE STENTS

A stent is a small tube, usually metal or plastic, that is inserted into a duct, vessel, or canal to maintain patency and relieve symptoms associated with cancer that is causing obstruction. These stents are usually placed with microsurgical techniques. **Common stents** include:

- **Pancreatic stents**: These open the bile duct to allow drainage in order to reduce jaundice and associated discomforts, to reduce pain, and to improve digestion.
- **Duodenal stents**: These are placed to maintain patency of the duodenum, which is often obstructed with pancreatic cancer, as an alternative to stomach bypass surgery and/or to relieve nausea and vomiting. Patients may be restricted to soft foods and fluids after the procedure.
- **Liver stents**: These are placed in the bile duct system to allow bile to drain into the small intestine in order to relieve jaundice and symptoms of liver failure.
- **Colonic stents**: These stents are placed to relieve colorectal blockage and relieve symptoms of bowel obstruction.
- **Ureteral stents**. These stents can be used to prevent urinary retention when ureters are obstructed.

Complications of stents may include infection, perforation, hemorrhage, and migration of the stent. Over time, obstruction may recur, especially with malignancies.

Palliative Radiation

Palliative radiation is used to reduce pain and symptoms. Most palliative radiation is done with external beam radiation therapy. **Radiotherapy** uses include:

- **Bone pain**: Radiotherapy may be utilized to reduce tumor mass, such as with multiple myeloma and bony metastasis, and to reduce pain and risk of fractures, with relief often occurring within days of treatment.
- **Pericardial effusions**: Radiotherapy is most effective in reducing effusions with radiosensitive tumors (leukemias, lymphomas).
- **Hemoptysis associated with lung cancer**: Radiotherapy can control hemoptysis in up to 80% of patients with inoperative lung cancer.
- **Spinal cord compression**: Radiotherapy is the primary treatment to relieve compression and reduce symptoms.
- **Brain tumor**: Radiotherapy may reduce the size of the tumor and associated symptoms, such as headaches and nausea.

Radiation does pose some risks of adverse effects that must be considered in relation to quality of life. Depending on the site of radiation, adverse effects may include fatigue, local skin irritation and burns, hair loss, GI upset (nausea, vomiting, dysphagia, diarrhea), dysuria, depressed immune system, and anemia.

Palliative Chemotherapy

Palliative chemotherapy is used primarily to reduce symptoms and pain by decreasing tumor size, which reduces compression of surrounding tissues, and to prolong life when cancer is advanced. Many chemotherapeutic agents are available, and adverse effects associated with use vary widely but can include nausea and vomiting, anorexia, hair loss, weakness, fatigue, and impaired immune system. **Palliative chemotherapy** is often given in conjunction with palliative radiation. Patients should be well-informed before deciding on a course of palliative chemotherapy and should understand how many cycles will be needed (usually 2 full cycles are given before deciding whether the treatment is effective), how long the cycles will be, what type of adverse effects to expect, what reduction in symptoms is anticipated, and how long studies show that the treatment prolongs life. If the prolongation of life and symptom relief is minimal, the trade-off for decreased quality of life must be considered.

Palliative Sedation

Palliative sedation differs from physician-assisted suicide in that it is primarily intended to provide comfort and alleviate suffering, and the hastening of death that may occur is a secondary effect while the primary purpose of physician-assisted suicide is to bring about a patient's death (even though it is also intended to provide comfort and alleviate suffering). These are legal distinctions. In most states, physician-assisted suicide is illegal, but the US Supreme Court has upheld the rights of individuals to have **palliative sedation** to alleviate symptoms. Midazolam (Versed) 0.5-6.0 mg/hr intravenously is often used for palliative sedation for patients who are highly agitated and in severe uncontrolled pain. Midazolam is a very short-acting benzodiazepine with action beginning within 5 minutes and peaking at 20-60 minutes. Propofol, another IV agent, is also used, with starting doses of 0.25 mg/kg/hr. Palliative sedation is indicated for patients when other medications and therapies have been unable to control their refractory symptoms, such as intractable pain, severe nausea and vomiting, feeling of suffocation, and seizures.

Counseling, Psychological Therapy, and Cognitive Behavioral Therapy

Both patients and their families may benefit from **counseling and psychological therapy**, which may allow them to express feelings and concerns that might otherwise remain hidden. Counseling may help patients/families come to terms with death, dying, and limitations and changes brought about by illness. Grief and bereavement counseling is especially helpful for family members after a patient has died. Pastoral counseling, often carried out by chaplains, pastors, and priests, may facilitate spiritual assessment and provide spiritual support. Psychological therapy may help to treat depression brought about by illness, and specific psychological techniques, such as visualization, relaxation exercises, and cognitive behavioral therapy, may help patients better control pain and reduce stress and anxiety.

Cognitive-behavioral therapy (CBT) focuses on the impact that thoughts have on behavior and feelings and encourages the individual to use the power of rational thought to alter perceptions and behavior. Individuals are assigned "homework" during the sessions to practice new ways of thinking and to develop new coping strategies. The therapist helps the individual identify goals and find ways to achieve them.

Cancer Diets

Cancer diets have been developed based on the premise that some foods "feed" cancer and others kill cancer cells although evidence-based support that the diets alter outcomes is lacking. Some people pursue diet therapy in place of traditional treatments while others use the diet in addition to other treatments. Many utilize a primarily vegan (plant-based) diet, which is usually lacking in vitamin B_{12}. While diets differ somewhat, basic concepts include:

- Avoiding refined carbohydrates (sugar, white flour) and milk products
- Avoiding fatty acids, fried foods, fast foods, and processed foods
- Avoiding alcohol, caffeine, nicotine, and chemicals
- Avoiding meats, such as beef and poultry (purported to interfere with the immune system)
- Avoiding cooking/overcooking and pasteurization (purported to destroy nutrients)
- Utilizing organic fruits and vegetables in order to avoid ingestion of pesticides
- Encouraging raw fruits, raw vegetables, seeds, whole grains, and nuts

Complementary and Alternative Therapies

Complementary Therapy

Complementary therapies are often used, either alone or in conjunction with conventional medical treatment. These methods should be included if this is what the patient/family chooses, empowering the family to take control of their plan of care. Complementary therapies vary widely and most can easily be incorporated. The **National Center for Complementary and Alternative Medicine** recognizes the following:

- **Whole medical systems**: Chinese medicine (acupressure, acupuncture), naturopathic and homeopathic medicines, and Ayurveda
- **Mind-body medicine**: Prayer, artistic creation, music and dance therapy, biofeedback, focused relaxation, and visualization
- **Biological medicine**: Aromatherapy, herbs, plants, trees, vitamins and minerals, and dietary supplements
- **Manipulation**: Massage and spinal manipulation
- **Energy medicines**: Magnets, electric current, pulsed fields, Reiki, qi gong, and laying-on of the hands

Precautions

The use of alternative and complementary therapies should be thoroughly discussed by patients and their physician. Patients should be encouraged to use therapies that are shown to have a beneficial, complementary effect on conventional medical treatment. These therapies include the use of massage, superficial stimulation, relaxation, distraction, hypnosis, and guided imagery.

- Encourage patients to practice the techniques until they are proficient in their use to give them a chance to prove their value.
- Teach the patient how the therapies work to encourage the patient to believe in them to contribute to the placebo effect.
- Caution the patient against abandoning current medical treatment.
- Inform the patient of the high cost of alternate therapies that can divert needed funds and result in little or no benefit.
- Provide the patient with resources in the form of books, pamphlets, and informative websites that prove the results of scientific research so that they can evaluate alternative therapies for themselves.

Whole Medical Systems

Whole medical systems are different philosophies and methods of explaining and treating health and illness. Some systems include:

- **Homeopathic medicine**: This European system uses small amounts of diluted herbs and supplements to help the body to recover from disease by stimulating an immune response.
- **Naturopathic medicine**: This is a European system that uses various natural means (herbs, massage, acupuncture) to support the natural healing forces of the body.
- **Chinese medicine**: Centers on restoring the proper flow of life forces within the body to cure disease by using herbs, acupressure and acupuncture, and meditation.
- **Ayurveda**: This is an Indian system that tries to bring the spirit into harmony with the mind and body to treat disease via yoga, herbs, and massage.

Essential Oils and Cupping

Essential oils (concentrated oils from plants) are either inhaled (aromatherapy) or diluted and applied to the skin. Essential oils are believed to reduce stress, aid sleep, improve dermatitis, and aid digestion. Commonly used essential oils include eucalyptus, lavender, lemon, peppermint, rosemary, rose, and tea tree. Oils may cause skin irritation when applied to the skin.

Cupping is an ancient practice still used in Southeast Asia and the Middle East to reduce pain, promote healing, and improve circulation. With dry cupping, cups are heated by placing something flammable (such as paper or herbs) inside the cup and setting it on fire to heat the cup, which is then immediately placed on the back along the meridians (generally on both sides of the spine) to form a vacuum that draws blood to the skin and causes circular bruises believed to heal that part of the body. Wet cupping includes leaving the heated cup in place for three minutes, removing it, making small cuts in the skin, and then applying suction cups again to withdraw blood. Cupping should be avoided in children under 4 and limited to short periods in older children.

Acupuncture

Alternative systems of medical practice include acupuncture, homeopathy, and naturopathy. **Acupuncture**, an ancient Oriental practice, uses stainless steel or copper needles inserted into superficial skin layers at points where energy or life force called *qi* is believed to occur. The needles are supposed to restore balance and the flow of *qi*. The NIH has recognized the effectiveness of acupuncture for certain side effects of other cancer treatments, such as nausea, vomiting, and pain. However, there is no documented scientific evidence to support the principles expounded. Acupuncturists are certified through either formal coursework or apprenticeships, and there is also board certification in this area for physicians. The needles used are classified as class II, which means they have manufacturing and labeling requirements.

Herbal Remedies and Regulations

In the United States, most **herbal preparations** are classified as dietary supplements. That means that they are not subject to the same rigorous manufacturing, safety, efficacy, and control practices as pharmaceutical drugs. Herbal supplements are only governed by the Dietary Supplement and Health Education Act (DSHEA). As long as no specific disease treatment or curative claims are made, the supplement can be marketed without limitation and safety concerns must be pursued by the FDA after the fact. Nevertheless, some herbal remedies have been undergoing clinical trials in the US to substantiate their health-enhancing or traditional/historical or international use claims. However, the focal point of these studies is still only on the effectiveness of the specific supplement. In Europe, there has been some movement toward greater regulation and licensing of herbal products, but not to the extent of formal drug regulations.

Toxicities Associated with Herbal Remedies

Use of herbal preparations has been associated with a variety of **toxicities**, primarily in categories such as cardiovascular problems, hypersensitivity reactions, disorientation, gastrointestinal problems, and liver malfunction. Because quality control measures are relatively lax for these remedies, contamination from infectious agents and toxic metals can potentially cause other side effects. Many of these herbal medicines **interact with conventional drugs**, thus altering their pharmacodynamics. For example, St. John's wort, which is primarily used for depressive disorders or as a sedative, interacts with a wide range of traditional pharmacologic agents and suppresses their levels in the bloodstream. Kava kava, made from dried roots of a type of pepper bush, is used as a sedative, but it also has been associated with hepatic failure and via interactions with several other drugs can actually induce a comatose state. Ginseng is an Asian remedy touted for its curative properties in a number of diseases. However, it can react with steroidal drugs and induce shaking and manic episodes. These are just a few examples of potential dangers.

Non-Pharmaceutical Pain Relief

Non-pharmaceutical methods to relieve pain that can be used exclusively or combined with medications include massage, heat, cold, electrical stimulation, distraction, relaxation, imagery, visualization, and music. Other **alternatives or adjuncts to pain medication** include hypnosis, magnets, acupuncture, acupressure, and therapeutic touch. Herbs, aromatherapy, reflexology, homeopathic medicine, and prayer may also be accepted by the patient. Any method that the patient feels may help that isn't harmful should be used to help get relief.

Mind-Body Medicine for Pain and Disease

Mind-body medicine (prayer, artistic creation, music and dance, biofeedback, relaxation, and visualization) can help distract people from pain or other symptoms if they are able to concentrate on the method. This can result in the transfer of less painful stimuli to the brain by stimulating the **descending control system**. These methods work if the patient can use them to create alternate sensations in the brain, but will not work if the patient is unable to concentrate due to intense pain.

Relaxation that occurs as a result of using these methods helps to reduce muscular tension that can make pain worse and reduces fatigue caused by chronic pain. Relaxation has been proven to be the most helpful after surgery. Postoperative patients report a greater feeling of control over their pain and tend to request fewer opioids to control pain. Biofeedback can help patients to recognize the feelings of both tension and relaxation and provide a way to indicate their success in managing muscle tension.

Use of Visualization

There are a number of methods used for **visualization** to reduce anxiety and promote healing. Some include audiotapes with guided imagery, such as self-hypnosis tapes, but the patient can be taught basic **techniques** that include:

- Sit or lie comfortably in a **quiet place** away from distractions.
- Concentrate on **breathing** while taking long slow breaths.
- **Close the eyes** to shut out distractions and create an image in the mind of the place or situation desired.
- Concentrate on that **image**, engaging as many senses as possible and imaging details.
- If the mind wanders, breathe deeply and **bring consciousness back** to the image or concentrate on breathing for a few moments and then return to the imagery.
- End with positive imagery.

Sometimes, patients are resistive at first or have a hard time maintaining focus, so **guiding** them through visualization for the first few times can be helpful.

STIMULATION OF THE SKIN TO REDUCE PAIN

Skin, muscles, fascia, tendons, and the cornea contain **nociceptors** that are nerve endings that respond to painful stimuli. Massage, transcutaneous electrical nerve stimulation (TENS), heat and cold provide stimulation to other nerves that transfer only sensation, not pain. These signals block some of the transfer of the nociceptor impulses:

- **Massage** not only sends alternate sensation to the brain, but also results in relaxation that decreases the muscular tension that contributes to pain.
- **TENS** works well on incisional and neuromuscular pain by providing a gentle electrical stimulation that overrides the painful impulses from the area and may stimulate endorphins.
- **Heat therapy** increases blood flow and oxygen to promote healing and stimulates neural receptors, decreasing pain. Heat also helps loosen tense muscles that may be contributing to pain.
- **Cold therapy** decreases circulation and reduces production of chemicals related to inflammation, thereby reducing pain.

TEMPERATURE-CONTROLLED THERAPIES

METHODS OF HEATING AND COOLING

There are a number of different ways to **heat** (thermotherapy) or **cool** (cryotherapy) for **healing**:

- **Conduction**: Conveyance of heat, cold, or electricity through direct contact with the skin, such as with hot baths, ice packs, and electrical stimulation.
- **Convection**: Indirect transmission of heat in a liquid or gas by circulation of heated particles, such as with whirlpools and paraffin soaks.
- **Conversion**: Heating that results from converting a form of energy into heat, such as with diathermy and ultrasound.
- **Evaporation**: Cooling caused by liquids that evaporate into gases on the skin with a resultant cooling effect, such as with perspiration or vapo-coolant sprays.
- **Radiation**: Heating that results from transfer of heat through light waves or rays, such as with infrared or ultraviolet light.

SUPERFICIAL HEAT

Superficial heat with externally applied heat sources penetrates only the superficial layers of the skin (1-2 cm after about 30 minutes), but it is believed to relax deeper muscles by reflex, decrease pain, and increase metabolisms (2-3 times for every 10 °C increase in skin temperature). Therapeutic temperature range is 40-45 °C. **Superficial heat modalities** include:

- **Moist heat packs** placed on the skin and secured by several layers of towels to provide insulation, applied for 15-30 minutes.
- **Paraffin baths** (52-54 °C) with the hand, foot, or elbow dipped 7 times, cooling between dippings, and then wrapping with plastic and towels for 20 minutes.
- **Fluidotherapy** uses hot-air warmed (38.8-47.8 °C) cellulose particles into which a hand or foot is submerged for 20-30 minutes.

Passive and active range of motion exercises are done after superficial heat treatment. Contraindications include cardiac disease, peripheral vascular disease, malignant tumor, bleeding, and acute inflammation.

Deep heat differs from superficial heat in that the heat is generated internally using ultrasound, short wave, and microwave diathermy rather than applied to the surface of the skin. Deep heating has penetrance to 3-5 cm.

THERAPEUTIC ULTRASOUND

Ultrasound treats soft-tissue injuries (such as myositis, bursitis, and tendinitis) with sound waves (frequency 0.8-3 MHz). Ultrasound utilizes a **piezoelectric crystal** that vibrates, producing sound waveforms, which are transmitted from the transducer through a gel substance into the tissue. The sound waves bounce off of the bone in an irregular pattern that causes an increase in temperature in the connective tissue, such as collagen fibers. Temperatures of the tissue may increase up to 43.5 °C, increasing metabolism in the area, neural conduction, as well as blood flow. Ultrasound is used to **decrease both contractures and scarring**. During treatment, the transducer passes in a circular motion about the skin surface, staying in contact with the gel medium. If a distal limb is submerged in water, the treatment is given with the head of the transducer 0.5-1.0 in from the skin surface. Treatment is followed by range of motion exercises, passive and active. Contraindications are similar to other heat-producing modalities and include peripheral vascular disease, but ultrasound may be used over metal prostheses.

TENS

Transcutaneous electrical nerve stimulation (TENS) uses electrical stimulation to stimulate **peripheral sensory nerve fibers** to reduce acute or recurrent pain. TENS machines may be 2-lead or 4-lead and have adjustments for both frequency (1-20 Hz) and pulse width (50-300 μs, 10-50 mA). Stimulation can be intermittent or continuous. TENS units are small and battery-powered with wires and adhesive electrodes attached so that they can be worn while the person goes about usual activities. The positioning of the electrodes and the settings depend upon the site and type of injury, following guidelines provided by the manufacturer. The TENS machine can be used for a number of hours, but if used for days at a time, it will be less effective. TENS treatment is contraindicated with demand pacemakers and should not be used on the head or neck or over irritated skin.

Patient Care: Symptom Management

Systems Review

System-Based Physical Examination

A system-based physical examination is carried out methodically, moving from one system to another to ensure that all body systems are reviewed. The examination begins with a patient and family history and then a general survey that includes assessment of psychosocial status, substance abuse, domestic partner violence, measurements (height, weight), and vital signs as well as assessment of pain level and nutritional assessment. **System-based physical examination** utilizes inspection, palpation, percussion, and auscultation. While the order may vary somewhat, the usual order of examination is:

- Skin, nails, and hair
- Head, face, and neck
- Eyes, ears, nose, mouth, and throat
- Breasts and regional lymph nodes
- Thorax and lungs
- Heart and neck vessels
- Peripheral vascular/lymphatic system
- Abdomen
- Musculoskeletal system (may include functional assessment)
- Genitourinary system
- Anus, rectum, and prostate

Elements of Systems Review

General	Normal weight, changes in weight, sleeping patterns, malaise, weakness, and fever
Head	Frequency or occurrence of headaches, head injuries. Frequency of upper respiratory infections, nasal stuffiness, discharge, itching, hay fever, sinus congestion, and nosebleeds. Condition of teeth and gums, last dental exam, hoarseness, bleeding gums, sore tongue, and frequency of sore throats
Neck	Swollen lymph nodes, stiffness, and goiter
Eyes	Vision (contacts, glasses), redness, tearing, visual disturbances, glaucoma, cataracts, and macular degeneration
Ears	Hearing, vertigo, tinnitus, earaches, and discharge
Skin	Rashes, texture changes, jaundice, nevi, dryness, and lesions
Breasts	Masses, nipple discharge, changes in nipple, date of last mammogram, and frequency of SBE
Cardiac	Heart problems, hypertension, heart murmurs, chest pain, paroxysmal nocturnal dyspnea and prior ECGs or heart tests
Respiratory	Cough, sputum, dyspnea, hemoptysis, bronchitis, COPD, asthma, TB, pleurisy, and last chest x-ray and/or PPD
Gastrointestinal	Dysphagia, heartburn, appetite, nausea, vomiting, regurgitation, indigestions, frequency and character of stools, abdominal pain, food allergies/intolerances, flatus, jaundice, and hepatitis, liver, or gallbladder problems
Urinary	Frequency, nocturia, polyuria, pain or burning, hematuria, urgency, incontinence, changes in urinary stream, urinary infections, and calculi
Peripheral/Vascular	Leg pain, cramping, varicose veins, and phlebitis
Gynecological	Age at menarche/menopause, regularity, frequency, and duration of menses, bleeding between periods/after intercourse, discharge, premenstrual tension, postmenopausal symptoms, itching, masses, gravida/para/abortus, contraception, and sexual problems
Musculoskeletal	Pains, stiffness, arthritis, gout, backaches, inflammatory changes, and limitations in mobility
Neurologic	Fainting, seizures, blackouts, paresis/paralysis, change in sensation (numbness, tingling), tremors, and involuntary movement
Hematologic	Bruising, bleeding, anemia, and past transfusions/reactions
Endocrine	Thyroid disease, heat/cold intolerance, diabetes, polyuria/polydipsia, excessive hunger, and excessive perspiration
Psychiatric	Mood/anxiety disorders, nervousness, tension, cognitive impairment

System-Specific End Stage Disease Progression

NEUROLOGIC SYMPTOMS

End-stage disease progression of neurologic disorders varies, but there are some commonalities:

- **Progressive weakness or disability**: Ambulatory patients may progress to wheelchair bound or bedridden. Patients may be unable to manage personal care or any ADLs, such as eating, toileting, and bathing, without assistance. While range-of-motion and other exercises may help, the changes are usually not reversible, so the caregiver may need assistance to provide care.
- **Speech impairment**: The patient's speech may be difficult to understand or the patient may lose the ability to communicate verbally. Assistive devices such as computerized systems may help, and the patient may be able to communicate through picture or letter boards.
- **Dysphagia**: The patient may choke easily and eventually lose the ability to swallow. Initially, the dysphagia may be controlled through changes in diet (soft or pureed foods) but eventually the patient may need a feeding tube to maintain nutrition and hydration.
- **Respiratory distress**: Positioning and oxygen administration may relieve respiratory distress, but those with severe impairment may require intubation and ventilation.

MYOCLONUS

Myoclonus is characterized by jerking muscle contractions. Myoclonus is common after opioid administration and mild twitching is usually not of major concern, but moderate or more pronounced myoclonus may progress to seizures. Reducing dosage, utilizing opioid rotation, or changing to an equianalgesic should relieve symptoms in one to two days. In addition to opioids, myoclonus may be associated with AIDS dementia, hypoxic conditions, administration of quinolones, placement of an intrathecal catheter, and neurological impairment following brain surgery. Myoclonus can be very tiring, especially if it occurs nocturnally and interferes with sleep. If myoclonus is very mild, a benzodiazepine (clonazepam, diazepam, midazolam) at bedtime may keep jerking from awakening the patient. Baclofen may also help reduce myoclonus. Protective padding should be placed about the patient (on side rails and assistive devices).

ENCEPHALOPATHY

Encephalopathy is a degenerative condition of the brain, characterized by alterations in mental status, often with confusion, memory loss, and personality changes. Patients may exhibit physical symptoms as well, such as ataxia, seizures, and tremors. Encephalopathy may be caused by lack of oxygen (anoxic, hypoxic) or disease process, such as infection, liver failure, kidney failure, brain tumors, brain abscess, alcohol withdrawal, vitamin deficiency, (B-1), chemical or alcohol toxicity, increasing intracranial pressure, and hypoglycemia. Management includes identifying and treating the underlying cause as some cases of encephalopathy may reverse with appropriate treatment, which can vary widely. The Glasgow Coma Scale may be utilized to assess level of consciousness. Patients should be protected from injury and oriented frequently. Some patients may benefit from administration of oxygen. Patients should usually be positioned with the head elevated to reduce pressure.

APHASIA

Aphasia is the loss of ability to use or understand written and spoken language because of damage to the speech center of the brain caused by brain tumors, brain injury, or stroke. The speech pathologist should assess the patient and provide guidance in communicating with the patient. There are different types of aphasia:

- **Global**: Difficulty understanding and producing language in speaking, reading, and writing although patients may understand gestures. Use pictures, diagrams, and gestures to convey meaning. Picture charts are useful.
- **Broca's**: Can understand language but has difficulty producing language to varying degrees. Speak slowly and clearly, facing the person, and be patient. Picture charts may be useful to help the patient communicate.
- **Wernicke's**: Difficulty understanding language but can understand gestures and is able to produce language although with some impairment, such as incorrect words or sounds. Patients may be able to write or use letter boards to assist communication.

Dysphagia

Dysphagia may occur in any phase of swallowing:

- **Oral phase**: Difficulty chewing and swallowing, tends to drool liquids and food; food remains in the mouth after the meal.
- **Pharyngeal phase**: Chokes while swallowing and often regurgitates food into the nose during the meal or immediately afterward. Breath sounds and voice may be gurgling after eating because of incomplete swallowing, and patients may feel as though food is caught in the throat.
- **Esophageal phase**: Has reflux and regurgitates food frequently after eating, difficulty swallowing solid foods. Patients rarely cough or choke but may feel as though food is caught in the chest.

If the patient may aspirate, the most appropriate referral is to a speech pathologist. The speech pathologist is able to assess the strength of the mouth, including the lips, the tongue, the palate, and the jaw, and may suggest preventive measures, including positioning, exercises, and diet modifications. In some cases, a feeding tube may be considered or withdrawal of food and fluids in the case of a dying patient.

Comfort Needs of Neurological Patients

Comfort needs of neurological patients include:

- **Physical**: Includes positioning, assisting with mobility, providing assistive devices and training, preventing thirst and hunger, providing adequate nutrition, controlling pain, managing muscle spasms and spasticity or other symptoms, managing bowel and bladder, carrying out skin care, managing adverse effects of drugs, and preventing complications
- **Psychosocial**: Includes helping patient make adjustments to disability, encouraging independence and decision making, addressing depression, reducing uncertainty, providing up-to-date information, encouraging friends and family to participate, helping patient explore sexuality concerns, recognizing stages of grief, being supportive and nonjudgmental, providing patient and family with lists of resources, collaborating with the patient in all aspects of care, and supporting spirituality
- **Environmental**: Includes maintaining comfortable temperature (heat, air-conditioning, blankets, fans), providing adequate light (ambient and artificial), controlling noise, avoiding clutter, maintaining cleanliness, ensuring safety and access (ramps, grab bars, safety rails, shower seats), and ensuring access to transportation

CARDIAC SYMPTOMS

End-stage disease progression of cardiac disorders often includes the following:

- **Dyspnea**: Opioids often help to relieve dyspnea. Other interventions include positioning the patient with head of bed elevated, using a fan aimed toward the patient's face, administering oxygen, and avoiding NSAIDS (which may reduce the effects of diuretics and other drugs). If dyspnea is related to pulmonary edema, diuretics and vasodilators may provide relief.
- **Pain**: This may be cardiac or edema-related, affecting the chest or the entire body. Opioids are generally the drugs of choice to relieve pain related to end-stage disease.
- **Fatigue and depression**: Relieving other symptoms and providing both physical and emotional support may help to reduce fatigue and depression.
- **Fluid retention**: Elevating the legs to improve circulation and administration of diuretics and vasodilators (as for dyspnea) may provide some relief.
- **General weakness**: Patients will become bedbound as the condition progresses and unable to attend to ADLs without assistance.

ANGINA

Impairment of blood flow through the coronary arteries leads to ischemia of the cardiac muscle and **angina pectoris**. Angina pain frequently occurs in males with crushing pain substernally, radiating to the neck and down the left arm or both arms. Females, whose symptoms may appear less acute, may experience nausea, shortness of breath, and fatigue. Stable angina episodes usually last for less than 5 minutes and are exercise-induced episodes caused by atherosclerotic lesions blocking more than 75% of the lumen of the effected coronary artery. They usually resolve by decreasing activity level and administering nitroglycerine. Unstable angina (preinfarction or crescendo angina) is a progression of coronary artery disease and occurs when there is a change in the pattern of stable angina. The pain may increase, may not respond to a single nitroglycerine, and may persist for more than 5 minutes.

- **Nitroglycerine**: Administered sublingually, 0.3-0.6 mg, repeated every 5 minutes up to 3 times. Avoid with myocardial infarction.
  - Adverse effects: May cause headache, flushing, dizziness, orthostatic hypotension, and palpitations.
  - Interactions: Avoid with erectile dysfunction drugs (sildenafil, tadalafil, vardenafil).

DYSRHYTHMIAS

Cardiac dysrhythmias include:

- **Bradyarrhythmia** (pulse rates that are abnormally slow because of impaired conduction)
  - Complete atrioventricular block (A-V block) may be congenital or a response to surgical trauma.

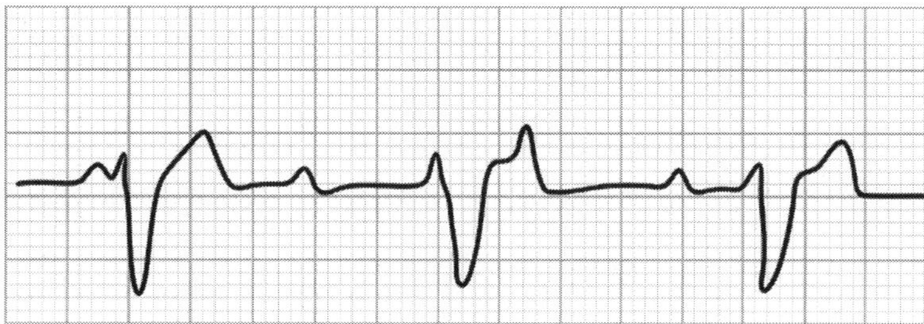

- Sinus bradycardia may be caused by the autonomic nervous system or a response to hypotension and decrease in oxygenation.

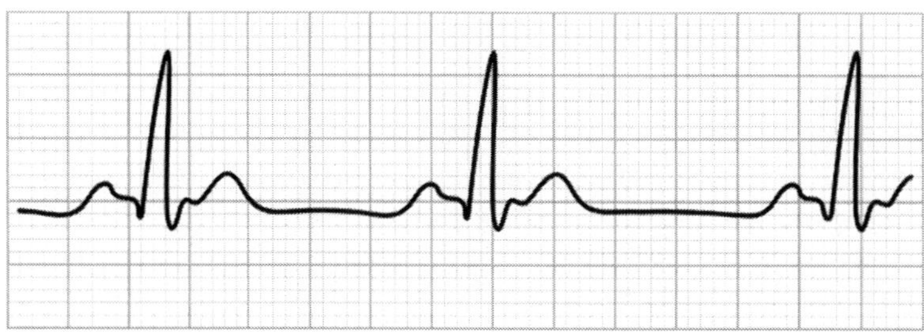

- Junctional or nodal rhythms often occur in post-surgical patients when absence of P wave is noted, but heart rate and output usually remain stable. Unless there is compromise, usually no treatment is necessary.

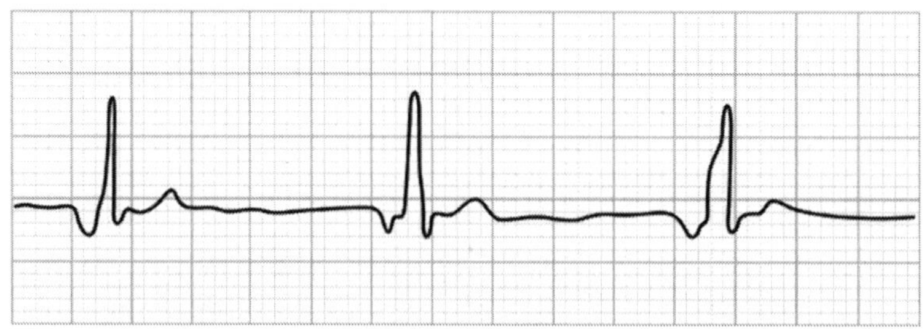

- **Tachydysrhythmia** (pulse rates that are abnormally fast, originating in the atria or ventricles)
  - Sinus tachycardia is often caused by illness, such as fever or infection.

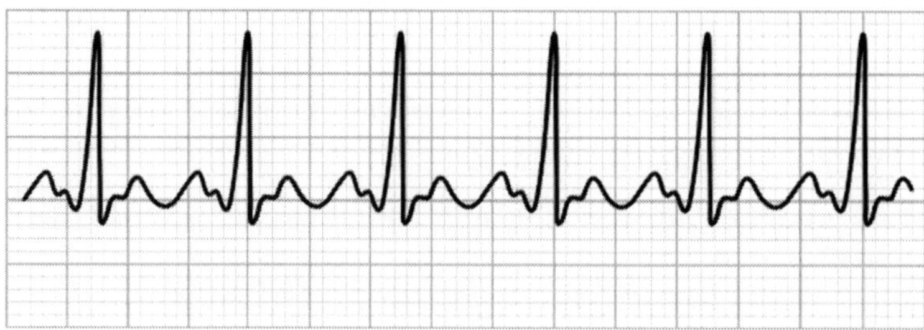

  - Supraventricular tachycardia (200-300 bpm) may have a sudden onset and result in congestive heart failure.

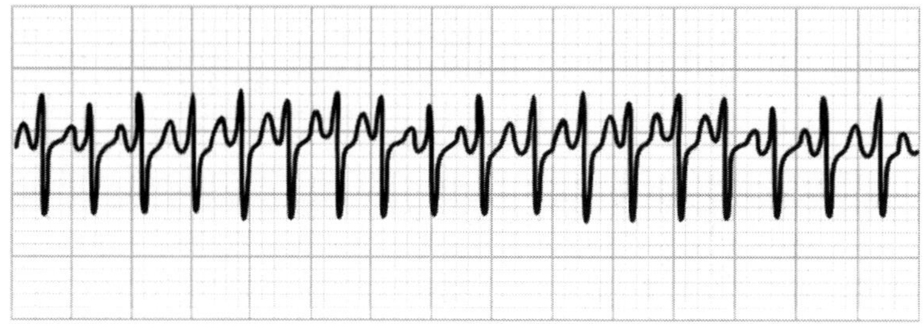

- Atrial fibrillation, atrial flutter, ventricular fibrillation, and PVCs may occur.

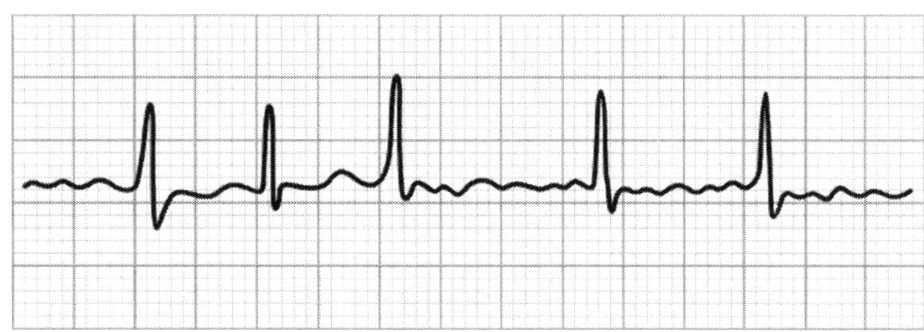

Management of dysrhythmia is usually with medications such as beta-blockers (tachydysrhythmia) or atropine (bradydysrhythmia), cardioversion, insertion of a pacemaker, and cardiac monitoring.

Edema

Edema is a result of excess fluid gathering within the tissues (interstitially). Capillary filtration exceeds lymph drainage, creating a fluid imbalance. The resulting fluid retention causes swelling, decreased skin mobility, tightness, tingling, decreased strength, mobility, and discomfort ranging from aching to severe pain. Skin can change color or even burst from the pressure. Edema is generally assessed according to the pitting scale.

- 1+ edema means the fluid buildup is barely detectable. The depression when pressure is applied is 2 mm and rebounds immediately.
- 2+ edema shows a slight indentation of 4 mm when pressed upon and takes less than 15 seconds to rebound.
- 3+ edema shows a deep indentation of 6 mm when pressed upon that takes 10 to 30 seconds to rebound.
- 4+ edema creates a depression of at least 8 mm when pressed upon and takes more than 20 seconds to rebound.

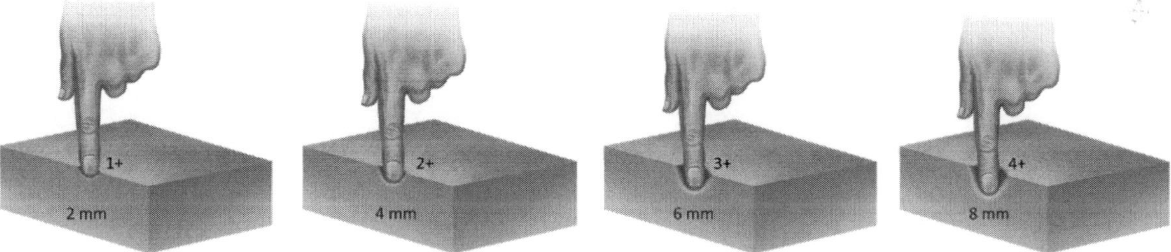

Left untreated, edema can transition to lymphedema. Management usually includes treating underlying condition, diuretics (hydrochlorothiazide, furosemide), elevation of limbs, and good skin care.

Pulmonary Symptoms

End-stage progression of pulmonary disorders often includes:

- **Dyspnea**: Patients with hypoxemia may need supplementary oxygen, and opioids may help to relieve the sensation of breathlessness (air hunger). Patients often breathe more easily with the head of the bed elevated with a fan aimed at the patient's head. Patients may benefit from diuretics (for pulmonary edema) or bronchodilators.
- **Pulmonary cachexia syndrome**: This syndrome comprises anorexia, weight loss, fat and muscle wasting, and weakness. The patient begins to appear emaciated and increasingly frail. Patients may benefit from nutritional supplementation and small, frequent meals. Some medications may improve appetite, such as progestational agents, corticosteroids, cannabinoids, and metoclopramide.
- **Anxiety and depression**: Some patients may benefit from relaxation techniques but others may require medications, such as SSRIs.
- **Cough**: Upright position and cough medicines may help produce some relief.
- **Stress incontinence (associated with cough)**: Patients should limit drinks containing caffeine and may need incontinence products.
- **Chest pain**: Some patients may need opioids to relieve discomfort.

Dyspnea

Dyspnea is common in hospice and palliative care patients. For patients already receiving morphine, increasing the dose by 2.5 mg may relieve the sensation of breathlessness. Opioid-naïve patients may benefit from 5 mg morphine orally every 4 hours. Providing oxygen (2-4 L) usually only provides some relief if the dyspnea is associated with hypoxia, such as with COPD, although the oxygen may help reduce anxiety. Elevating the head of the bed should be done routinely, but that alone may be ineffective for severe dyspnea. Directing the airflow of an electric fan toward the patient's face may make the patient feel less anxious about the shortness of breath. Cheyne-Stokes respirations are commonly found in dying patients. As the lungs become less effective and more congested, gas exchange is poor, and carbon dioxide levels increase. This increase usually triggers respiration, but as brain function decreases, this function is impaired, so respirations may deepen and then become shallower and irregular with periods of apnea that may last for up to a minute in a repeating cycle.

Sleep Apnea

Obstructive sleep apnea results from passive collapse of the pharynx during sleep, often associated with narrow or restricted upper airway (micrognathia, obesity, enlarged tonsils). Patients often snore loudly with cycles of breath cessation caused by apneic periods up to 60 seconds, occurring at least 30 times a night despite continued chest wall and abdominal movements, indicating automatic attempt to breathe. ECG changes may indicate bradydysrhythmia during apnea and tachydysrhythmia when breathing resumes. Hypoxemia or hypercarbia may persist during waking hours.

Central sleep apnea involves apneic and hypopneic episodes without obstruction and usually results from cardiac or neurological disorders that cause impairment of ventilation. Snoring is usually mild, and individuals may complain of insomnia because they awaken frequently. Chest wall and abdominal movements do not occur during apneic periods with this breathing-related sleep disorder. Cheyne-Stokes respirations may be present (apnea, 10-60 seconds of hyperventilation, followed by another period of apnea). Treatment for both types includes head elevation and use of CPAP or BiPAP during sleep.

COUGH AND SECRETIONS

Cough is common in patients with advanced heart failure, lung cancer, various other cancers, cystic fibrosis, asthma, COPD, and HIV/AIDS and may be related to infection, inflammation, pulmonary edema, and increased secretions. **Cough** may result from the direct effects of tumors or from treatment, such as radiotherapy. Treatment depends on the underlying cause but may include nonopioid antitussives (dextromethorphan, benzonatate) and inhaled anesthetics (lidocaine, bupivacaine) for non-productive cough. Productive cough is most often treated with chest physiotherapy, oxygen, suctioning, expectorants, and mucolytics. Opioids (such as codeine) may also decrease coughing.

As patients near death, they are unable to cough to clear **secretions** that begin to pool in the oropharynx and bronchi, resulting in rales (death rattles). Because the sound is often distressing to family members, an anticholinergic (glycopyrrolate or atropine) may be given subcutaneously to relieve respiratory distress. A hyoscine hydrobromide transdermal patch is also available, but action is slower, 12 hours compared to 1 minute for injections. Elevating the head of the bed or turning the patient to the side may also relieve rattling.

HEMOPTYSIS

Hemoptysis is the expectoration of blood from the lower respiratory tract. It occurs frequently in patients with advanced cancer due to metastasis or infection. An additional common cause in the United States is bronchitis. The initial assessment needs to distinguish this condition from gastrointestinal and nasopharyngeal bleeding. Patient complaints typically include a persistent blood-producing cough, dyspnea, wheezing, chest pain, fever, night sweats, and weight loss. The severity of hemoptysis is determined by the amount of blood produced within a 24-hour period. Mild hemoptysis is the production of less than 20 mL of blood within that time period. Moderate hemoptysis requires expectoration of 20-200 mL. Massive hemoptysis is 200-600 mL of blood expectorated within a 24-hour period. Massive hemoptysis occurs in fewer than 5% of cases, but it is life threatening and associated with an 85% mortality rate. The primary risk is asphyxiation from blood clots in the airway.

MANAGING RESPIRATORY ISSUES THROUGH THE BREATHES PROGRAM

The **BREATHES program** is used to manage respiratory symptoms in older palliative care patients:

B	**Bronchospasms**	Consider the use of albuterol nebulizers or steroids.
R	**Rales/crackles**	Reduce fluid intake through fluid restriction and discontinuation of IV therapy. Consider using diuretics at a dosage of 20-40 mg/day of furosemide or 100 mg daily of spironolactone.
E	**Effusion**	Determine the presence of a pleural effusion by physical examination and chest x-ray. Treatment options such as thoracentesis or chest tube should be considered.
A	**Airway obstruction**	Assess for aspiration risk and provide preventative measures, such as pureed meals, thickened liquids, and keeping the patient upright during and after meals.
T	**Tachypnea and breathlessness**	Do frequent medication assessments, provide treatments for anxiety as needed. Opioids may reduce the respiratory rate and create feelings of breathlessness and anxiety. Providing cool, moving air may also help reduce feelings of breathlessness
H	**Hemoglobin**	If the hemoglobin is low, consider a blood transfusion.
E	**Education**	Educate and support the patient and family.
S	**Secretions**	If secretions are copious, provide pharmacological treatment.

Gastrointestinal Symptoms

End-stage progression of gastrointestinal disorders may vary according to the type of disorder but may include:

- **Anorexia or difficulty eating**: Patients may benefit from supplementary feedings, small frequent meals, parenteral nutrition, or feeding tubes. Oral foods may require modification, such as in consistency (soft or pureed). Some may tolerate only bland foods.
- **Ascites**: This may result in abdominal pressure and shortness of breath. Patients may need to be positioned with the head elevated. In some cases, paracentesis may relieve symptoms for a short period but fluid tends to recur.
- **Constipation or diarrhea**: Diet modifications (increased fiber and fluids, prune juice) may help alleviate constipation, and antispasmodics or anti-secretory drugs may reduce diarrhea.
- **Bowel obstruction**: Abdomen may become hard and distended. If the patient is not a candidate for surgery, such as colonic stenting, an NG tube may help relieve symptoms temporarily. A venting gastrostomy may be placed to reduce discomfort as well as nausea and vomiting.
- **Pain**: Opioids are often needed to relieve pain, especially associated with bowel obstruction.
- **Nausea and vomiting**: Antiemetics may provide some relief.

Nausea and Vomiting

Nausea and vomiting are common with hospice and palliative care patients occurring in about half of patients with terminal cancer. Asking the patient to do deep breathing and controlled swallowing may help to control the gag/vomit reflex. Other measures include serving cold or room temperature foods rather than hot, restricting intake of fluids during meals, and elevating the head or lying flat (varies with individuals) for at least 2 hours after eating. Patients may benefit from 5 or 6 small meals per day rather than 3 large meals. Fluids should be taken in small amounts (sips) throughout the day rather than in a large volume. Antiemetics are routinely administered to help control nausea and vomiting. Nursing management includes oral hygiene after emesis, control pain, reducing odors, and ensuring clothes are not tight fitting. Other interventions include marijuana, self-hypnosis, relaxation exercises, biofeedback, distraction, desensitization, acupuncture, acupressure, and music therapy.

Bad Taste and Xerostomia

Patients nearing end of life often have a very **bad taste** in their mouths. Strategies to increase patient intake include avoiding highly spiced hot foods and food odors, rinsing the mouth with a salt and soda mixture before eating, using a straw to drink liquids to minimize contact with taste buds, drinking very cold liquids, and eating cold or room-temperature food.

Xerostomia (dry mouth) is a common problem that exacerbates a bad taste and may result from medications, radiotherapy, or disease. Tests to assess xerostomia:

- **Cracker test**: Patient eats a dry cracker. If the patient is unable to chew and swallow the cracker without drinking liquid, the test is positive. Some versions have the patient try to eat 6 crackers in one minute.
- **Tongue blade test**: Tongue blade is placed flat on a patient's tongue. Because xerostomia results in pasty thickened saliva, if the tongue blade sticks to the tongue, the test is positive.
- **Saliva measurement** (stimulated or unstimulated): Mouth is swabbed or patient spits repeatedly into a container for a set duration.

Pilocarpine is a nonselective muscarinic that increases saliva production, but it may result in increased perspiration, nausea, flushing, and cramping. Saliva substitute may provide partial relief.

Intractable Hiccups

Hiccups are involuntary contractions of the diaphragm and chest wall that occur intermittently, usually at a rate of 4-6 per minute. A **hiccup bout** is an episode that lasts up to two days. Intractable hiccups may last indefinitely or recur repeatedly, exhausting the patient and making it difficult to eat, drink, or sleep. Additionally, the jerking motion may exacerbate a patient's pain. Intractable hiccups may be associated with gastric distention (most common), irritation of the phrenic or diaphragmatic nerves, brain tumors, and hyponatremia. Intractable hiccups usually do not respond to the common strategies, which include eating a spoonful of sugar, doing the Valsalva maneuver, and drinking water. Various medications may be used to attempt to control hiccups, depending on the cause: antacids, anticonvulsants, calcium channel blockers, corticosteroids, tricyclic antidepressants, and muscle relaxants. Vagal nerve stimulation through ocular compression, gentle carotid massage, or digital rectal stimulation may be effective in some cases. If the hiccups are associated with diaphragmatic irritation, chlorpromazine 25 mg orally or rectally TID may be effective. In some cases, a cervical phrenic nerve block may provide relief.

Genitourinary Symptoms

Neurogenic Bladder

Neurogenic bladder is bladder dysfunction from lesions of peripheral or central nervous system. Neurogenic bladder may result from stroke, brain tumor, supraspinal lesions, spinal cord lesions, multiple sclerosis, peripheral nerve lesions (diabetes, herpes), Alzheimer's disease, and Parkinson's disease. Nerve damage can cause an underactive bladder that is unable to contract effectively to empty the bladder or an overactive bladder that contracts frequently and ineffectually. **Symptoms** vary:

- **Underactive**: This is characterized by incontinence, dribbling, straining or inability to urinate, and retention. Usually treated with intermittent catheterization. While Foley catheters pose a risk of increased infection, this is not a primary concern in the dying patient, and insertion of the Foley catheter to control incontinence is a comfort measure and may reduce skin irritation.
- **Overactive**: This is characterized by bladder spasms, frequency, urgency, dysuria, urinary tract infection, and fever. Treatment includes antibiotics for infection, absorbent pads, pelvic floor muscle exercises, bladder training, and anticholinergic/antispasmodic drugs (oxybutynin chloride), TCAs, and Beta-3 adrenergic receptors (Mirabegron).

DIAPERS MNEMONIC FOR CAUSES OF URINARY INCONTINENCE

The DIAPERS mnemonic describes the causes of acute urinary incontinence.

D	**Delirium**	Acute delirium and the related confusion may cause urinary incontinence.
I	**Infection**	A urinary tract infection can cause or worsen incontinence.
A	**Atrophic urethritis**	Atrophic urethritis creates irritative voiding symptoms and stress incontinence.
P	**Pharmacy**	Medications such as opioids, sedatives, antidepressants, antipsychotics, and antiparkinsonian drugs can reduce contractility and increase urinary retention, overflow, and stress incontinence.
E	**Excessive urine production**	Chronic disease states such as diabetes mellitus cause polyuria and affect smooth muscle and nerve involvement.
R	**Restricted mobility**	Immobility and restricted accesses to appropriate toileting facilities lead to urinary incontinence.
S	**Stool impaction**	Stool impaction can result in urinary retention, urinary tract infection, and incontinence.

MUSCULOSKELETAL SYMPTOMS

PATHOLOGICAL FRACTURES

Pathological fractures occur as a result of weakening or abnormality of the bone rather than direct trauma. The most common bones affected are the vertebrae, pelvis, proximal humerus, and proximal femur. In the hospice and palliative care patient, pathological fractures most often result from advanced osteoporosis, from bony metastasis (most commonly from the prostate, breast, or lung), and from multiple myeloma or another tumor affecting the bone. Signs and symptoms include acute pain at the fracture site, swelling of soft tissue (sometimes present before the fracture), and muscle spasms. Treatment may require surgical repair (such as femur fractures) or fracture immobilization (cast) to allow healing. Some patients may undergo radiotherapy to reduce cancerous lesions, but radiotherapy may delay bone healing. Patients usually require analgesia and muscle relaxants if they are experiencing muscle spasms. Muscle relaxants include carisoprodol, cyclobenzaprine, or methocarbamol. Patients should have a diet with adequate protein, calcium, phosphorus, and magnesium to promote healing.

MUSCLE SPASMS

Muscle spasms can result in painful cramps, especially in the muscles of the calf. Muscle spasms may result from pathological fractures, dehydration, impaired peripheral circulation, spinal cord injury, neuromuscular disease (multiple sclerosis, amyotrophic lateral sclerosis, Huntington's disease), and electrolyte abnormalities, particularly deficiency of potassium or magnesium. Stroke patients may have muscle spasms on the affected side, with spasticity often occurring within 48 hours, leading to contractures, so range of motion exercises and proper positioning are essential. Numerous medications may also cause muscle spasms, including diuretics (furosemide, hydrochlorothiazide), donepezil, statins, raloxifene, neostigmine, asthma medications (albuterol), and nifedipine. The first step in managing muscle spasms is to identify the cause and determine if that can be modified. Encouraging hydration and stretching the muscles may provide some relief. Some patients may benefit from muscle relaxants and application of heat or cold. Patients with muscle spasms associated with spinal cord injury may have some relief from antispasmodics, such as baclofen, dantrolene, or tizanidine.

Skin and Mucus Membranes

Pruritus and Xerosis

Pruritus (itchy skin) is a common finding in hospice and palliative care patients and may be associated with many different diseases (endocrine, hepatic, neurological, hematological, and oncologic) as well as dehydration, infections, and drugs. **Xerosis** (dry skin) may occur because of aging, chemotherapy, or radiation, and applying a moisturizer may help reduce itching. Most opioids can cause pruritus, but morphine, which causes more histamine release, is more likely to cause pruritus than other opioids such as fentanyl, codeine, and oxymorphone. If itching is mild, an antihistamine given concurrently may control itching, but in some cases discontinuing the morphine and switching to another drug or rotating between morphine and another drug may be necessary. Application of cold may help relieve itching to a localized area, but heat often increases itching. Topical antipruritics, such as hydrocortisone, may relieve itching but are not practical if itching is generalized. Management depends on the cause and may include propofol, local anesthetics, and androgenic steroids.

Stomas

Stomas may be fecal or urinary and constructed from the small intestine, colon, bladder, or ureters. The stoma should be assessed for color (red if from intestines and pale pink if from ureter or bladder), size, and shape. If the stoma appears blue-tinged, this indicates ischemia. The stoma may protrude at times or retract but should be at or slightly above skin level. Urostomies should have a continuous flow of urine, but colostomies may have intermittent flow, depending on the site of the stoma. The stoma should be carefully wiped clean with water. Superficial bleeding usually stops spontaneously, but severe bleeding may occur with liver disease, anticoagulant therapy, steroid therapy, or a bleeding mesenteric vessel. Other complications may include prolapse, mucocutaneous separation, retraction, stenosis, and direct trauma. The correct size and shape of pouching system is essential to preventing irritation of the skin about the stoma. Peristomal complications can include candidiasis, folliculitis, and contact dermatitis.

Pressure Ulcers

Pressure ulcers result from pressure or pressure with shear and friction over bony prominences. The **National Pressure Injury Advisory Panel (NPIAP) stages** include:

- **Stage I**: Intact skin with non-blanching reddened area
- **Stage II**: Abrasion or blistered area without slough but with partial-thickness skin loss
- **Stage III**: Deep ulcer with exposed subcutaneous tissue. Tunneling or undermining may be evident with or without slough
- **Stage IV**: Deep ulcer, full thickness, with necrosis into muscle, bone, tendons, or joints
- **Suspected deep tissue injury**: Skin discolored, intact, or blood blister
- **Unstageable**: Eschar or slough prevents staging prior to debridement

Patients should be placed on pressure reducing support surfaces and turned at least every two hours, avoiding the area(s) with a pressure ulcer. Wound care depends on the stage of the wound and the amount of drainage, but includes irrigation, debridement when necessary, antibiotics for infection, and appropriate dressing. Patients should be encouraged to have adequate protein and iron in their diets to promote healing and to maintain adequate hydration.

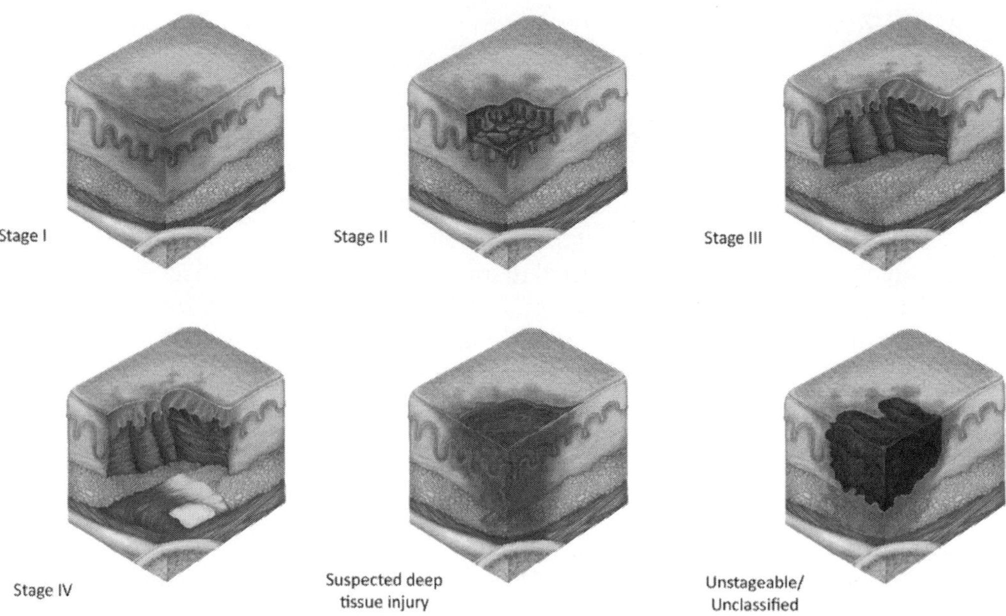

Fungating Tumors

Fungating tumors are those that are rapid growing and erupt in a mass through the skin, often with irregular surface, nodules, and necrotic tissue. These tumors are often very vascular and bleed easily and have copious foul-smelling drainage. They are also often very painful, and the odor is distressing to the patient and family members. Careful irrigation of the wound should be done and dressings applied as necessary. Metronidazole, in gel or solution, has proven to be an effective topical treatment to control infection and odor in fungating and necrotic tumors as it is effective against a wide range of anaerobic bacteria. The solution is used to irrigate the wound, and the gel is applied directly to the tissue. Various treatments (surgery, radiotherapy, chemotherapy) may be tried to reduce the size of the tumor, but healing is unlikely. The patient should receive adequate analgesia to control pain and should receive emotional support.

Mucositis

Mucositis is inflammation of mucous tissue and can occur throughout the gastrointestinal tract as an adverse effect of chemotherapy, other drugs, and radiotherapy. Signs and symptoms usually occur within 10 days of onset of treatment and may persist for 6 weeks or more. The entire mucosa may become inflamed, edematous, infected, and painful:

- Oral inflammation (stomatitis) is common and may result in oral lesions, halitosis, and difficulty eating and drinking because of pain. Good oral care is essential to prevent infection. Special antibiotic or antifungal mouth rinses may be used if infection (such as candidiasis) occurs. Sucking on ice chips or lozenges may relieve discomfort.
- Intestinal inflammation may result in severe diarrhea, treated with antidiarrheal medications, rehydration, and electrolyte replacement.
- Rectal inflammation may result in ulceration, bleeding, and severe pain. Rectal treatment may include steroid suppositories.

Patients who also have neutropenia have increased risk of developing septicemia. Preventive treatment includes benzydamine (for radiotherapy to head and neck) and ranitidine or omeprazole (for chemotherapy). Topical pain relievers, analgesics, and corticosteroids may reduce discomfort.

FISTULAS

A fistula is an abnormal opening or channel connecting two structures. There may be multiple branches from a fistula rather than just one channel. Care strategies include:

- **Skin protection**: Low output fistulas may need only skin barriers and easily changed absorbent dressings. Creases, folds, and depressions may need to be filled with skin barrier paste, wafers, or powder before solid barriers are applied. Solid barriers last as long as they remain intact, liquid skin sealants last up to 24 hours, and skin powders or pastes last up to 24 hours.
- **Drainage control**: If drainage cannot be contained with an absorbent dressing, then ostomy appliances with solid skin barriers and pouches are indicated. The barrier should extend at least 1.5 inches around the perimeter of the fistula. The barrier must adhere to even skin to avoid drainage getting under the barrier, so the opening may need to be enlarged. Pouching systems with barriers that can be cut to fit usually work best. If drainage is extensive, a bedside drainage bag may be used. Very large wounds (more than 4 inches) may require a custom pouching system.

NUTRITION AND METABOLIC CHANGES

NUTRITIONAL ISSUES ASSOCIATED WITH ADVANCED DISEASE

Nutritional issues are a concern with advanced disease. Patients almost always begin to eat and drink less at the end of life, often stopping altogether a few days before death. This is a normal progression, but there is still some debate as to when and if it is appropriate to use tube or parenteral feedings and IV fluids. The decision often rests with the patient or family, but there is little evidence that these interventions improve quality of life or death. Issues commonly associated with nutrition and advanced disease include:

- **Dehydration**: Intake may be hampered by somnolence, nausea, and decreased sensation of thirst.
- **Nausea and vomiting**: Patients may be unable to eat or retain food.
- **Weakness**: The effort to eat and drink may be more than the patient can manage.
- **Bad taste in mouth**: Food may taste metallic or bitter.
- **Xerostomia**: Dry mouth can make it difficult to chew and swallow.

NUTRITION INTERVENTIONS

Generally, the patient receiving hospice or palliative care should be permitted to eat whatever the patient desires rather than focusing solely on nutritional concerns. However, fatigue is a major concern impacting **nutrition**. Education should be provided about the importance of proper nutrition and adequate energy-providing foods when appropriate. It may be helpful to recommend nutritious, high-protein, nutrient-dense foods as snacks and small, frequent meals rather than large meals as well as adequate fluid intake and frequent oral hygiene. Protein supplements may also be suggested. Eggs or protein powder can be added to many foods to increase protein intake. For example, custards can be prepared with double or triple the usual number of eggs without affecting palatability. People with nausea often avoid meat products and those that can cause gas, such as beans. Simply telling patients to eat better is not usually enough to overcome the negative effects of nausea on diet. Chilled dietary supplement drinks, such as Ensure, may be added to the diet if the patient can tolerate them.

Dehydration

Dehydration is common, especially as patients near death. Symptoms are based on the level of dehydration:

- **Mild (5% loss)**: Dizziness, lethargy, reduced skin turgor, dry mucous membranes, and orthostatic hypotension
- **Moderate (10% loss)**: Confusion, resting hypotension, tachycardia, and oliguria or anuria
- **Severe (>15% loss)**: Occurs when total body water decreases but sodium does not; characterized by marked hypotension and anuria as well as symptoms associated with lesser dehydration

Dehydration may result from inadequate fluids, excess water loss, NG suctioning, drugs, diarrhea, vomiting, and fever. Increased fluids may alleviate dehydration in palliative care patients, but patients normally stop taking fluids as they near death, resulting in dehydration and drying of the mucous membranes of the mouth. Frequent mouth care and moistening of the mucous membranes can alleviate mouth discomfort. The mouth may be swabbed with artificial saliva, such as Salivart. As airways dry, secretions lessen, and the ability to cough is reduced. The death rattle also begins to lessen. IV fluids may relieve dehydration but prolong dying.

Anorexia and Cachexia

Almost all patients with terminal cancer or other serious illnesses experience anorexia and cachexia (muscle wasting). In fact, there is little that has been able to reverse anorexia and cachexia when people are in advanced stages of disease, and telling patients they must eat to live only adds to stress. However, some strategies can help to slow the process. Patients often do better when they eat small amounts every hour or two and supplement their diet with nutritional drinks such as Ensure to increase calories and nutrients. The nurse should explore dietary preferences with the patient, trying to find foods that the patient feels like eating, although this can prove challenging and may vary from day to day. Other strategies include lifting dietary restrictions, supplementing food with added protein and calories, avoiding hot food (to reduce odor), accommodating patient preferences for eating schedule and types of foods, allowing alcoholic beverages if the patient desires them, avoiding weighing the patient or stressing weight loss, and never forcing the patient to eat or drink.

ELECTROLYTE IMBALANCES

Sodium 135-145 mEq/L	**Hyponatremia**: <135 mEq/L. Critical value: <120 mEq/L. Causes: Inadequate sodium intake or excess loss, diarrhea, vomiting, NG suctioning, severe burns, fever, SIADH, and ketoacidosis. **Hypernatremia**: >145 mEq/L. Critical value: >160 mEq/L. Causes: Renal disease, diabetes insipidus, and fluid depletion.
Potassium 3.5-5.5 mEq/L	**Hypokalemia**: <3.5 mEq/L. Critical value: <2.5 mEq/L. Causes: Diarrhea, vomiting, gastric suction, and diuresis, alkalosis, starvation, and nephritis. **Hyperkalemia**: >5.5 mEq/L. Critical value: >6.5 mEq/L. Causes: Renal disease, adrenal insufficiency, metabolic acidosis, severe dehydration, burns, hemolysis, and trauma.
Calcium 8.2-10.2 mg/dL	**Hypocalcemia**: <8.2 mg/dL. Critical value: <7 mg/dL. Causes: Hypoparathyroidism and occurs after thyroid and parathyroid surgery, pancreatitis, renal failure, inadequate vitamin D, alkalosis, magnesium deficiency and low serum albumin **Hypercalcemia**: >10.2 mg/dL. Critical value: >12 mg/dL. Causes: acidosis, kidney disease, hyperparathyroidism, prolonged immobilization, and malignancies
Phosphorus 2.4-4.5 mEq/L	**Hypophosphatemia**: <2.4mEq/L. Causes: Severe protein-calorie malnutrition, excess antacids with magnesium, calcium or albumin, hyperventilation, severe burns, and diabetic ketoacidosis. **Hyperphosphatemia**: >4.5 mEq/L. Causes: Renal failure, hypoparathyroidism, excessive intake, and neoplastic disease, diabetic ketoacidosis, muscle necrosis, and chemotherapy
Magnesium 1.6-2.6 mEq/L	**Hypomagnesemia**: <1.6 mEq/L. Critical value: <1.2 mg/dL. Causes: chronic diarrhea, chronic renal disease, chronic pancreatitis, excess diuretic or laxative use, hyperthyroidism, hypoparathyroidism, severe burns, and diaphoresis. **Hypermagnesemia**: >2.6 mEq/L. Critical value: >4.9 mg/dL. Causes: renal failure or inadequate renal function, diabetic ketoacidosis, hypothyroidism, and Addison's disease.

ASTHENIA AND FATIGUE

Asthenia is characterized by loss of strength and weakness, while fatigue is characterized by feeling tired and exhausted after little or no exertion. Asthenia and fatigue are often experienced together in hospice and palliative care patients because of the debilitating effects of advanced disease and chronic pain or as a consequence of treatment, such as chemotherapy and radiation. In some cases, asthenia and fatigue may relate to inability to sleep well at night. The patient should be carefully assessed to determine the cause of fatigue and any aggravating or alleviating factors. Stimulant medications, such as methylphenidate, pemoline, or dextroamphetamine, and methylprednisolone may be helpful for some patients. If fatigue is associated with depression, an antidepressant may relieve symptoms. Treating severe anemia may also relieve fatigue. Fatigue may not be reversible with end-stage disease, but patients should be provided with supportive care and frequent opportunities to rest.

LYMPHEDEMA

Lymphedema is the accumulation of lymph in the soft tissue because of damage to the lymph nodes, such as following radiation or excision. Over time, the tissue becomes distended, hard, painful, and fibrotic. Any limb can be affected, and lymphedema of the arm is common after surgery and treatment for breast cancer. Pressure bandaging and stockings and avoiding dependent positioning can help to reduce swelling and discomfort. With lower extremity lymphedema, there is an increased risk of fungal infection of the toes, so antifungal powder should be applied routinely and the patient should be advised to wear cotton socks and breathable shoes (such as canvas). Signs of fungal infection include redness, itching, and peeling of skin. Antibiotics are given for infections, which are common complications because of stasis and accumulated debris in tissues. Antibiotics may be given prophylactically if patients have repeated infections.

Nutrition Assessment

NUTRITIONAL ASSESSMENT

Nutritional assessment should be done within the first 24 hours of care for hospitalized patients and at the first visit for others to ensure that nutritional requirements are met. The history and physical exam should include the following information about the previous 3 months:

- Changes in food intake, including number of meals eaten daily
- Weight loss (or gain)
- Episodes of depression or stress that may relate to dietary intake

A sample of a usual daily menu should be developed. Additional **screening** should include:

- Daily number of protein, fruit, grain, and vegetable servings
- Usual fluid intake, including type, amount, and frequency
- Method of feeding, independent or assisted
- Mobility
- Mental status
- Body mass index (BMI), mid-arm circumference, and calf circumference
- Living status (independent or dependent)
- Prescription and non-prescription drugs
- Pressure sores or other wounds or skin problems

PHYSICAL ASSESSMENT FOR NUTRITIONAL DEFICIENCY

The physical assessment is an important part of nutritional assessment to determine malnutrition or problems with self-feeding:

- Hair may be dry and brittle or thinning.
- Skin may show poor turgor, ecchymosis, tears, pressure areas, ulcerations, abrasions, or other compromises.
- Mouth may show dry mucous membranes. Lips may have cheilosis, cracking at the corners, and scaly lips (riboflavin deficiency). Gums may be swollen or bleeding, teeth loose or needing care, or poorly fitting dentures. Tongue may be inflamed, dry, cracked, or have sores.
- Nails may become brittle. Spoon shaped or pale nail bed indicates low iron.
- Hands may be crippled or arthritic, making eating difficult.
- Vision may be compromised so that people can't see to prepare food or have difficulty feeding themselves.
- Mental status may be impaired to the point that people can't understand diet instructions or prepare or eat meals.
- Motor skills may decrease, including hand-mouth coordination or ability to hold utensils.

Psychosocial, Emotional, and Spiritual

MALADAPTIVE BEHAVIORS

Six maladaptive behaviors that patients and families dealing with life-threatening illnesses may exhibit are:

- **Denial**: A way for the person to reject the reality of the situation they find themselves in. It is a refusal to accept physical, psychological, and emotional knowledge they do not want to believe in or deal with. Denial may be transiently adaptive when it is brief, securing only a little more time to gather the emotional reserves necessary for successful coping.
- **Guilt**: An unreasonable feeling of responsibility for negative influences or consequences over which the person may or may not have control.
- **Depression**: A mental state of hopelessness and despair. A severe loss of happiness and motivation.
- **Avoidance**: Withdrawal or turning away from actions or consequences associated with negative stimuli.
- **Decathexis**: Withdrawing prior feelings of affection for and attachment to a person or object, typically in anticipation of an impending loss.
- **Aggression**: Hostile behavior, whether physical or verbal, meant to be demeaning, destructive and increase negative emotions in those around them.

MANAGING EMOTIONAL STATES IN PATIENTS

DENIAL AND ANGER/HOSTILITY

Denial and anger/hostility are very common first reactions to bad news, and some patients are unable to get past these emotional states:

- **Denial**: Patients may act stunned and immobile or detached and unable to respond appropriately. In the beginning, denial serves as a protective mechanism that allows the patient to cope, but as time passes patients may become increasingly resistive to information and treatment, attempting to carry on as though everything is normal or blaming symptoms on minor problems, such as "heart burn." The nurse should remain patient and supportive, and repeat information as many times as needed while avoiding forcing the patient to "face the truth."
- **Anger and/or hostility**: Some patients may lash out at others and express overt hostility. Others may blame themselves or others for their conditions. Some patients are resentful they are ill and may complain loudly and often about medical care and healthcare providers. The nurse must not respond in anger or take patient statements personally but should remain calm and supportive while alert to the risk of physical attack.

FEAR

Fear is a common feeling among hospice and palliative care patients, and while some fears may be irrational, many are realistic, so identifying the patient's fear and developing strategies to alleviate those fears are important to the patient's sense of wellbeing:

Fears	Strategies
Pain	Maintaining adequate pain control and preventing breakthrough pain is essential, as is giving the patient some degree of control over decisions about pain control.
Treatments	Provide accurate information about what treatments entail and what type of discomfort and adverse effects to expect, especially in relation to surgery, chemotherapy, and radiotherapy.
Change of self-image	Provide patients with information about expected physical changes (loss of hair, amputation, scars) and prostheses (wigs, breast prosthesis, limb prosthesis) and other methods (clothing, makeup) to disguise or modify physical changes.
Costs	Provide information about costs and resources for financial and other assistance.
Dependency	Encourage the patient to remain independent in decisions or care to the degree possible and provide emotional support to the patient and caregiver.
Dying	Encourage the patient to express feelings and carry out a life review.

GUILT

Guilt is a common emotion associated with hospice and/or palliative care:

- **Patients** often feel guilty about leaving family behind. They may regret actions that they have taken or failed to take and feel guilty about being a burden, especially if they depend on family for caregiving, and about the cost of care. The nurse should take time to listen to the patient and help the patient focus on positive things the patient has provided for the family.
- **Family members** may feel that they have not done enough to help or may begin to regret harsh thoughts or things they have said. They may wish the patient would die to end suffering or relieve them from caregiving, but then feel guilty about wishing the patient's death. Some may feel guilty about placing a patient in hospice care or that they were not present when the patient died. The nurse should listen and support the family, reassuring them that the feelings that they have experienced are normal and that it's not unusual for patients to wait until family are gone to die. Some may benefit from a support group.

ANXIETY

Peplau's four levels of anxiety include:

1. **Mild**: Feelings include increased motivation, sharpened senses, alertness, enlarged perceptual field, restlessness, irritability, and hypersensitivity to sensory input, but the client can still solve problems, and learning is effective. Client may experience GI upset ("butterflies").
2. **Moderate**: The perceptual field narrows to a specific task and attention is selective. The client speaks rapidly in a high pitch and experiences muscle tension, diaphoresis, pounding pulse, headache, dry mouth, GI upset, and frequent urination.

3. **Severe**: The perceptual field continues to narrow, and the client cannot complete tasks, solve problems, or learn effectively. The client feels fear, dread, or horror and experiences severe headache, GI upset, trembling, rigidity, vertigo, pallor, tachycardia, and chest pain. Actions may be ritualistic.
4. **Panic**: Perceptual field focuses on self, not responding to environmental stimuli. The client experiences perceptual distortions, is unable to think rationally or recognize danger, and may be suicidal. The client may have disorganized personality, delusions, hallucinations, and inability to speak. The client may run or remain immobile.

Suffering

There are multiple aspects of **suffering** in which an individual can feel pain or distress. It encompasses emotional, spiritual, and physical aspects of life and affects the whole person. Suffering must be addressed from a comprehensive, holistic perspective while recognizing that it is not always possible to find the source, or entirely resolve all suffering. Identifying suffering involves careful observation, and different disciplinary perspectives can be helpful in making an accurate assessment. Issues surrounding suffering must be adequately addressed or the suffering is more likely to compound rather than diminish over time. However, it is not necessary for the caregiver to give, or even have, answers to the difficult questions that may arise. Rather, the primary intervention requires in reassurance of non-abandonment and continued support while the patient seeks answers for themselves. Religious or spiritual counseling is often useful as well.

Hope

Multiple factors can affect an individual's **outlook during a terminal illness**. Among these are the opportunity and ability to experience one or more meaningful relationships. All individuals need to feel that they are needed and an important part of the lives of their loved ones. Maintaining contact with family and close friends is thus crucial. In addition, maintaining feelings of lightheartedness, delight, joy, or playfulness will also help the individual identify and express positive personal attributes. They will be more accepting of themselves and others if they are able to identify courage, determination, serenity, and positive esteem within themselves. Spiritual beliefs and participation in spiritual rituals can provide a further sense of meaning to their life. The individual can thereby better focus their energies on achieving short-term, positive goals by which to provide direction to their lives, and allowing them to continue to share meaningfully with others. In the final stages of a terminal illness, individuals who have maintained a feeling of hope and other positive feelings are able to look toward their eventual death with greater peace and serenity.

In assessing whether or not an individual is experiencing exaggerated or unrealistic hope, determine if the hope is either too broad or too dismissive in nature, such as a complete denial of the disease process itself or a persistent belief in a cure when none is available. If the hope is unlikely to be realized, how determined is the individual to their course of belief? Is he or she able to acknowledge the possibility of a negative outcome? Or does the individual claim a sure knowledge of what will happen, rather than expressing realistic hopes and fears? Those experiencing unrealistic hope are more likely to engage in reckless behaviors and to ignore or dismiss worsening symptoms or warning signs. Such unrealistic hope may alienate the individual from family and friends, ultimately creating isolation. Is the person's level of hope impeding their ability to place their personal affairs in order or to acknowledge and properly grieve their own loss? Realistic hope allows for the wish of a miracle, even while preparing for the likelihood of a loss. Realistic hope becomes more, rather than less, accepting over time.

Coping Mechanisms

Coping mechanisms are important for people to deal effectively with stress (often associated with loss), and those who have overcome trauma and/or loss over the course of their lifetime tend to utilize the most effective strategies. Those with ineffective coping skills may express anxiety, anger, and agitation (which may interfere with decision making) and may develop depression and physical ailments, such as anorexia, weight loss, nausea, urinary and bowel problems, and sleep disturbance. **Coping mechanisms** include:

- **Avoidance**: Finding means to avoid stressors or reduce their impact is sometimes possible.
- **Problem solving**: Actively searching for a way to reduce stress or cope with it can promote self-assurance.
- **Physical activity**: An exercise program can often increase feelings of wellbeing and allow people to cope more effectively.
- **Spirituality**: About 90% of older adults are religious, with 50% attending religious services, and religion/spiritual endeavors can provide emotional support and a positive outlook to help people cope.

Task-Oriented Coping

Some people cope best with dying by focusing on the tasks that must be completed throughout the process. These **tasks** may be summarized as follows:

- **Physical tasks**: Bodily needs must be met and physical distress minimized in ways that are consistent with the patient's values and beliefs.
- **Psychological tasks**: The patient must feel a sense of dignity. They will seek reassurance and satisfaction in their lives, as well as security and autonomy.
- **Social tasks**: Interpersonal relationships must be nurtured and sustained, and past conflicts resolved and forgiveness expressed in order to fully address the social and relational implications of dying.
- **Spiritual tasks**: Sources of spiritual energy must be identified, developed, and reaffirmed in order to secure a continuing hope and purpose to their existence.

Coping Assistance

Many factors influence a patient's coping abilities, including the patient's disability, socio-demographic characteristics, personality, and the social and physical environment. Patients who lack self-efficacy (belief in one's abilities to cope) and hope may have difficulty coping or may utilize coping strategies, such as avoidance, that may be counterproductive. **Coping assistance** may include:

- Educating the patient about coping strategies
- Helping the patient come to terms with the condition through encouraging patient to share experiences and through active listening
- Utilizing strategies to promote self-awareness (education, feedback, counseling, rating tasks)
- Providing positive reinforcement
- Providing opportunities for the patient to make decisions and to be as independent as possible
- Helping the patient to establish order in his or her life through pacing, planning, and prioritizing
- Providing a home-based education program for the patient and family
- Encouraging small successes to help instill hope
- Enhancing support systems through encouraging friends and family to participate in rehabilitation
- Establishing a therapeutic relationship with the patient

Suicidal Ideation

Patients with chronic and/or terminal illnesses are at increased risk of **suicidal ideation** because they no longer want to live with pain, they do not want to become or remain a burden to family, they do not want to become dependent on others, they are lonely and frightened, they are exhausted from caregiving, and/or they suffer from depression or mood disorders.

- **Passive suicidal ideation** involves wishing to be dead or thinking about dying without making plans while active suicidal ideation involves making plans.
- Those with **active suicidal ideation** are most at risk. People with suicidal ideation often give signals, direct or indirect, to indicate they are considering suicide because many people have some ambivalence and want help. They may, for example, have a sudden change in mood, talk about dying, begin to give things away, stop taking medications, and/or become increasingly withdrawn. Others may act impulsively or effectively hide their distress.

A **suicide risk assessment** should be completed and documented upon admission, with each shift change, at discharge, or any time suicidal ideation is suggested by the individual. Interventions include asking the patient about suicidal ideation, discussing feelings, making a safety plan, treating pain more effectively, and helping to resolve problems.

SLEEP DISTURBANCES

Sleep disturbances are common among hospice and palliative care patients, especially those with cancer, and may be associated with anxiety and depression, medications (corticosteroids, chemotherapeutic agents), pain, and other medical conditions (ALS, obstructive or central sleep apnea, restless legs syndrome, diabetes, arthritis, CHF, coronary artery disease, GERD, asthma, thyroid disorders, and renal failure). **Insomnia** is most common although some patients (especially those depressed) may sleep excessively and remain **somnolent**. Management begins by identifying and treating the underlying cause when possible:

- **Pharmacologic treatment**: Includes benzodiazepines (estazolam, quazepam, temazepam, flurazepam, lorazepam, triazolam), non-benzodiazepine receptor agonists (zaleplon, zolpidem, eszopiclone), melatonin-receptor agonist (ramelteon), and tricyclic antidepressants (amitriptyline, doxepin, mirtazapine, trazadone).
- **Non-pharmacologic treatment**: Includes exercise regimens, cognitive-behavioral therapy, education about the effects of medication, and complementary therapies, such as aromatherapy, massage, self-hypnosis, mindfulness, and relaxation and visualization exercises. Some patients may benefit from better sleep hygiene and resetting the sleep-wake cycle by avoiding excessive napping or taking a short daily nap, setting a regular time for sleep, limiting fluid intake before bed (if nocturia present), avoiding caffeine in the afternoon and evening, and keeping the bedroom quiet and peaceful.

INTIMACY/RELATIONSHIP ISSUES

Intimacy/relationship issues may arise between hospice and palliative care patients and their significant others:

- **Dynamics of dependency**: Role reversal may occur as the person who was previously dominant (such as the primary wage earner) may become dependent on the other person for financial support and/or caregiving. This may cause guilt, resentment, depression, and anger (on both parts). A stay-at-home parent may have to seek employment, and this can become stressful, especially if the person lacks marketable skills.
- **Impotence, decreased libido**: Pain, medications, progression of disease, and depression can all impair the patient's interest in or ability to engage in sexual intercourse.
- **Lack of privacy**: Patients who are hospitalized in an acute, long-term care, or hospice facility often have little privacy, especially if they share a room with another patient.

The nurse should discuss intimacy/relationship issues with patients and significant others, encouraging them to express their feelings and providing resources, including information about alternative methods of expressing intimacy, such as through cuddling, massage, or oral sex. When possible, the nurse should assist the patient to achieve some privacy, such as through bed curtains or signs on the door.

CULTURAL ISSUES

Each person is entitled to receive an individualized full assessment and personalized care. The nurse should first assess his or her own background, values, and beliefs in order to consciously avoid placing biases upon the patient. Obtain further knowledge in order to understand the background of the patient being addressed, and show acceptance of differences even when they may diverge from the nurse's own comfort zone and culture. Nurses should also acknowledge differences concerning end-of life care and be sensitive and open to the individual patient's beliefs rather than trying to predict behavior or impose ideas. Assumptions regarding care, needs, or beliefs should not be made based on assumptions arising from a patient's race or ethnicity.

Culture is a set of learned and shared experiences among a group and is continuously changing. Culture is not based on heredity or genes. Culture may guide behavior, but not all members of a group follow the same cultural traditions or beliefs. Members of a cultural group may have divergent personal beliefs that are variations of the whole tradition. Individuals become members of a cultural group when they adopt the group's basic beliefs and values. Smaller groups may realign themselves with a larger or more dominate culture through **acculturation. Ethnicity** describes a similarity in ancestry, history, and/or language that a group has in common. Members of an ethnic group may share social, political, and cultural backgrounds. Not everyone who shares ethnicity will relate to or feel they belong with the rest of the group. Ethnic groups can house several different cultural groups. **Race** is a term often used to define human differences through genetic and biological means, but it is not scientifically supported.

Culturally competent behavior goes beyond knowing general culture-based facts; it is a dynamic process of being aware of and showing respect for cultural differences of all types. It begins with being aware of one's own beliefs and not letting them interfere with the care provided. Just as each nurse brings his or her own individual background, beliefs and practices to the caring experience, each patient and family has their own unique contributions to the world and environment of the care plan. Cultural competence is providing knowledgeable care that corresponds with the patient and family's own cultural background. The nurse provides a complete and unbiased, sensitive assessment of the patient's background and beliefs, obtains further knowledge as necessary, then coordinates and executes a plan of care that is meaningful to the patient and the family regardless of the care provider's own beliefs.

C. M. Fong proposed the mnemonic **CONFHER** to summarize an assessment model to ensure culturally sensitive care.

- **C**ommunication: Identify the patient's primary language and comprehension level.
- **O**rientation: Ask to whom the patient relates. Find out their ethnic identity and identify their value orientations and acculturation.
- **N**utrition: Find out the patient's food preferences and restrictions. Ask the patient about their feelings, associations, and meanings behind food.
- **F**amily relationships: Identify the family structure, dynamics, and goals.
- **H**ealth and health beliefs: Discuss the patient's personal beliefs and health behaviors.
- **E**ducation: Identify the patient's cognitive style. Find out about their formal education, occupation, or profession.
- **R**eligion: Discuss the patient's spiritual beliefs and practices. Find out if the patient relates to a higher power and if they have a religious preference.

Hospice and Palliative Care Emergencies

AUTONOMIC DYSREFLEXIA

Autonomic dysreflexia can occur with central cord lesions at or above T6 and can result in encephalopathy and shock if undiagnosed and untreated. Autonomic dysreflexia occurs after the initial spinal shock has resolved. Onset is often very sudden and constitutes a medical emergency. Common causes include distended bladder, fecal impaction, pressure sores, tight clothing, hyperthermia, and other painful stimuli.

Symptoms

- Hypertension, severe pounding headache, increased ICP, and/or rupture of cerebral vessel
- Bradycardia, other cardiac arrhythmias
- Diaphoresis, piloerection, flushing of skin below level of injury and pallor above
- Nasal congestion
- Blurred vision, spots in visual field
- Seizures

Treatment

- Elevate head immediately to reduce blood pressure.
- Identify and rectify cause (check bladder, bowels, skin, clothing, temperature).
- If related to bladder distention, catheterize and drain the bladder slowly.
- If initial treatment is not successful in reversing symptoms, then give medications (IV antihypertensives, such as hydralazine, and antispasmodics).

SEIZURES

Common causes of seizures at the end-of-life include brain tumors, medications (TCAs, phenothiazines, butyrophenones, opioids), and infection. In hospice and palliative care patients, the most common types of **seizures** include:

- **Simple partial (focal)**: Unilateral motor symptoms including somatosensory, psychic, and autonomic
- **Aversive**: Eyes and head turned away from focal side
- **Sylvan (usually during sleep)**: Tonic-clonic movements of the face, salivation, and arrested speech
- **Tonic-clonic (general)**: Occurs without warning
    - Tonic period (10-30 seconds): Eyes roll upward with loss of consciousness, arms flexed, stiffen in symmetric tonic contraction of body, apneic with cyanosis and salivating.
    - Clonic period (up to 30 minutes, but usually ~30 seconds). Violent rhythmic jerking with contraction and relaxation. May be incontinent of urine and feces. Contractions slow and then stop.

During a seizure, the patient should be unrestrained but positioned on the side to prevent aspiration. Anticonvulsants or other drugs (phenytoin, carbamazepine, phenobarbital, valproic acid, divalproex, midazolam) may be administered to prevent or control seizures. The seizure should be timed, and the patient protected from harm.

HEMORRHAGE

Hemorrhage may be internal (hemorrhagic stroke, GI bleeding) or external (bleeding wound, tumor) and may be associated with disease (leukemia, disseminated intravascular coagulopathy, AIDS, uremia), clotting disorders (thrombocytopenia), tumor necrosis (eroded vessels), trauma (penetrating injuries), and medications (warfarin, NSAIDs, beta-lactam antibiotics, aspirin). Symptoms (pallor, hypotension, tachycardia) are usually evident with acute rapid hemorrhage when about 20% of blood volume is lost because the body is not able to compensate for the loss. Hemorrhage may be treated aggressively or palliatively, depending on the patient's condition and advance directive and the site/extent of bleeding, but steps are generally taken to **control bleeding**:

- Apply pressure dressing to control external bleeding.
- Provide fluid resuscitation.
- Stop anticoagulant drugs and administer reversal agents.
- Treat coagulopathy.
- Carry out invasive interventions: surgery, radiotherapy, embolization, endoscopic procedures (balloon tamponade, lavage), and cryosurgery.
- Apply hemostatic agents, dressings.
- PPIs and H2 receptor antagonists (gastric bleeding).
- Administer tranexamic acid.
- Administer blood products, such as packed red blood cells.

SVCS

Superior vena cava syndrome (SVCS) is the result of a **partial occlusion of the superior vena cava**, which results in decreased venous blood flow from the head and neck to the right atrium. The blockage may result from cancerous growths. This is considered an emergency condition marked by headache, facial edema, hoarseness, dyspnea, and swollen arms. In situations of rapid onset, the loss of circulation can be life threatening. The severity and timing of symptom onset can be gradual or acute. Patients may report subtle signs such as swelling in the morning hours, or increasing discomfort with bending forward or stooping. The most common complaint is dyspnea. Other physical findings can include vein distention in the neck and chest, a ruddy complexion or cyanosis, tachypnea, stridor, orthopnea, hoarseness, nasal stuffiness, periorbital and conjunctivae edema. As symptoms progress, cerebral edema will occur, potentially leading to stupor, coma, seizures, or death.

Support, Education, and Advocacy

Advance Care Planning

Patients' Rights

The rights of patients and their families in relation to what they should expect from a healthcare organization are outlined in standards of both the Joint Commission and the National Committee for Quality Assurance. Rights include:

- Respect for the patient, including personal dignity and psychosocial, spiritual, and cultural considerations
- Response to needs related to access and pain control
- Ability to make decisions about care, including informed consent, advance directives, and end of life care
- Procedure for registering complaints or grievances
- Protection of confidentiality and privacy
- Freedom from abuse or neglect
- Protection during research and information related to ethical issues of research
- Appraisal of outcomes, including unexpected outcomes
- Information about organization, services, and practitioners
- Appeal procedures for decisions regarding benefits and quality of care
- Organizational code of ethical behavior
- Procedures for donating and procuring organs/tissue

Confidentiality

Confidentiality is the obligation that is present in a professional-patient relationship. Nurses are under an obligation to protect the information they possess concerning the patient and family. Care should be taken to safeguard that information and provide the privacy that the patient deserves. This is accomplished through the use of required passwords when family call for information about the patient and through the limitation of who is allowed to visit. The nurse should not assume that family members can be apprised of an older adult's health information without that person's consent. There may be times when confidentiality must be broken to save the life of a patient or others, but those circumstances are rare. The nurse must make all efforts to safeguard patient records and identification. Computerized record keeping should be done in such a way that the screen is not visible to others, and paper records must be secured.

HIPAA

HIPAA regulations are designed to protect the rights of individuals regarding the privacy of their health information. The nurse must not release any information or documentation about an individual's condition or treatment without consent, as the individual has the right to determine who has access to personal information. Personal information about the individual is considered **protected health information (PHI)**, and consists of any identifying or personal information about the individual, such as health history, condition, or treatments in any form, and any documentation, including electronic, verbal, or written. Personal information can be shared with the spouse, legal guardians, those with durable power of attorney for the individual, and those involved in care of the individual, such as physicians, without a specific release, but the individual should always be consulted if personal information is to be discussed with others present to ensure there is no objection. Failure to comply with HIPAA regulations can make a nurse liable for legal action.

Review Video: HIPAA
Visit mometrix.com/academy and enter code: 412009

ADVANCE DIRECTIVES, DNR, AND DURABLE POWER OF ATTORNEY

In accordance to Federal and state laws, individuals have the right to self-determination in health care, including decisions about end-of-life care through **advance directives** such as living wills and the right to assign a surrogate person to make decisions through a **durable power of attorney**. Patients should routinely be questioned about an advanced directive as they may present at a healthcare organization without the document. Patients who have indicated they desire a **do-not-resuscitate (DNR)** order should not receive resuscitative treatments for terminal illness or conditions in which meaningful recovery cannot occur. Patients and families of those with terminal illnesses should be questioned as to whether the patients are hospice patients. For those with DNR requests or those withdrawing life support, staff should provide the patient palliative rather than curative measures, such as pain control and oxygen, and emotional support to the patient and family. Religious traditions and beliefs about death should be treated with respect.

Hospice and Palliative Care Benefits

ADVOCATING FOR HOSPICE AND PALLIATIVE CARE

The nurse can advocate for hospice and palliative care by:

- Joining professional organizations and participating in activities
- Writing articles (journals, newspapers, magazines) regarding hospice and palliative care
- Speaking in public forums (community meetings, social gatherings) about the importance of hospice and palliative care
- Utilizing social media
- Mentoring and coaching other nurses to help them become proficient in hospice and palliative care
- Completing continuing education courses in the field in order to remain current
- Discussing the role of nurses in hospice and palliative care with physicians
- Addressing administration and the board of directors regarding patient care and professional needs
- Developing training courses for other staff members
- Participating in development of community information resources, such as pamphlets
- Representing the profession in an ethical manner

BARRIERS ACROSS HEALTH CARE SETTINGS

Barriers across health care settings include:

- **Geographic**: Some areas, especially rural, lack adequate healthcare resources, such as hospice and palliative care programs, hospitals, clinics, and physicians. Providing services is often not cost-effective for organizations.
- **Financial/insurance**: Many people lack financial resources to pay for adequate insurance coverage and cannot afford out-of-pocket payment for services.
- **Transportation**: People who do not have motor vehicles or no longer drive are at a disadvantage in accessing health care. Public transportation is not available in many areas and can be expensive for those on limited income.
- **Education/health literacy**: People with limited education or those who are functionally illiterate may lack the health literacy needed to understand their health needs or the healthcare services that are available.
- **Fear/anxiety**: People may fear medical care itself or fear hearing bad news, but both types of fears can prevent people from accessing the medical care that they need.

Initiating, Developing, and Fostering Hospice and Palliative Care Services

Strategies to initiate, develop, and foster hospice and palliative care services include:

- Providing continuing education credit for palliative care and hospice training sessions
- Visiting physicians, nurse practitioners, hospitals, and other health care providers and organizations to disseminate information
- Hosting an open-house or other event to publicize the services
- Budgeting for marketing expenses
- Tracking results of marketing activities
- Emphasizing collaboration and partnerships with other healthcare organizations
- Publishing a newsletter for healthcare professionals and community members
- Placing ads and/or public service announcements in local newspapers, television, and radio
- Sponsoring conferences regarding palliative and hospice care
- Reviewing potential barriers
- Providing excellence in patient care and services
- Serving as a referral source
- Utilizing social media in a responsible manner to market services

Application of Business Strategies to Hospice and Palliative Care

Organizations that provide hospice and palliative care often benefit from application of **business strategies**:

- **Internal review**: Determine what unique characteristics the organization has that can provide an advantage over other organizations. This includes measurements across all aspects of the organization to determine current status in relation to other organizations.
- **External review**: Assess community needs and determining where deficits occur to identify opportunities for provision of additional services. Determine the organization's market and resources as well as any obstacles the organization faces.
- **Growth initiatives**: Planning should look at opportunities for expansion, addition of staff, and addition of services.
- **Cost-benefit analysis**: Services, supplies, and equipment should be assessed in terms of return on investment, and cost-cutting measures taken where they do not impact the quality of service, such as buying in bulk and using different vendors.
- **Planning**: The organization should develop a comprehensive plan for the future and the direction the organization wants to take.

APPLICATION OF MARKET ANALYSIS TO HOSPICE AND PALLIATIVE CARE

Market analysis is done to determine both the current status of the market for a product or service and the future potential. Market analysis includes assessment of the following:

- **Size of the market and demand**: Current data about sales from government, industry, surveys, and major producers of similar products or services
- **Marketing trends**: Regulations, social factors, environmental factors, innovations, and any factors that may affect sales
- **Growth rate of market**: Based on analysis of historical data and current sales data as well as developments that may impact growth positively or negatively
- **Opportunity assessment**: In terms of competition
- **Profitability**: Assessment of influencing factors (Porter), including buyer and supplier power, barriers to market entry, possible threat of competitive substitute products/services, and company rivalry
- **Cost structure**: Determining value and costs
- **Methods of distribution**: Existing and emerging
- **Necessary factors**: Resources, access to distribution, technology

APPLICATION OF MAXIMIZED REIMBURSEMENT TO HOSPICE AND PALLIATIVE CARE

Methods to maximize reimbursement include:

- Timely recording of information and sending of claims
- Utilizing care managers to determine the most cost-effective care plan
- Utilizing standardized billing codes (CPT, ICD)
- Ensuring that the healthcare provider's National Provider Identifier (NPI) is present on all claims
- Updating systems promptly when new coding (such as ICD-10) and billing regulations (such as pay-for-performance) are issued rather than waiting for the end of the grace period so that problems can be identified and corrected early
- Ensuring that the present on admission (POA) Medicare Severity-Diagnosis Related Group (MS-DRG) diagnosis is correct to avoid a different discharge diagnosis
- Monitoring quality of care to prevent complications and reduce costs related to the Do Not Pay List
- Sending claims in the correct form and to the correct address for different entities, such as insurance companies, Medicaid, or Medicare

PROMOTING CONTINUITY OF CARE

Many forces disrupt the **continuity of care**. In some cases, physicians (or advanced care nurses) no longer follow patients from the home to the in-patient facility because care at each level is managed by different health care providers, such as hospitalists. While this has some advantages, patients are often cared for by healthcare providers who don't actually know them or their history, so the most important factor in promoting continuity of care is communication. Case managers and discharge planners are critical to improving continuity of care by ensuring that all parties understand patients' needs and that patients and families understand their rights and responsibilities. Healthcare providers must make sure that patients have signed appropriate releases of medical records so that information can be shared. Hospice and palliative care organizations need to establish partnerships and good working relationships with other providers of healthcare services.

Facilitating Safe Passage

Facilitating safe passage is part of caring practice that ensures patient safety, in a broad sense, from a variety of perspectives:

- Giving appropriate medications and treatment without errors that endanger the patient's health is essential.
- Providing information to the patient/family about treatments, changes, conditions, and other aspects related to care helps them to cope with situations as they arise.
- Preventing infection is central to patient safety and includes staff using proper infection control methods, such as handwashing.
- Knowing the person requires the nurse to take the time and effort to understand the needs and wishes of the patient/family.
- Assisting with transitions involves not only helping the patient/family cope with moving from one form of treatment, or one unit to another but also with transitions in health, such as from health to illness, or from illness to death.

Health Insurance Options

Types and Characteristics of Health Insurance

Types and characteristics of health insurance include:

- **HMO**: With health maintenance organizations (HMOs), a primary care provider (PCP) coordinates care and referrals to a network of healthcare providers. The individual has little choice and requires a referral from the PCP to see a specialist. Plans may provide preventive care but may also require co-payments and a deductible.
- **PPO**: With a preferred provider organization (PPO) an individual can choose to see any healthcare provider, including specialists, in a network of healthcare providers. The individual is not usually required to select a PCP but may have to pay co-payments and a deductible, depending on the plan. Individuals can usually see healthcare providers outside of the network but reimbursement is typically lower, so the individual may have to pay part of costs.
- **EPO**: The exclusive provider organization (EPO) is similar to a PPO in that the individual can see any physician within a network except that the individual does not have the option of seeing a healthcare provider outside of the network except in emergency situations.
- **POS**: Point of service plans (POSs) are combined HMOs and PPOs. The individual has a PCP within a network, and the PCP makes referrals, but the individual can see out-of-network healthcare providers. The individual must pay part of cost to see out-of-network providers.
- **HDHP**: High deductible health plans (HDHPs) may be HMOs, PPOs, or EPOs but are characterized by a high deductible before the insurance begins to reimburse for care. People with low-income often select this option to avoid catastrophic costs but may end up with large bills for healthcare services.

MEDICARE

Medicare, a federal health insurance program for those who have Social Security or bought into Medicare, provides payment to private healthcare providers, such as physicians and hospitals, but limits reimbursement. Physicians receive 80% of usual customary and reasonable (UCR) fees if they accept Medicare assignment. If they do not, they can charge up to 115% of what Medicare allows. Patients are responsible for the remaining 20% or up to 115% if the physicians do not accept Medicare. Parts include:

- **Medicare A**: Hospital insurance covers acute hospital care, limited nursing home care, and home health care as well as hospice care for the terminally ill. There is no premium for this part.
- **Medicare B**: Medical insurance covers physicians, advance practice nurses, laboratory, physical and occupational therapy. Patients must pay an annual deductible as well as monthly payments.
- **Medicare D**: The prescription drug plan covers part of the costs of prescription drugs at participating pharmacies. It is administered by private insurance companies, so monthly costs and benefits vary somewhat.

MEDICAID

Medicaid is a combined federal and state welfare program authorized by Title XIX of the Social Security Act to assist people with low income with payment for medical care. This program provides assistance for all ages, including children. Older adults receiving SSI are eligible as are others who meet state eligibility requirements. The Medicaid programs are administered by the individual states, which establish eligibility and reimbursement guidelines, so benefits vary considerably from one state to another. Older adults with Medicare are eligible for Medicaid as a secondary insurance. Expenses that are covered include inpatient and outpatient hospital services, physician payments, nursing home care, home health care, and laboratory and radiation services. Adults who are legal resident aliens are ineligible for Medicaid for 5 years after attaining legal resident status. Some states pay for preventive services, such as home and community-based programs aimed at reducing the need for hospitalization.

TRICARE

Tricare is the health care program serving active military, retired military, and their spouses and dependents. Tricare provides a number of different plans, depending upon location and eligibility. For those with Medicare, Tricare becomes the secondary insurer. If patients choose to opt out of Medicare (such as those with no insurance or private insurance), Tricare pays the amount equivalent to a secondary insurer (20% of allowable), and the patient is responsible for the rest. By law, all other insurances must pay before Tricare. Patients may access care at military treatment facilities (MTF) on space-available basis, but must enroll in Tricare Plus to receive primary care at MTFs. Those eligible for both Tricare and Veterans Affairs (VA) programs may receive care at VA medical facilities if the service is covered under Tricare and the facility is part of the Tricare network. It is important to note, the VA cannot bill Medicare, so costs not covered by Tricare must be paid by the patient even if the patient has Medicare coverage.

Coverage for Hospice Care

While palliative care may be utilized during all stages of illness, **hospice care** is for the terminally ill, usually within the last 6 months of life (two 90-day periods) although this may be extended by physician authorization every 60 days. Medicare patients must be eligible for Medicare A, and a physician must certify that the patient is terminal with life expectancy ≤6 months. The patient (or responsible family member) must agree to receive Hospice care rather than regular Medicare, requiring that the patient receive palliative rather than curative treatment. The goal of hospice care is to maintain the person in the home environment, so the patient is provided home health aides and homemakers, durable goods (dressings, adult diapers, under pads), pain management, case management, counseling, and social worker assistance. Routine home care is intermittent and must comprise 80% of total care. In-home continuous care is available during crisis for short periods. In-patient hospice (often beds assigned in a skilled nursing facility) may be used for 4-5 days for symptom management and/or a 5-day respite period for caregivers.

Causes of Lapses in Health Care Coverage Related to Hospice and Palliative Care

Lapses in health care coverage related to hospice and palliative care most often result from lack of insurance or limitations of insurance:

- **High deductibles**: To save money on premiums, some people opt for insurance policies with high deductibles, resulting in thousands of dollars in costs before insurance coverage begins.
- **Lack of insurance**: Some people have no insurance because they are unable to afford it or simply choose to gamble that they won't need it, but they may end up with huge medical bills and may not be eligible for Medicaid assistance.
- **Home health care**: Patients may need care in the home but lack qualifying hospital stays for Medicare coverage or lack insurance for home health care.
- **Hospice benefits**: Patients may not qualify for hospice benefits because their life expectancy is greater than 6 months, they don't have Medicare coverage, or their insurance does not cover hospice care.

Cost of Drugs

The cost of drugs is one of the most expensive aspects of medical care for patient, so patients sometimes can't afford treatment. Even those with insurance drug coverage or Medicare D may have considerable costs, especially with non-generic drugs. There is much pressure from drug representatives to prescribe new drugs, and patients are often influenced by direct-to-consumer advertising, but the ACHPN can help the patient ensure that drugs are prescribed based on evidence. Additionally, the cost versus benefit of drugs must always be considered. It is the responsibility of the ACHPN to act in the best interests of the patient and to educate the patient about drugs. If a less expensive drug is as effective as a more expensive or newer drug, then the ACHPN and patient should request that the less expensive drug be prescribed. The ACHPN should educate people about the use of generic drugs as a cost-saving measure because, in most cases, these are as effective as non-generic.

Patient Needs and Patient Safety

Financial Assistance

Financial Issues

Even with insurance and Medicare, patients may incur huge medical costs for medications alone, and if they need nursing care at home or in a facility, the costs can range from $6,000 to over $12,000 monthly, quickly depleting savings. Medicare strictly limits hospital and extended care stay as well as home health care. When a patient is no longer improving, such as with terminal illness or Alzheimer's disease, their care is not paid for until they are eligible for hospice care, and that has limitations too. Long-term care is not provided by Medicare or most insurance policies unless the insurance is especially intended for that purpose, and these policies are costly. This leaves patients and families with financial burdens that they sometimes cannot pay.

Financial Assistance Organizations

Numerous local, state, and national **organizations** are available to provide hospice and palliative care patients with financial assistance. Organizations include:

- **Patient Advocate Foundation**: Provides assistance for co-pays and transportation expenses for cancer patients and has aid programs specifically for those with metastatic breast cancer and multiple myeloma.
- **Partnership for Prescription Assistance**: Provides information about free or low-cost prescription drugs.
- **PAN Foundation**: Offers financial assistance to pay medical costs through 60 disease-specific programs.
- **Healthwell Foundation**: Provides financial assistance through the Emergency Cancer Relief Fund.
- **CancerCare**: Has a financial assistance program that assists with costs of transportation, home care, child care, and co-payments. Breast cancer patients can receive financial assistance for medications, lymphedema supplies, and durable medical supplies.
- **The Samfund**: Provides twice yearly grants to assist young (21-39) cancer patients with living expenses, tuition, education, medical bills, and various other health-related expenses.

Providing Cost-Effective Quality Care

It's important for the nurse to consider not only the cost-benefit (savings) of interventions but also the cost-effectiveness. A **cost-benefit analysis** uses average cost of problem (such as infection) and the cost of intervention to demonstrate savings. A cost-effective analysis, on the other hand, measures the effectiveness of an intervention rather than directly measuring the monetary savings. Each year, about 2 million nosocomial infections result in 90,000 deaths and an estimated $6.7 billion in additional health costs. From that perspective, decreasing infections should reduce costs, but there are human savings in suffering as well, and it can be difficult to place a dollar value on that. If each infection adds about 12 days to hospitalization, then a reduction in infection by 5 would be calculated as $5 \times 12 = 60$ fewer patient infection days and increased health and wellbeing.

Community Resources Helpful for Hospice or Palliative Care Patient

Community resources that may be helpful for the hospice or palliative care patient include:

- **Home health agencies**: These can provide homebound patients with medical treatment, monitoring, and personal care (bathing) and referral to other needed services, such as a social worker.
- **Volunteer agencies**: These vary but may include faith-based or other volunteers who will visit, assist with shopping and/or cooking, transport patients, sit with patients, or carry out other non-skilled activities to support the patient and family.
- **Medical supply companies**: Patients may need a wide variety of assistive devices, including small items such as grab/reach tools, tub rails, and grab bars, and larger devices, such as wheelchairs, walkers, lifts, and hospital beds.
- **Educational resources**: These may include libraries (medical and general), podcasts, videos, national organizations (such as the Alzheimer's Association), and internet sources.
- **Support groups**: Local hospitals, senior centers, and organizations often provide a variety of support groups for both patients and family/caregivers, such as support groups for those with cancer.
- **Meal programs**: Home meal delivery may be necessary.

Community/Internet Resources Available to Support Patients and Families

Community/internet resources available to support patients and their families include:

- **Association of Cancer Online Resources (ACOR)**: Provides information and internet support groups for patients and families as well as information about diseases and treatment.
- **American Cancer Society**: Provides support groups and assistance with non-medical expenses, such as durable medical equipment, transportation costs, and hair replacement wigs. The "Look Good, Feel Better" program provides assistance with techniques to minimize physical changes caused by treatment.
- **Group Loop**: Provides an online support group for teens living with cancer including discussion boards, personal blogs, and video journals.
- **National Children's Cancer Society (NCCS)**: Provides financial assistance for non-medical expenses.
- **Ronald McDonald House**: Provides living accommodations for families, care mobiles, and family rooms (in hospitals).
- **Sibshops**: Provides workshops for siblings.
- **Songs of Love Foundation**: Provides free personalized songs for children and teens with severe illness.
- **Starlight Foundation**: Provides personalized entertainment experiences for children with life-threatening illness.
- **13Thirty Cancer Connect**: Provides online support for teens and young adults
- **CancerCare**: Provides limited financial assistance (transportation costs, co-payments), information about managing costs, and links to various resources.

Environmental Considerations

Environmental factors should be assessed within the actual environment if at all possible. If not, careful questioning and drawing of diagrams and approximate floor plans with the patient—or asking the patient to do drawings—can be useful, especially when showing the patient needed modifications. Family members may also assist with the assessment, providing useful information. Some patients, especially the elderly, may be reluctant to admit that the home is cluttered or that they are unable to maintain the home environment in a sanitary condition. Brochures and handouts about home safety and assistive devices should be provided to the patient as well as contact names and telephone numbers for equipment needed in the home. A checklist should be compiled of all necessary changes or additions, with specific details, such as "Install 18-inch grab bar across from toilet." In some cases, a social worker or occupational therapist should visit the patient.

Environmental Adaptations

Adaptations needed in the environment may vary widely for the hospice or palliative care patient:

- **Access issues**: If the patient needs to use a wheelchair, furniture may need to be moved, doorways widened, and wheelchair ramp installed. If the bathroom is difficult to access (upstairs, not wheelchair accessible), a bedside commode may be needed. Items may need to be moved or placed so they are easier to reach.
- **Safety issues**: Grab bars may need to be installed in bathrooms, hallways, and stairways and scatter rugs removed. Lighting may need to be improved. Patients may need assistive devices, such as wheelchairs, canes, and walkers. If patients are confused/disoriented/wandering, the home may need door latches, movement alarms, and other safety devices.
- **Equipment issues**: The patient may need a hospital bed or other equipment to facilitate care or relieve symptoms, and this can involve changes in wiring, moving furniture, and sometimes changing rooms.

Environmental Risk Factors

When assessing a patient, it is important to consider that certain environmental factors may place the patient at increased risk or may be a factor in disease. There are a number of different types of environmental factors:

Factors	Examples	Effects
Toxic chemicals	Lead, arsenic, muriatic acid, sulfuric acid, ammonia, lime	May result in poisoning (lead, arsenic) or burns (acids, ammonia, lime)
Physical objects	Guns, cars, knives, equipment	Accidents, gunshot wounds, stabbings, various injuries
Biological organisms	Bacteria, fungi, viruses	Infections
Temperature variations	Heat, cold	Burns, dehydration, heat stroke, hypothermia, frostbite
Ambient noise	Sirens, loud music, traffic noise, work-related noise	Hearing loss/deafness
Psychosocial	Increased stress	Anxiety, hypertension

Environmental Assessment

Environmental assessments are very helpful when developing a care plan to provide for care and safety. **Rooms should be assessed** according to their function:

- Entryway should be free of obstacles and surfaces even. Handrails and/or ramps may be needed for those who are unsteady or wheelchair bound.
- Stairs/steps should have handrails, non-skid surfaces, and contrast markings for each step.
- Living area should be comfortable and furniture arranged for convenience. Chairs should be firm enough for people to stand from easily.
- Bedrooms should have a night light and phone near the bed. Bed should be positioned close to the nearest bathroom if possible and at the appropriate height for easy access and appropriate firmness.
- Bathrooms may require grab bars, hand-held shower, and elevated toilet seat, tub seat.
- Kitchen may need items moved for convenient access as well as a sturdy step stool. Unsafe equipment/tools should be removed.

Additional Environmental Considerations to Assess

Some elements of environmental assessment are not specific to rooms in the house but are general needs that must be met in order for people, especially the elderly or disabled, to remain safe:

- Environmental hazards such as piles of papers or trash on the floors, loose carpet or rugs, and cluttered pathways can cause falls and must be cleared, organized, or repaired.
- Lighting should be adequate enough for reading in all rooms and stairways.
- Heat and air conditioning must be adequate. The young and the elderly are especially susceptible to heat and cold injury.
- Sanitation should ensure that health hazards do not exist, such as from rotting food or infestations of cockroaches or rodents.
- Animals should be cared for adequately with access to food, water, toileting, and routine veterinary care.
- Smoke/chemicals in the environment may pose a hazard, such as exposure to cigarette smoking or cleaning materials.

Psychosocial, Spiritual, and Cultural Needs

Spiritual Assessments

HOPE Mnemonic

HOPE is a simple mnemonic used as a guideline for the spiritual assessment:

H	Hope	What sources of hope (who or what) do you have to turn to?
O	Organized	Are you a part of an organized religion or faith group? What do you gain from membership in this group?
P	Personal	What spiritual practices (prayer, meditation) are most helpful?
E	Effects	What effects do your beliefs play on any medical care or end-of-life issues and decisions? Do you have any beliefs that may affect the type of care the health care team can provide you with?

FICA Mnemonic

FICA is another abbreviated spiritual assessment tool:

F	Faith	Do you have a faith or belief system that gives your life meaning?
I	Importance	What importance does your faith have in your daily life?
C	Community	Do you participate and gain support from a faith community?
A	Address	What faith issues would you like me to address in your care?

SPIRIT Mnemonic

SPIRIT (Maugens) is a mnemonic used for a spiritual assessment tool:

S	Spiritual	Do you have a formal religious affiliation?
P	Personal	Which practices and beliefs do you personally accept and practice? Does spirituality play a part in your daily life?
I	Integration	Do you participate in a spiritual community and receive support from that community?
R	Ritual	Are there specific practices and restrictions in your religious convictions that would affect your healthcare choices?
I	Implication	Are there aspects of your spirituality you would like me to keep in mind during your care?
T	Terminal events	As you prepare for the end of life, how does your faith affect the decisions you make or how you feel about death?

Spiritual Care at the End of Life

The patient's basic beliefs should be assessed in order to provide holistic care as the end of life approaches. **Spiritual care** must be provided according to the patient's religion and/or philosophy of choice, and must remain unbiased from the caregiver's own beliefs. If the patient does not wish to have spiritual counseling, it should not be pressed upon them. Advice and comfort can be provided by anyone known to the patient. Spiritual care is intended to relieve spiritual suffering and to explore answers to significant questions that the patient and family may have. Even those who do not have a formal religion affiliation or philosophical practice may experience questions and may search for meaning and comfort at the end of life.

The caregiver must assess prior and present religious affiliations, along with individual beliefs about God and the afterlife. The information must include devotional practices, rituals, and routines, and identify the degree of involvement and support available from the patient's chosen religious community. This spiritual assessment opens the door for effective spiritual caregiving, and it allows patients and their families to access spiritual coping strategies and support mechanisms. The holistic assessment addresses the patient's ability to resolve meaningful spiritual questions, identifying deeper understandings and retaining hope, strength, and peace. Questions can include the patient's interpretation of the meaning and purpose of their life, the role of family, and personal strengths and connections to various spiritual communities and to nature. Provisions should be made to explore spiritual relationships and to provide support for loss and crisis, as desired by the patient and family.

Addressing Emotional and Spiritual Health

Strategies to address emotional and spiritual health include:

- Remain observant and note both verbal and nonverbal communication.
- Address the patient by the surname unless asked to do otherwise, avoiding terms such as "honey" and "dear."
- Take the time to converse with the patient before broaching serious subjects.
- Use a pleasant and soft tone of voice when talking with the patient.
- Note indications of spiritual beliefs, such as Bibles, Korans, offering bowls, prayer beads, rosaries, and religious symbols as well as prayers, meditation, chants, signs of the cross, and fasts.
- Ask the meaning of unfamiliar symbols or items.
- Respect personal space, including noting how close the patient and family members stand to others.
- Avoid judgmental statements or attitudes toward traditions and practices that are different from those common to Western culture.
- Assist with religious or spiritual rituals and practices if requested.
- Ask the patient and family members if their needs are being met and about what issues are important to them.

Life Completion and Search for Meaning

Life Completion and Closure

Developmental landmarks associated with **life completion and closure** include:

- A sense of completion in all affairs, including worldly, community, and interpersonal relationships with family and friends. The individual must feel that they have taken care of all unfinished business.
- They feel a satisfaction in life and work. After reflecting on their lives, patients can accept themselves and their accomplishments as fulfilling and worthwhile.
- They can experience feelings of love and acceptance for self and others: pursuing worthiness, forgiveness, gratitude, closure, and resolution of past hurts and wrongs to bring about peace and satisfaction.
- The patient is able to identify a general understanding of the meaning and finality of life.
- They express a willingness to move forward into the unknown, accepting death and saying goodbye.

Visual Life Review Projects

When the patient is ready for a life review, the nurse can suggest that he or she begins by looking at **old photos** and **home movies**. These are often a source of happiness and encourage recitation of memories and favorite times during family life. Most people are apt to take photographs of happy times. Provide a photo album or scrapbook for the patient and family to put together. The album offers an opportunity for patients to relive fond memories with the family, and they can review it independently when family and friends are unavailable. Life review is also helpful for the family after the patient has died. Remember that very young children think death is reversible, and may need to be reminded again and again that someone in the pictures is not coming back. Emphasize that the person who died did not go away because they were angry with the child, and that the doctors could not prevent the death.

Journaling or Telling a Life Story

The end-stage patient and family need to review their life together to identify its meaning. Obtain a **journal** and writing materials for the patient. If the patient wants newspaper clippings to include in the journal, contact a librarian about how to obtain them. The patient may initially be hesitant to review his or her life with others, but as trust is built, will probably do so willingly. Ask the family for their assistance because they shared many of the events with the patient and may have supplemental information. Use the hospice's program resources and guides to assist the patient and family in capturing their memories. If the patient is too weak to write, borrow a tape recorder or get a volunteer to take dictation. The patient may want to preserve favorite memories as a gift for family members, or write explanations, and this is therapeutic for all concerned.

Legacy Interventions at End-of-Life

Legacy interventions are those that promote a life review on the part of the patient at the end-of-life and create a memory product for survivors. **Legacy interventions** include:

- **Encouraging life talk**: The patient and family talk about the patient's life, such as favorite activities, vacations, friends, and special memories.
- Providing **artistic opportunities**: The patient and family can share feelings/memories through drawings, paintings, and music.
- Creating a **scrapbook**: This may include pictures, drawings, certificates, diplomas, awards, and other things that are important to the patient.
- Creating a **video journal or audiotape journal**: A smart phone or other video/audio recording device may be used to record messages to family members or memories.
- **Story/poetry writing**: Some patients may want to write a story or poem that expresses their feelings.
- Making **handprints or fingerprint jewelry**: Kits are available to save handprints of children, and a fingerprint can be memorialized in silver or other metal.

Creating an Audio or Video Legacy

End-stage patients want to ascribe meaning to their lives. Life review happens in most cultures. Ask a librarian to inspire the patient with an autobiography from an author with the same cultural and spiritual background. If the patient wishes to leave an **audio legacy**, obtain the resources from the recreation director or occupational therapist. Schedule recording for a time when the patient has the most energy and will be able to participate fully. If the patient desires to create a video for family or friends, make certain the patient is groomed appropriately. Find out how to disguise illness with makeup through Look Good Feel Better, which donates complimentary tool kits and teaches patients how to use hair alternatives, prosthetic clothing, and cosmetics. Help the patient call family members or friends to arrange a film debut. If they cannot attend in person, ask the IT manager how to broadcast the movie over an internet connection.

Phone Calls and Internet Chats

End-stage patients may miss family and friends who do not live locally, or are unable to be physically present. Facilitate communication between the patient and family members or friends because saying a final goodbye is psychologically important for closure. Modern technology makes long-distance communication simple, while requiring little energy expenditure from the patient, and the instantaneous communication brings much comfort. If the patient does not have their own communication devices, arrange time for the patient to use one of facility's devices to communicate with family and friends, ideally corresponding to the time of day when the patient has the most energy, even if that means interrupting the patient's usual schedule.

Patient's and Family's Search for Meaning and Hope

Cultures and families vary in how they perceive illness and disability, and this may profoundly affect the patient's **search for meaning and hope**. It's important to understand the patient's cultural belief system about what causes disease or disability. Likewise, it's important to know how to respond and to show respect for traditions, such as the use of healers. Some cultures attach stigma to some types of diseases, and these attitudes may be difficult to overcome if they are not acknowledged. The patient's family, spiritual, and cultural values should be incorporated into the plan of care. Family members may experience severe stress resulting from the patient's impairment and should be included whenever possible in care decisions and interventions and allowed to express their own feelings of loss and concern. All family members are impacted when one member faces impairment, and family systems may be strained if members are not adequately prepared for helping or caring for the patient, especially after discharge.

Strategies that help the patient/family manage disease and find meaning and hope include:

- **Coaching**: Nurses acting as coaches are responsible for assisting patients to obtain the information and confidence they need to participate actively in the management of their own healthcare. The coach works in collaboration with the patient to provide support in self-management as well as emotional support. The coach conducts follow-ups with the patient and helps the patient navigate the healthcare system.
- **Motivating**: The nurse can encourage patients to change behavior by appealing to their own sense of motivation. Motivating may include the use of motivational interviewing, which focuses on establishing an empathetic relationship with the patient and utilizes open-ended (yes/no) questions, affirmations (expression of empathy), reflective listening, and summary.
- **Negotiating**: It is important to take the time to deliberate with a patient to determine the best course of action. The nurse should present the pros and cons of treatment and provide clear explanations as to why a particular treatment may be indicated, taking into consideration the needs, desires, and concerns of the patient.

Caregiver/Family Self-Care Activities

Caregiver Support in Terminal Illness

The nurse must understand that terminal illness and death involve the entire family. The family's response to an illness will depend on the stage of life that they are in as well as the basic family relationships and dynamics. Nurses should help reduce both physical and emotional burdens placed on the **caregiver** and other family members. They should provide the knowledge and skills needed to enhance the patient's comfort. The nurse should also provide access to additional caregiver support resources. Interventions and referrals might include respite care, social worker assistance, occupational therapy, and referrals to help simplify tasks and conserve energy, along with referral for an aide to help with patient ADLs. The nurse is responsible for frequent assessment of the caregiver's health and his or her ability to provide care, as well as watching for signs of neglect and abuse. The nurse strives to help the family develop healthy ways to cope as they prepare for the impending death.

Caregiver Assessment and Interventions

Assessing caregiver ability begins with asking the caregiver about the skills the person has, what the caregiver feels comfortable doing, and what areas the caregiver needs assistance. This shows respect for the caregiver and allows the caregiver to express concerns. The best method of assessing the actual **skills** is to work with the caregiver and observe, providing positive feedback during the process. Rather than criticizing ("Don't pull your spouse under the arms"), a better approach is focus on the caregiver's needs ("Let me show you how to move your spouse without risking injuring your back"). Assessment should include not only the caregiver's knowledge and physical ability to provide care but also the caregiver's **emotional ability, resources available, values, and perceptions**. It's important to know if the caregiver is willing to provide care or is doing so out of necessity, as this may affect the caregiver's sense of wellbeing and the patient-caregiver relationship.

Promoting Family Self-Care Activities

The nurse can promote family self-care activities by:

- Assessing the need for care and the strengths and weaknesses of the family
- Educating the family about the burdens and benefits of provision of care
- Providing demonstrations and practice to help the family gain confidence in provision of care
- Engaging the patient and family in development of the plan of care so they feel some degree of control
- Serving as a mentor and resource for the family
- Modeling appropriate care
- Educating the family about the importance of personal time and respite
- Providing information about respite services
- Assisting family with coping strategies, such as relaxation and visualization
- Discussing risks for increased stress, such as inadequate sleep, poor diet, lack of exercise, and failure to care for personal health issues
- Assisting family members to set personal goals (such as taking a daily walk or nap)
- Helping family create a problem list and possible solutions

Caregiver Fatigue

Caregiver fatigue is very common and can relate to physical or emotional fatigue. The nurse should discuss issues of **caregiver fatigue** early in the care process if possible so that the caregiver is aware of the effects of stress and overwork. Caregivers often get inadequate sleep and become exhausted from the constant demands of patient care and have no idea where to turn for help. The nurse should address signs of fatigue directly ("You look exhausted") to encourage the caregiver to discuss problems. If the patient is under hospice care and is eligible for respite care, the nurse can help to facilitate this. The nurse can also provide the caregiver with information about community resources that may help to reduce the burden of care, such as Meals-on-Wheels, volunteers, adult day care, and caregiver support groups, and should assess the environment to determine if accommodations would be helpful.

Caregiver Support Programs

Home Meal Delivery Programs

Home meal delivery programs (such as Meals-on-Wheels) provide nutritious meals for homebound adults (often restricted to older adults). The programs usually serve meals 5-7 days a week with home delivery, often by volunteers. Meals are usually low cost ($2-4 per meal) but this varies with program. Most programs deliver one hot meal a day and may provide food for one or two other meals (such as a sandwich for dinner and cold cereal for breakfast the next day). Requirements and age restrictions vary with some serving those ≥60 and others ≥65. People with temporary disabilities may be restricted in length of service. Some programs are intended for those with low incomes, but others do not have income restrictions. Most programs provide little choice in menu but may offer low fat, low salt, or low carbohydrate diets. Many home meal delivery programs have waiting lists because the need outpaces the number of programs.

Home Health Agencies

Home health agencies provide intermittent care in the home environment or assisted-living facilities. Home health care can include nursing care (assessment, medications, and treatment), social workers, speech pathologists, physical and occupational therapists, and certified nurse aides (personal care). Home health agencies may provide professionals to draw blood for lab tests and administer intravenous fluids. Home health care allows patients to be sent home earlier from acute hospitals and skilled nursing facilities and is more cost effective than in-patient care. Many Home Health Agencies include hospice care. Some insurance companies pay for home health care, and Medicare pays for care with requirements: Patients must be homebound, in need of skilled care <7 days/week or <8 hours each day over a period of ≤21 days. Those eligible may receive home health aide services, but total hours of care may not exceed 28-35 hours/week (depending on need). Medicare pays a set amount for each episode of care (60-day period), depending on the health care condition.

Adult Daycare

Adult daycare is an option to provide caregiver respite and to allow caregivers to continue with employment. Daycare programs are generally intended for older adults who require some type of supervision and/or assistance. The focus of daycare programs may be on:

- Social interaction
- Medical assistance
- Alzheimer care

Most adult daycare programs have some type of nursing supervision and nursing care to assist with toileting, medications, eating, walking, and social activities and are open during usual daytime hours (such as from 8 AM to 5 PM) and provide 1 or 2 meals and snacks, sometimes at extra cost. Costs may vary widely, with costs typically higher for those that provide specialized services. Costs are usually not covered by health insurance or Medicare although some long-term care policies may provide coverage. If the program is licensed as an Alzheimer's program, Medicaid may cover some costs.

Principles of Hospice and Palliative Education

LEARNING STYLES

Not all patients are aware of their preferred learning style. A range of teaching materials/methods that are age appropriate and relate to all three learning preferences—visual, auditory, kinesthetic—should be available. Part of assessment for teaching involves choosing the right approach based on observation and feedback. Often presenting learners with different options gives a clue to their preferred learning style. Some individuals have a combined learning style:

Visual learners	**Learn best by seeing and reading**: Provide written directions, picture guides, or demonstrate procedures. Use charts and diagrams. Provide photos and videos.
Auditory learners	**Learn best by listening and talking**: Explain procedures while demonstrating and have the learner repeat. Plan extra time to discuss and answer questions. Provide audiotapes.
Kinesthetic learners	**Learn best by handling, doing, and practicing:** Provide hands-on experience throughout teaching. Encourage handling of supplies/equipment. Allow the learner to demonstrate. Minimize instructions and allow the person to explore equipment and procedures.

LEARNING PRINCIPLES

YOUNG ADULTHOOD

Young adulthood encompasses the ages of 20-40 during which people are usually in the cognitive stage of formal operations and psychological stage of intimacy vs. isolation. **Young adults** tend to be autonomous and self-directed and have intrinsic motivation to learn. Their personal experience may enhance or interfere with their learning. Young adults tend to be competency-based leaners who are able to make decisions and analyze critically. The provider should assess learner motivation and try to identify obstacles to learning and support systems. Teaching strategies include:

- Utilize problem-centered learning.
- Allow people to learn at their own paces and draw on experiential learning.
- Encourage people to participate actively.
- Utilize roleplaying, hands-on practice, and immediate application.
- Keep materials and presentations well organized and clear.
- Recognize the social roles of learners.
- Encourage self-directed learning.
- Focus on health promotion.

MIDDLE-AGED ADULTHOOD

Middle-aged adulthood encompasses the ages of 41-64 during which people are in the cognitive stage of formal operations and the psychological stage of generativity vs stagnation. **Middle-aged adults** tend to be at the peak of their careers with a well-developed sense of self although they may have concerns about physical changes. They may explore alternative lifestyles, question achievements, and reexamine values and goals. They may desire change but still have confidence in their abilities. The provider should assess learner motivation and try to identify obstacles to learning and support systems. Teaching strategies include:

- Be flexible but organized and efficient.
- Assess and recognize potential technology gaps.
- Encourage people to utilize experiential learning.
- Review study skills.
- Relate learning to life concerns.
- Provide reassurance and positive reinforcement.
- Modify approaches for physical disabilities or impairments.

Older Adulthood

Older adulthood is age 65 and older, during which the person is in the cognitive stage of formal operations and the psychological stage of ego integrity vs. despair. The provider should encourage participation from **older adults**, assess coping mechanisms, and provide supplementary materials to reinforce learning. Teaching strategies include:

- Spend a little time getting to know the person so the person is more relaxed and receptive to learning.
- Determine what information is critical and what is non-essential.
- Evaluate the person's learning style and previous knowledge about the topic.
- Plan ample time for each session of instruction.
- Ensure that sessions are closely spaced to reinforce learning.
- Provide the person ample time to practice.
- Allow the person to guide the pace of the session as much as possible and encourage feedback.
- Prepare age-appropriate handouts at an accessible reading level with large-size font.
- Provide materials (pencil, paper) in case the patient wants to make notes.
- Be supportive, patient, and enthusiastic.

Therapeutic Environment Conducive to Learning

Factors to consider when establishing a therapeutic environment conducive to learning include:

- **Temperature**: The temperature should be comfortable for the patient. If the room temperature cannot be adjusted, then a fan or extra blankets may be used to ensure patient comfort.
- **Lighting**: The lighting should be at an adequate level to view materials but should not be glaring or excessively bright.
- **Noise**: The environment should be as free of extraneous noise as possible. A quiet space is ideal, but if that's not possible, the door to the room should be closed.
- **Comfort**: The patient should receive adequate analgesia because pain is very distracting. Additionally, the patient and family should be in positions of comfort. For example, the patient may be most comfortable sitting in bed or in a comfortable chair.
- **Timing**: The provider should discuss the best time with the patient and family. If the patient has pain, then learning is usually optimal during the time the pain is best controlled. Patients should exhibit readiness to learn.

Characteristics of Formal Education

Formal education is planned and developed to meet particular needs, such as educating patients about pain control and the use of a PCA. Planning includes carrying out a needs assessment and then developing a syllabus and materials in support of the topics that is appropriate for the students. Characteristics common to **formal education** include:

- **Setting**: Formal education usually takes place in a classroom or specified area.
- **Timing**: Classes are scheduled on specific dates and times.
- **Structure**: An instructor presents material and leads the class. The instructor should be credentialed, certified, or qualified to teach the material.
- **Materials**: May include overhead projection, equipment, books, pamphlets, handouts, videos, and audio recordings.
- **Assessment**: Some type of assessment is normally included, such as a test or a return demonstration.
- **Class size**: While formal education is usually directed at a group, the size may vary, and in some cases a formal education module may be utilized for individuals.

Characteristics of Informal Education

Informal education takes place outside of the classroom and is generally unplanned and follows no particular format. Informal education most often occurs in the course of conversation with a patient and family members. While informal education is not planned in the same way as formal education, being knowledgeable and educated about disease and patient concerns prepares the nurse when opportunities for informal education occur. Characteristics of **informal education** include:

- **Setting**: Informal education can take place anywhere.
- **Timing**: It often happens as an immediate response to patient's questions and needs and to observations.
- **Structure**: Patient or family and instructor (nurse) have a reciprocal exchange.
- **Materials**: Usually those on hand, such as equipment being used during the exchange, although the nurse may offer to provide additional materials.
- **Assessment**: The nurse can assess through informal questioning: "Did you understand?" or "Do you have any more questions?"
- **Class size**: Informal education almost always happens as one-on-one exchanges although in some cases family members or others may be present and participate.

Readiness to Learn

Learner characteristics related to readiness to learn should be assessed because if people are not ready, instruction is of little value. Often readiness is indicated when people ask questions or show interest in procedures. There are a number of factors related to **readiness to learn**:

- **Physical factors**: There are a number of physical factors than can affect ability. Manual dexterity may be required to complete a task, and this varies by age and condition. Hearing or vision deficits may impact ability. Complex tasks may be too difficult for some because of weakness or cognitive impairment, and modifications of the environment may be needed. Health status, age, and gender may all impact the ability to learn.

- **Experience with learning**: People's experience with learning can vary widely and is affected by their ability to cope with changes, their personal goals, motivation to learn, and cultural background. People may have widely divergent ideas about what constitutes illness and treatment. Lack of English skills may make learning difficult and prevent people from asking questions.
- **Mental/emotional status**: The support system and motivation may impact readiness. Anxiety, fear, or depression about the condition can make learning very difficult because people cannot focus on learning, so the nurse must spend time to reassure them and wait until they are emotionally more receptive.
- **Knowledge/education**: The knowledge base of patients, their cognitive abilities, and their learning styles all affect their readiness to learn. The nurse should always begin by assessing what knowledge the people already have about their disease, condition, or treatment and then build from that base. People with little medical experience may lack knowledge of basic medical terminology, interfering with their ability and readiness to learn.

Selection of Teaching Methods

There are many teaching methods, and the nurse must prepare, present, and coordinate a wide range of educational workshops, lectures, discussions, and one-on-one instructions on any chosen topic. All types of classes may be needed, depending upon the purpose and material:

- **Educational workshops** are usually conducted with small groups, allowing for maximal participation. They are especially good for demonstrations and practice sessions.
- **Lectures** are often used for more academic or detailed information that may include questions and answers but limits discussion. An effective lecture should include some audiovisual support.
- **Discussions** are best with small groups so that people can actively participate. This is good for problem solving exercises.
- **One-on-one instruction** is especially helpful for targeted instruction in procedures for individuals or for those who need additional assistance.
- **Computer/internet modules** are good for independent learners but may be valuable supplements to traditional classroom presentations, especially if they are interactive.

Teaching Tools Available for Patient Education

Teaching tools include:

- **Print materials**: Print materials may be provided before, during, or after class and can include books, journals, and copies of articles, handouts, reference cards, and posters.
- **Electronics/audio-visual**: Computer-assisted learning modules, tablet applications, and podcasts are especially valuable for independent study. Videos and audio-recordings may be used independently or to supplement a class presentation. For example, videos may be used for demonstrations if equipment is not available or to show how to use equipment.
- **Display**: Various types of displays can be used, including whiteboards, electronic whiteboards, flipcharts, and slide show presentations.
- **Internet resources**: Databases, NIH/CDC sites, Medline can provide excellent reference materials. Government sites often offer brochures and pamphlets for free download.
- **Equipment**: Medical equipment can be used to teach, such as mannequins and simulations.
- **Guest speakers**: Physicians, advance practice nurses, social workers, infection control nurses, administrators, risk managers, and substance abuse counselors all may serve as guest speakers.

Educational Needs of Caregivers

The caregiver of the hospice or palliative care patient needs specific education in a number of areas:

- **Stress**: The caregiver should be aware of the indications and effects of stress on the individual, patient, and family members, methods of dealing with stress, and when to ask for help.
- **Community resources**: Needs may be many and varied, and the caregiver often needs assistance from outside agencies.
- **Patient care**: The caregiver should understand basic patient care, such as assisting the patient with bathing, dressing, transferring, and taking/administering medications. The caregiver should also receive education regarding appropriate diet and nutrition, wound care, and any other necessary medical care (such as catheter care).
- **Signs/symptoms of imminent death**: Family members need to know what to expect when death nears, such as increasing incontinence or lack of urinary output and sleeping, death rattle, mottling of skin, Cheyne-Stokes breath, increased confusion, and hallucinations (seeing decreased relatives). This knowledge helps reduce fear and better prepares family members to cope with the changes and to know when to seek help from professional caregivers.
- **End-stage disease progression**: Both the patient and family should be prepared for changes that may occur and should know how to deal with these changes. For example, if a patient is expected to have increased dyspnea, patient and family should be aware of options for oxygen supplementation and optimal positioning to relieve symptoms.
- **Pain and symptom management**: Patients and their families need to understand the patient's right to control of pain and other negative symptoms and should know, step-by-step, how to manage them and what resources are available to help, including medications or other treatments that may alleviate symptoms and any equipment (such as a hospital bed or wheelchair) that may be of use.

Hospice vs. Palliative Care

It is important to be able to educate the patient and family on the differences between hospice care and palliative care.

Hospice care	Palliative care
Duration: Hospice care is intended for the last 6 months of life.	Duration: Palliative care is intended for throughout the illness.
Patients have a terminal medical condition.	Patients have a serious medical condition.
In-home care is covered through Medicare hospice benefit without need for qualifying hospital stay.	In-home treatment is not usually covered by Medicare unless patient has qualifying hospital stay.
Care is usually provided in home environment.	Care is usually provided in inpatient facility but can be provided at home.
Treatment focuses on comfort and pain control and preparation for death.	Treatment focuses on comfort and pain control.
Patients forego life-saving treatment.	Life-saving treatment may continue.
Age: Those qualified for Medicare part A are usually 65 or older, although some insurance plans may provide coverage for younger individuals.	Age: Any age can qualify, although services may or may not be covered by insurance.

BENEFIT VS. BURDEN OF TREATMENT OPTIONS

Patients and their families must be educated on the benefits and burdens of various treatment options at the end of life.

Treatments	Benefits	Burdens
Hydration	Prevents thirst, prevents drying of mucus membranes, and provides reassurance/comfort to family.	May increase death rattle, increase nausea and vomiting, increase pulmonary and generalized edema, prolong the dying process (minimally) and hasten breakdown of skin.
Turning, repositioning	Prevents pressure sores (although some breakdown of skin may be unavoidable) or worsening of existing sores, helps prevent infection and associated odor and exudate, and prevents contractures.	May increase pain and general discomfort and may be counter to the patient's desire to be left undisturbed, may increase dyspnea when positioned on the side.
Opioid administration	Relieves pain and perception of shortness of breath, and may relieve anxiety and fear of death.	May result in depressed respirations, hallucinations, impaired ability to communicate, loss of consciousness, increased constipation, and a hastening of the dying process.
Resuscitation efforts	Allow family to deny death is imminent.	Cause unnecessary suffering and prolong dying process
Supplemental nutrition	Relieve family's anxiety that the patient is hungry. Prolong life.	May cause nausea, vomiting. May increase tumor growth with cancer. May increase discomfort.
Active treatments (antibiotics, chemotherapy)	Prolong life. Relieve symptoms. Reassure family.	Prolong the dying process. Side effects may be severe (as with chemotherapy).
Glucocorticoids	Reduces intracranial pressure, increases appetite, controls pain, reduces fatigue.	Can result in insomnia, GI upset, delirium, depression, increased risk of infection and hyperglycemia, Cushing's syndrome, anxiety, increased risk of thromboembolism, myopathy, and interference with other medications.

Therapeutic Communication

Communicating with the Palliative Care Patient and Family

A vital role of the nurse in a palliative care setting is to facilitate **communication** and establish a trusting relationship with the patient and family. Communication takes place on many different levels and the message received may not always be that intended by the sender. In fact, as much as 80% of all communication takes place on the nonverbal level. Though the information can be overwhelming to the patient or family, most individuals expect honesty and truthfulness in their communications with a health care provider. Communication should establish the following: trust and openness, inclusion of the patient and family in all options and care decisions, assurances to the individual and family that they will be listened to and respected, and that they will not be ignored or abandoned. Nurses should avoid and resolve conflicts and allow patients and families to vocalize their needs, expecting them to be addressed. It is also important to extend this communication to the entire health care team to better facilitate understanding and continuity of care.

Communicating about Diagnosis and Progression of Disease

When communicating about a patient's **diagnosis and progression** of disease, the approach and the vocabulary depend on the receiver of the information. When communicating with professionals, such as physicians and other nurses, the information is usually provided in a factual and organized manner, using appropriate medical terminology and common abbreviations. However, when communicating with family members and patients, the nurse must consider the family or patient's age, condition, and ability to understand as well as readiness (physical and emotional) to learn and understand. Communication with the family and patient should always begin with asking what they know and what they want to know, followed by addressing the issues in language that they can understand. It's important to avoid focusing only on medical issues and not considering the emotional impact of information. The nurse should also avoid changing the subject to avoid sensitive discussions.

Adjusting Communication to Receiver Response

Adjusting communication to the receiver's response requires close observation of not only the words of a receiver but also nonverbal responses, such as body language, facial expression, and eye contact. The healthcare provider should avoid giving advice, asking for reasons, patronizing, giving false assurance, interrupting, or trying to force a response. **Common receiver responses** include:

- **Anger**: May be expressed directly or indirectly by criticizing care or particular caregivers or changing physicians. Remain calm, validate concerns, ask what the person needs/wants, and help make a plan for resolution.
- **Shame/guilt**: May be a response to a particular diagnosis, care needs, or belief in culpability. Reassure, express empathy without directly using the word "shame" or "guilt," provide factual information, and avoid all judgmental statements.
- **Fear**: May result from lack of information, bad news, unfamiliarity, or lack of control. Show compassion and empathy, provide clear and appropriate information, reassure, and provide support as needed.
- **Confusion**: May result from emotional overload, medications, and medical condition. Revisit, provide information in simple terms, and reassure.

Advance Care Planning

The nurse must remain attentive to the patient and recognize opportunities to discuss advance care planning, such as when a patient comments or asks questions about the future or prognosis. The discussion should not be hurried, so if necessary the nurse should set a time to have the discussion: "I see you have questions about the future. I'd like to sit down and talk about advance care planning with you this afternoon, if that's all right." A discussion of advance care planning should include:

- What advance planning means
- Cultural attitude toward advance care planning
- Different types of advance care planning
- Legal aspects (including those that are state-specific) and benefits to the patient
- How advance care planning affects treatment
- References for obtaining appropriate advance care documents
- Storing and maintaining advance care documents
- Emotional impact of advance care planning
- Right to opt out of advance care planning or to alter plans

Discussions Related to Resuscitation Efforts

Discussions related to resuscitation efforts are sensitive and should involve not only the patient but also close family members who may be in the position to make decisions if the patient is unable to do so. The patient and the family members may have very different opinions, and this needs to be discussed and resolved. It's important during the discussion about resuscitation to discuss all different aspects, including cardiopulmonary resuscitation, fluid resuscitation, and mechanical ventilation. Patients often believe making decisions about resuscitation is an all-or-nothing proposition; however, patients can specify the types of resuscitation they want. Some patients, for example, may be willing to undergo cardiopulmonary resuscitation efforts but are opposed to being maintained on mechanical ventilation. Any discussion of resuscitation should include the importance of having an advance directive in place although it is not, in fact, legally binding in all states.

Facilitating Patient and Family Conferences

The nurse should be alert to the need for a patient/family conference. Indications include:

- The patient and family have many questions about diagnosis, treatment, or prognosis.
- The patient and family members have differing ideas about end-of-life care.
- The patient will need one or more family members to provide care or other support.
- Family members have unrealistic expectations of the patient or vice versa.
- The patient and family members are involved in conflict.
- The patient and family members fail to communicate effectively.
- The patient or family members appear confused about the patient's condition or care issues.

Depending on the type of concern, the nurse should contact appropriate team members and consultants to participate in the patient/family conference, explaining the rationale for their participation. These members may include a spiritual advisor, physician, physical therapist, nurses, and pharmacist. It's important to elicit as much input as possible from the patient and family members, stressing that the purpose of the conference is to assist rather than direct.

SPIKES Strategy for Providing Sensitive Information

The SPIKES strategy (Beale et al.) can be used as a guide to providing sensitive information (bad news) to the patient and family:

S	**S**et up interview	Make a plan for delivering news and arrange for a private space and presence of significant others (such as spouses or children).
P	Assess patient **p**erception	Question the patient/family about what they know about the disease and discover any misperceptions.
I	Obtain **i**nvitation	Ask the patient/family directly if they want information and how much and respect their decisions, remaining available for questions.
K	Provide **k**nowledge	Provide sensitive information or bad news slowly rather than quickly so the patient and family have time to digest the information. Ask if they have questions and avoid technical jargon. Consider psychosocial implications as well as cultural differences.
E	Address **e**motions	Respond to the patient's/family's feelings and emotional response. Attempt to identify emotional response (sad, depressed, angry, confused) and acknowledge (move closer, touch patient, express regret, verbally respond).
S	**S**trategy/ **S**ummary	Ask if the patient and family are ready to discuss a treatment plan. Present treatment options if "yes" and set up a later time to discuss if "no."

Use of Interpreters

Healthcare agencies that are federally funded are required to provide free **interpretive services** for clients speaking commonly encountered foreign languages. The patient must be informed that an interpreter will be made available to them. In order to ensure appropriate care and communication, a third-party interpreter who is trained in medical terminology, fluent in both languages being used, and is familiar with the ethics and HIPAA regulations of acting as an interpreter is the best option. Meeting these requirements ensures compliance with federal guidelines. Family members cannot be required to serve as interpreters unless the client specifically requests a family member to act in this capacity. In emergency situations it is appropriate to use whatever means are readily available to assist in communicating with the patient.

Grief and Loss Support/Bereavement Services

Basic Tenets in Relation to Death and Dying

Roman Catholicism

Roman Catholics often pray with a rosary and may ask for the Sacrament of the Sick. Symbols such as crosses, holy water, and pictures and statues of saints hold significance.

Orthodox/Conservative Judaism

After death, the body is cleaned and wrapped in a linen shroud. Embalming is considered a desecration of the body, and cremation is never done because the body must contact the earth, and the body is never displayed. Family should be with the patient at the time of death and the body should be attended while awaiting burial, and those in attendance should not eat or drink in the presence of the body. Mourning practices are carried out to comfort the living and demonstrate respect for the dead. Organ donation is permitted and considered a good deed.

Judaism

For a Jewish patient, all mirrors should be covered at the time of death. A prayer for the dead, called the Kaddish, is recited and the body receives a special washing. There is an urgency to complete the burial process within 24 hours of the death. This should occur before sundown in that same time frame. The only exception is if it interferes with Sabbath. The Jewish faith also observes *shiva*— the seven-day grieving period after the burial of a loved one. During this time the mourners do not work. Mourning for a parent lasts one year. Kosher foods are required.

Hinduism

After death, the body is cleansed and adorned. Cremation is practiced to free the soul from the body and the existence on earth. However, unnamed babies and untouchables (low caste) have traditionally been buried. Individuals may decide about organ donation. Hindus believe the soul experiences many lifetimes and that life unfolds according to *karma.*

Buddhism

Buddhists believe that the soul stays with the body for some time after death, so family members may wish to leave the deceased undisturbed for a period of time to allow the soul time to leave the body in peace. Buddhists believe that the soul experiences multiple lifetimes to learn necessary lessons and that actions in a previous lifetime influence the current life, including illnesses, and that death is a natural part of the transition from one life to another. Buddhists are usually cremated. Individuals may decide about organ donation.

Islam

Islamic tradition forbids cremation of the body or embalming. Traditionally, the body is bathed with water (with genitals covered) usually by members of the family who are of the same gender or are a spouse or parent of a minor child. The body is then wrapped in a shroud, usually plain white cloth with 3 pieces used for males and 5 for females. Funeral prayers (*Janazah*) are said during a gathering of people to honor the dead. Burial should be within 24 hours and to at least a depth of 5 feet. Organ donation is generally permitted.

Rando's Six R's

Rando (1984) described **six active grieving tasks** ("grief work") of the bereaved. The six Rs include:

- **Recognizing**: The person must recognize the degree of loss and accept that the loss is real.
- **Reacting**: The person actively experiences the emotional response to the loss.
- **Recollecting and re-experiencing**: The person reviews memories of the person who has died, re-experiencing events.
- **Relinquishing**: The person accepts that the loss has caused the world to change and that there is no return from that reality.
- **Readjusting**: The person begins to grieve less, returning to daily life and feeling less overwhelmed with loss.
- **Reinvesting**: The person accepts the changes that the loss has brought and begins to actively reenter the world, form new associations and relationships, and make new commitments.

Bereavement

Bereavement occurs after the death of a family member, friend, or someone to whom a person identifies closely. It is a time of mourning and is part of the natural grieving process, but some people are not able to move past the grieving process and may suffer signs related to severe depression, such as poor appetite, insomnia, and other symptoms, such as chest pain, that may mimic physical illnesses. Some may enter a stage of denial or anger that interferes with their daily activities and work. People suffering bereavement may present with vague and varied complaints. A careful history is important. Treatment varies according to the needs of the individual. In some cases, SSRIs (such as Prozac) may provide temporary relief, but the client should be referred for psychological counseling, bereavement services, or psychiatric care, depending upon the severity of symptoms.

Assessing for Complicated Bereavement

Families should be assessed for the risk of **complicated bereavement**, which may indicate the need for counseling to help individuals cope. Complicated bereavement can result in prolonged periods of mourning, depression, and negative impacts of social interactions and health. Risk assessment begins with family interview and may include specific tools, such as the Bereavement Experience Questionnaire, and the Bereavement Risk Index. Indications that a person is undergoing traumatic grief include a duration of at least 60 days of the following:

- Avoiding reminders of or talking about the deceased
- Exhibiting signs of depression and negative feelings about the future
- Feeling numb, dazed, shocked
- Having feelings of incompleteness, as though part of self has also died
- Expressing anger, bitterness, and blame associated with the death
- Withdrawing from social or occupational roles
- Exhibiting impaired functioning (careless dress, cluttered home, poor hygiene)
- Losing sense of trust in others and security
- Assuming negative behaviors (smoking, drinking) of the deceased

Factors that Influence Bereavement Process

Factors that influence the bereavement process include:

- **Type of death**: Sudden unexpected death can be much harder to cope with than death after an extended chronic illness during which the bereaved has had time to come to terms with the fact that the patient is dying. Suicide can be especially traumatic because the bereaved may have feelings of guilt or may anguish over failing to save the person.
- **Support system**: Bereaved who lacks a strong support system may be unable to express feelings or come to terms with them.
- **Age of bereaved**: Young people may feel abandoned and angry while older people may focus on feelings of loneliness and loss.
- **Secondary losses**: Death may mean a sudden loss of income (such as with the death of the head of a household) or a sudden increase in responsibilities (need to get a job, necessity of maintaining a home and caring for children alone). Friendships may falter.

Postmortem Care and Services

Postmortem Decomposition

The process of postmortem decomposition begins almost immediately after death. **Livor mortis** occurs as the blood vessels become more permeable and red blood cells begin to break down, resulting in the pooling of blood and staining of tissue that occurs in dependent parts of the body (**lividity**). The skin may appear splotchy within 4-5 hours, but lividity with bluish-purplish-red discoloration is very evident by 5-6 hours. The discoloration remains after compression by about 12 hours and, as red cells break down, a marbling discoloration occurs, and Tardieu spots (tiny dark spots) result from capillary rupture. When lividity occurs, the rest of the body takes on a grey hue. The color of the lividity may vary depending on the cause of death, and the face is often deep reddish-purple in those with cardiac-related death. While liver mortis is occurring, the body also goes through rigor mortis, muscle contracture and stiffening, and algor mortis, cooling of the body to ambient temperature.

Rigor Mortis

Immediately after death, the body tends to be flaccid. However, changes occur within a few hours. **Rigor mortis** is an exaggerated contraction of muscles that occurs 2-6 hours after death when stores of **adenosine phosphate (ATP)**, which is necessary for muscle relaxation, are depleted. Rigor mortis is progressive, beginning with the internal organs and progressing to small muscles in the head and neck (such as the eyelids) and on to larger muscles in the trunk and extremities. Rigor mortis may be more pronounced in those with large muscles while those who are thin and frail may have less rigor mortis. Ambient temperatures may affect the onset and duration of rigor mortis with high temperatures speeding and low temperatures slowing the changes. Chemical activity usually peaks around 12 hours after death and persists for around 18 hours following this peak, but it may persist for another 48 hours or more before the muscles relax.

Algor Mortis

Normal body temperature is about 37 °C, but when body functions cease at death, **algor mortis** (cold death), a gradual decrease in body temperature, begins within approximately one hour, and the body starts to cool by about 1 °C every hour until it reaches **ambient temperature**. The exterior surface temperature cools more rapidly than the internal temperature, and the overall rate of cooling may vary depending on the patient's internal temperature at the time of death, the ambient temperature of the environment, the patient's size (muscle mass, fat), and the presence and thickness of clothing or blankets. High temperatures (internal or external) slow the cooling process. As the body cools, the skin loses elasticity and takes on a waxy appearance. This stage of the process of death ends when the temperature begins to rise again as part of **decomposition**, generally within 24 hours.

Death Vigil

A death vigil entails staying with a dying person and ensuring that the person is never left alone. In some cases, the death vigil may be over within hours, but other patients may die slowly over a number of days, and family members can become exhausted, so they should be encouraged to take turns sitting vigil or to take periodic rest periods. In some cultures, a death vigil means a large number of people are present, but in other cases only one or two close family members. In either case, the nurse and nursing assistant can support this practice by helping to make the room comfortable with adequate seating and encouraging friends/family to maintain a quiet and peaceful environment (low lights, soft music, limited conversation, and distractions). The provider should assist with any cultural traditions that the family desires and ask the family if they want a visit from a spiritual leader/advisor (such as a priest or shaman) and help with arrangements.

Postmortem Care

The body should be prepared in order to provide a clean, peaceful impression for those family members who desire an opportunity to say good-bye before transport to a funeral home. Kindly caring for the body shows respect to the family, the continued value of the deceased, as well as modeling grief-facilitating behaviors for others present. Religious or other rituals the family may find comforting should be encouraged, as should participation in the preparation of the body. Explain the process and what to expect as care is given. Unless otherwise indicated by protocol or the need for autopsy, any tubes, drains, and other medical devices should be removed. Bandages should be applied, as fluids may still be expressed. A waterproof pad or incontinence brief underneath the body is helpful for containing fluids. Packing of the vagina or rectum is unnecessary. Wash the body and comb the hair. Consider dressing the body in something normalizing. It should be noted that the body may "sigh" as it is rolled and the lungs are compressed. If the area is kept cool, the decomposition process will be slowed, allowing the family time to grieve.

Providing Support When Notifying Family and Coworkers at Time-of-Death

The provider should prepare to notify family and coworkers near and at the time of death by asking family members **before death is imminent** who should be notified in the event the patient's condition worsens and how that notification should be carried out (telephone, text) and should post this information prominently in the patient's **chart**. Because of HIPAA regulations regarding privacy and confidentiality, only those coworkers and friends that the patient and/or family have indicated should be notified can be contacted. (Health information remains protected under HIPAA for 50 years after a patient's death). If calling to notify a person of a death, the nurse should prepare the person first: "I'm sorry to say that I have some bad news." Then, the provider should briefly explain that the patient has died, avoiding euphemisms, which may be misunderstood and should answer any questions the person may have. The provider should express sympathy, "I'm so sorry for your loss," but avoid clichés such as, "He is in a better place."

Death Pronouncement

The death pronouncement itself is fairly straightforward, but it can be complicated by the presence of family members or friends, so the provider must remain sensitive to their needs and emotions. Protocols for **death pronouncement** may vary somewhat but generally include:

- Gather information from medical health record and staff members if not present at the time of death
- Identify the patient, verifying patient's ID number
- Description of the body's appearance and location
- Verbal and tactile stimulation utilized and lack of response
- Check of pupillary reflex and finding of fixed and dilated pupils
- Assessment of respiratory status and lack of breathing/lung sounds
- Assessment of cardiac status and lack of pulse noted on palpation and auscultation of apical pulse for at least 60 seconds
- Note and record the official time of death
- Note family and physician notifications
- File report to the CDC for those conditions that require notification if part of responsibility
- Describe notification of appropriate authorities for suspicious death or when regulations require notification of the medical examiner

Documentation Needed at the Time of Death

Documentation needed at the time of death includes:

- Deceased name, birthdate, address, and unique patient number
- Date and time of documentation
- Reason for attending to the deceased
- List of those present at time of death
- Description of circumstances, including location and complications or disease processes that may have contributed to death
- Outline of death confirmation according to established protocol
- Outcome of assessment and time of death
- Interactions with others present, including staff members and family members
- Specific notifications, such as of spouse, children, or physician
- Description of any special requests or concerns, such as cultural practices
- Discussion regarding organ donation and plans
- Plans for disposition of body (funeral home, autopsy, body/organ donation)
- Notification of medical examiner if required by circumstances/regulations
- Signature, including full name, role, any professional ID number, and contact information

Ethical Issues Related to End of Life

Promoting Autonomy

Autonomy is the ethical principle that the individual has the right to make decisions about his or her own care. In the case of children or patients with dementia who cannot make autonomous decisions, parents or family members may serve as the legal decision maker. The right of patients to make decisions about end-of-life care through advance directives, to refuse care, and to make informed consent was formalized in the Patient's Self-Determination Act (1991). However, with hospice and palliative care, the nurse must encourage active participation by patients and families and respect cultural differences that may impact decision-making. In some cultures, decisions are often made by the family or the head of the family rather than the individual. Additionally, there are limitations to autonomy. In most states, even if patients want physician-assisted suicide, the practice is illegal.

Decision-Making Models

Do no harm	This model is based on nonmaleficence, the requirement that the treatment provided does no harm; however, by their nature, some treatments can and often do harm patients, so the underlying intent and goal of treatment must be considered when making decisions. For example, CPR may be carried out to save a patient's life and done with correct technique but still result in rib fractures.
In good faith	The motive for a decision should be honest and fair and decisions made with sincere intention to do good even though the outcome may be negative. For example, EMS personnel may provide a treatment for a patient in good faith although the treatment later proves to be ineffective.
Patient's best interest	Making a decision in the patient's best interests includes considering the patient's or parents' (in the case of children) wishes, the best clinical judgment, the best choice of various options, the chances for improvement or decline, and religious or cultural preferences.

Promoting Beneficence

Beneficence is an ethical principle that involves performing actions that are for the purpose of benefitting another person. In the care of a patient, any procedure or treatment should be done with the ultimate goal of benefitting the patient, and any actions that are not beneficial should be reconsidered. While hospice and palliative care focuses on comfort needs rather than extension of life, all of the patient's needs must be considered. Beneficence applies not only to obligatory acts (such as medical treatments) but also to non-obligatory acts (such as taking time to sit and talk with a patient). The patients' physical needs and emotional needs should have equal importance in the provision of care. The nurse has a responsibility to promote beneficence in all aspects of the care plan and to actively work to prevent harm.

Promoting Veracity

Veracity refers to the obligation the healthcare provider has to tell patients and families the truth and to avoid lying or making misleading statements. The nurse should not purposefully withhold information that the patient is entitled to, such as when a medication or treatment error has occurred, although the reality is that patients are often not informed about such occurrences. In Western culture, the idea that people are entitled to truthful information about their condition is paramount and supported by law, but not all cultures view veracity in the same manner. In some cultures, bad news, such as a diagnosis of cancer, is routinely withheld from patients and telling them is considered cruel. The nurse should consider the cultural implications of veracity and discuss the issue with the patient and family members when appropriate, keeping in mind that although truth may be negative it should never be unkind.

Promoting Nonmaleficence

Nonmaleficence is an ethical principle that means healthcare workers should provide care in a manner that does not cause direct intentional harm to the patient:

- The actual act must be good or morally neutral.
- The intent must be only for a good effect.
- A bad effect cannot serve as the means to get to a good effect.
- A good effect must have more benefit than a bad effect has harm.

With provision of care to hospice and palliative care patients, the nurse must continually reevaluate patient care and treatments that may be beneficial initially but later negatively impact the patient's comfort needs. Nonmaleficence is a consideration when patients are receiving chemotherapy or radiotherapy that results in severe adverse effects. These effects must be balanced against the potential for long-term improvement in condition or prolonged survival, considering the patient's wishes.

Promoting Justice

Justice is the ethical principle that relates to the distribution of the limited resources of healthcare benefits to the members of society. This issue may arise when there are more patients than can be accommodated. Decisions should be made according to what is best or most just for the patients and not colored by personal bias. The nurse should apply the principle of justice in ensuring that all patients have equal consideration of their needs and that resources are distributed fairly; however, the realities of healthcare access (insured versus uninsured) present a challenge to upholding justice as some people can afford necessary care and others cannot. The nurse has a responsibility to try to compensate by helping people finding additional sources of financial assistance and supplies that they cannot otherwise afford. Some hospice and palliative care programs have fund raising programs so they can serve patients who lack adequate insurance and/or income.

Policies Regarding Donation of Organs and Tissue

People of any age can donate organs and/or tissue, including organs, stem cells, blood/platelets, tissue, and whole body. There are different types of **donations**:

- **Whole body**: Usually organs cannot be donated separately and the body is donated intact.
- **Donation after cardiac or brain death**: Solid organs must be transplanted 6-72 hours after removal although tissues can be frozen and banked.

Tissues and organs are screened for diseases that may infect the recipient. People who are HIV positive are restricted from donating. Some restrictions apply to patients who die of cancer although some organs can be donated if the cancer hasn't spread within the previous year. Patients with metastasis, primary cerebral lymphoma, or hematologic cancers cannot donate. People may indicate they wish to be organ donors, but family members often must make the decision after patient death. The request for donor organs should be made with sensitivity, and no one should be coerced into approving donation.

Suicidal Ideation

Suicidal ideation occurs frequently in patients with mood disorders or depression. While females are more likely to attempt suicide, males actually commit 3 times more suicides than female, primarily because females tend to take overdoses from which they can be revived while males choose more violent means, such as jumping from a high place, shooting, or hanging. Risk factors include psychiatric disorders (schizophrenia, bipolar disorder, PTSD, substance abuse, and BPD), physical disorders (HIV/AIDS, cancer, diabetes, stroke, traumatic brain injury, and spinal cord injury). Passive suicidal ideation involves wishing to be dead or thinking about dying without making plans while active suicidal ideation involves making plans. Those with active suicidal ideation are most at risk. People with suicidal ideation often give signals, direct or indirect, to indicate they are considering suicide because many people have some ambivalence and want help. Others may act impulsively or effectively hide their distress.

Euthanasia and Physician-Assisted Suicide

Euthanasia (mercy killing) is bringing about the death of someone deliberately and without legal standing in order to save them from suffering. This usually happens through the administration of high dose opioids although some people, usually family members, have resorted to more violent means, such as through gunshots or smothering. In some cases, euthanasia is carried out at the request of the patient, but it may be involuntary in other cases. Euthanasia is illegal in all states.

Physician-assisted suicide, on the other hand, requires that a patient be of sound mind and go through a legal process verifying that the patient's condition is terminal and the patient chooses to die. Physician-assisted suicide is legal in some form in California, Colorado, the District of Columbia, Hawaii, Maine, New Mexico, New Jersey, Oregon, Vermont, and Washington in the United States. In these states, physicians can order drugs that will bring about death.

Ethical Issues Related to Sedation of Hospice Palliative Care Patients

Palliative sedation (sometimes referred to as *terminal sedation*) is often used in the end-stages of dying to relieve severe pain and suffering. Patients usually receive analgesia along with a sedative so that they can die peacefully although they are no longer able to communicate with family members, so there is a tradeoff. There is concern among some people, especially those opposed to physician-assisted suicide, that sedation may hasten death and is, in fact, a method of slow euthanasia. However, most patients at this time are also unable to take food or fluids, and studies have shown that the addition of sedation does not hasten death and, in fact, may prolong life because the stress and exhaustion of experiencing severe pain or dyspnea is relieved. One concern is that there is no standard guideline for this type of sedation and practices vary.

Practice Issues

Standards of Practice

Nurse Practice Act

Each state has its own Nurse Practice Act, which is administered by the state Board of Nursing. The Nurse Practice Act outlines requirements for licensure and certification and delineates the scope of practice of nurses, including duties and delegation. Typically, licensure is granted to those who complete an accredited LVN/LPN or RN program and pass the nursing exam (NCLEX) or receive endorsement because of licensure in another state. RN programs may be 3-year hospital-based programs, associate degree programs, or bachelor's degree programs. Foreign-trained nurses may need to meet special requirements that are determined by the state Board of Nursing and included in the Nurse Practice Act. Advance practice nurses complete a master's or doctorate program. The Nurse Practice Act of each state provides the requirement for advanced practice certification and the professional designation. Additionally, the Nurse Practice Act outlines the requirements for relicensing or recertification, often including the need for continuing education. The Nurse Practice Act also includes provisions for disciplinary action.

Incorporating National Standards into Nursing Practice

Incorporating national hospital and palliative standards into nursing practice includes:

- Obtaining a commitment from administration and staff members
- Researching and identifying appropriate national standards and practice guidelines to apply to practice, such as those of the National Consensus Project
- Assessing current status to identify gaps in practice, such as through gap analysis
- Educating staff members about the standards and changes in practice needed to meet standards
- Establishing a timeline for training and implementation of practice guidelines to achieve standards
- Providing ongoing in-service training to ensure that standards are instituted properly and that staff members have necessary knowledge and skills
- Determining appropriate measurement tools to assess progress
- Conducting ongoing measures to evaluate implementation and outcomes
- Reviewing outcome measures to determine if gaps still remain
- Providing progress reports to administration and staff on a regular basis

National Consensus Project Guidelines

Major hospice and palliative care organizations have joined forces to form the **National Consensus Project**:

- American Academy of Hospice and Palliative Medicine
- Center to Advance Palliative Care
- Hospice and Palliative Nurses Association
- National Hospice and Palliative Care Organization
- Partnership for Caring: America's Voice for the Dying

The National Consensus Project published 8 clinical practice guidelines that outlined standards for palliative care, most recently updated in 2018. Practice **guidelines** include:

- Structure and Processes of Care
- Physical Aspects of Care
- Psychological and Psychiatric Aspects of Care
- Social Aspects of Care
- Spiritual, Religious, and Existential Aspects of Care
- Cultural Aspects of Care
- Care of the Patient Nearing the End of Life
- Ethical and Legal Aspects of Care

Each practice guideline contains a number of sub-guidelines with criteria for achieving that standard of care. For example, Structure and Processes of Care comprises 10 guidelines, such as Guideline 1.1 "Interdisciplinary Team."

Strategies for Self-Care and Stress Management

Stress Management Strategies

While it's not possible to eliminate all stress, nurses can learn to manage stress so it has less emotional and physical impact on their lives. **Stress management strategies** include:

- **Meditation/breathing exercises**: Slow in and out while repeating a word or phrase
- **Massage**: Self-massage or by others
- **Progressive relaxation techniques**
- **Visualization/positive thinking**: Use the power of the mind to imagine a more positive outcome.
- **Time management**: Establish priorities, make schedule, and delegate.
- **Exercise**: Increase activity and exercise 20-30 minutes daily.
- **Breaks**: Plan regular breaks from work or other activities, 5-15 minutes.
- **Snacks**: Prepare healthy snacks and avoid high sugar/high fat snack foods.
- **Hobbies or interests**: Find an outlet, such as reading, music, painting, or crafts.

Critical Incident Stress Management

Critical incident stress management (CISM) is a procedure to help people cope with stressful events, such as disasters, in order to reduce incidence of post-traumatic stress syndrome. CISM can also help the hospice and palliative care staff members cope with the stress of caring for dying patients:

- **Defusing sessions** usually occur very early, sometimes during or immediately after a stressful event, and are used to educate personnel who are actively involved about what to expect over the next few days and to provide guidance in handling feelings and stress.
- **Debriefing sessions** usually follow in one to three days and may be repeated periodically as needed. These sessions may include people who were directly involved as well as those indirectly involved. People are encouraged to express their feelings and emotions about the event. The six phases of debriefing include introduction, fact sharing, discussing feelings, describing symptoms, teaching, and reentry. Critiquing the event or attempting to place blame is not productive as part of the CISM process.
- **Follow-up** is done at the end of the process, usually after about week but this can vary.

Burnout

Burnout, a response to ongoing stress, is a pervasive problem in the nursing profession. Nurses often have excessive workloads and work long hours, often including unwanted overtime because of inadequate staffing. Nurses may feel that they have little control over their work and do not receive sufficient reward or support and feel that nurses are often treated unfairly or are victims of bullying in the workplace. Stress tends to build up over time, interfering with the nurse's ability to concentrate and to carry out duties effectively. Burnout is one of the leading causes for nurses abandoning the field of nursing for other occupations. **Stages leading to burnout** include:

- Fight or flight response: Withdrawal, discord
- Emotional reaction: Anger, shock, surprise
- Negative thinking: Despair, anger, depression, anxiety
- Physical reaction: Headaches, GI upset, backache
- No change in stressor or person: Increased stress
- Burnout: Extreme exhaustion

ASSESSMENT TOOLS FOR STRESS AND BURNOUT

The **Professional Quality of Life Scale (ProQOL)** consists of 30 statements about feelings, such as "I feel connected to others," and "I feel trapped by my job." Each item on the tool is scored as (1) never, (2) rarely, (3) sometimes, (4) often, and (5) very often. Ten questions assess satisfaction, 10, burnout, and 10 secondary traumatic stress. The ratings are totaled for each set of 10 questions and the level is assigned as low, average, or high depending on the score.

The **Life Stress Test** lists possible events, such as retirement (45 points), death of a close friend (37 points), and change in work hour (20 points), and assigns point values. The points for those that apply are totaled. Scores of 0 to 149 indicate low risk for developing stress-related illness; 150-299, medium risk; and 300 and greater, high risk.

The **Empath Test** has 25 statements, such as "You sense others' pain and sadness" and "You feel drained around certain people." Each statement is scored as (0) never, (2), sometimes, or (3) always and the scores totaled. Score of 25-50 is that of a true empath.

COMPASSION FATIGUE IN NURSES

Compassion fatigue can occur when people overly identify with the pain and suffering of others and begin to exhibit signs of stress as a result. These people are often empathetic, tend to place the needs of others above their own, and are motivated by the need to help others. **Indications of compassion fatigue** include:

- Blaming others and complaining excessively
- Isolating oneself from others and having trouble concentrating
- Exhibiting compulsive activities (gambling, drinking)
- Having nightmares, sleeping poorly, and exhibiting a change in appetite
- Exhibiting sadness and/or apathy
- Denying any problems and having high expectations of self and others
- Having trouble concentrating
- Questioning spiritual beliefs, losing faith
- Exhibiting stress disorders: tachycardia, headaches, insomnia, pain

Healthcare providers who exhibit compassion fatigue may need to take a break from work in order to recover some sense of self and may benefit from stress management programs, cognitive behavioral therapy, relaxation and visualization exercises, and physical exercise.

Quality Improvement in Hospice and Palliative Care

Performance Improvement Models

A number of different performance improvement models have been developed over the years. Evaluating and applying these models are part of strategic management and quality healthcare. In some organizations, one approach may be used, but often models are combined in various ways in order to meet specific needs. Planning and understanding how these models can facilitate change are important for those in leadership roles because, in order for these models to be effective, there must be cooperation and consensus across the organization. The various models share some like elements:

- The models focus on continuous improvement and are planned, systematic, and collaborative and apply to the entire organization.
- They share a common focus on identifying problems, collecting data, assessing current performance, instituting actions for change, assessing changes, team development, and use of data.

A model or models should be chosen that seem appropriate to the needs of the organization and to those who will work with the model.

CQI

Continuous Quality Improvement (CQI) emphasizes the organization and systems and processes within that organization rather than individuals. It recognizes internal customers (staff) and external customers (patients) and utilizes data to improve processes. CQI represents the concept that most processes can be improved. CQI uses the scientific method of experimentation to meet needs and improve services and utilizes various tools, such as brainstorming, multivoting, various charts and diagrams, storyboarding, and meetings. Core concepts include:

- Reaching quality and success is meeting or exceeding internal and external customer's needs and expectations.
- Problems relate to processes, and variations in process lead to variations in results.
- Change can be in small steps.

Steps to CQI include:

- Form a knowledgeable team.
- Identify and defining measures used to determine success.
- Brainstorm strategies for change.
- Plan, collect, and utilize data as part of making decisions.
- Test changes and revise or refine as needed.

PDCA Method of Quality Improvement

Plan-Do-Check-Act (PDCA) is a method of continuous quality improvement. PDCA is simple and understandable; however, it may be difficult to maintain this cycle consistently because of lack of focus and commitment. PDCA may be more suited to solving specific problems than organization-wide problems:

- **Plan**: Identifying, analyzing, and defining the problem, clearly defining it setting goals, and establishing a process that coordinates with leadership. Extensive brainstorming, including fishbone diagrams, identifies problematic processes and lists current process steps. Data is collected and analyzed and root cause analysis completed.
- **Do**: Generating possible solutions from which to select one or more and then implementing the solution on a trial basis.
- **Check**: Gathering and analyzing data to determine the effectiveness of the solution. If effective, then continue to Act; if not, return to Plan and pick a different solution. (*Study* may sometimes be used in place of *Check*: PDSA.)
- **Act**: Identifying changes that need to be done to fully implement solution, adopting the solution, and continuing to monitor results while picking another improvement project.

Gap Analysis

Gap analysis is a method used to determine the steps required to move from a current state or actual performance or situation to a new state or potential performance or situation and the "gap" between the two that requires action or resources. Essentially gap analysis answers the questions "What is our current situation?" and "What do we want it to become?" Gap analysis includes determining the resources and time required to achieve the target goal. **Steps to gap analysis** include:

- Assessing the current situation and listing important factors, such as performance levels, costs, staffing, satisfaction, and all processes
- Identifying the current outcomes of the processes in place
- Identifying the target outcomes for projected processes
- Outlining the process required to achieve target outcomes
- Identifying the gaps that are present between the current process and goal
- Identifying resources and methods to close the gaps

TQM

Total Quality Management (TQM) is one philosophy of quality management that espouses a commitment to meeting the needs of the customers at all levels within an organization. It promotes not only continuous improvement but also a dedication to quality in all aspects of an organization. Outcomes should include increased customer satisfaction and productivity, as well as increased profits through efficiency and reduction in costs. In order to provide TQM, an organization must seek the following:

- Information regarding customer's needs and opinions.
- Involvement of staff at all levels in decision making, goal setting, and problem solving.
- Commitment of management to empowering staff and being accountable through active leadership and participation.
- Institution of teamwork with incentives and rewards for accomplishments.

The focus of TQM is on working together to identify and solve problems rather than assigning blame through an organizational culture that focuses on the needs of the customers.

CHPN Practice Test #1

Want to take this practice test in an online interactive format?
Check out the online resources page, which includes interactive practice questions and much more: **mometrix.com/resources719/chpn-19006**

1. A 67-year-old terminally ill patient wishes to receive comfort care measures in his home. The patient's physician recommends placement in a hospice facility so that Medicare will cover the cost of hospice care. Which of the following statements most accurately describes the Medicare hospice benefit?

a. the Medicare hospice benefit applies to patients who have a life expectancy of 12 months or less.
b. the Medicare hospice benefit does not cover the cost of medications used to treat symptoms of terminal illness.
c. the Medicare hospice benefit covers the cost of hospice services in multiple settings, including the patient's home.
d. services provided under the Medicare hospice benefit vary from state to state.

2. A 24-year-old palliative care patient with terminal osteosarcoma takes oral narcotics regularly for the treatment of bone pain. Because of a misunderstanding at the pharmacy, his prescription for narcotic medication is filled 48 hours late, and he develops symptoms of opiate withdrawal, which is most consistent with which of the following?

a. psychological dependence (i.e., addiction) on narcotic medication
b. physical dependence on narcotic medication
c. tolerance to narcotic medication
d. underuse of prescribed narcotic medication

3. The primary goal of palliative sedation, also known as "terminal" or "total" sedation, in the patient with a terminal illness is

a. relief of intractable pain or suffering.
b. hastening of death.
c. improved oxygenation.
d. reduction in opioid medication doses.

4. A home hospice patient becomes progressively less mobile and is ultimately bed-bound. A common complication of immobility in the palliative care patient is

a. myoclonus.
b. pathological fractures.
c. pressure ulcers.
d. pruritus.

5. Assessment of a palliative care patient's spiritual or religious beliefs should encompass which of the following?

a. screening for spiritual beliefs that may conflict with the palliative care nurse's religious practices
b. encouraging the patient to join a religious community if they do not already belong to one
c. asking about spiritual customs or rituals around illness and death that are meaningful to the patient
d. assessing spiritual or religious beliefs only if the patient volunteers information about religion and spirituality

6. After the history, physical examination, and urinalysis, a useful initial tool in assessing urinary incontinence in the palliative care patient is

a. urodynamic testing.
b. a multiday bladder log.
c. spinal magnetic resonance imaging.
d. a trial of systemic hormone replacement therapy.

7. If an adult patient is concerned about the emotional effect of his terminal illness on his 7-year-old child, the hospice nurse should explain that

a. a 7-year-old child is not old enough to understand serious illness and death.
b. changing family routines will help the child come to terms with the illness.
c. there are age-appropriate ways to assist a child through the grieving process.
d. it is helpful to let the child overhear other family members talking about the death of the parent rather than having a direct conversation.

8. A benefit of using a pain assessment tool (e.g., pain scale) in the palliative care patient is the ability to

a. observe a trend in the patient's response to analgesic therapy.
b. treat the adverse effects of pain medications.
c. detect symptoms of drug withdrawal.
d. differentiate true pain from drug-seeking behavior.

9. Patients with AIDS most commonly die as a result of

a. malignancy.
b. heart failure.
c. opportunistic infections.
d. renal failure.

10. A terminally ill patient is showing decreased awareness of his surroundings, decreased oral intake of solids or liquids, and is no longer able to get out of bed. The most likely explanation for this constellation of findings is

a. loss of hope.
b. impending death.
c. depression.
d. urinary retention.

11. A 51-year-old hospice patient with metastatic breast cancer is experiencing severe pain in association with daily dressing changes of an ulcerating malignant skin wound. These pain episodes are consistent with

a. end-of-dose failure.
b. spontaneous pain.
c. incident pain.
d. psychic pain.

12. A 57-year-old patient with end-stage heart failure expresses sadness that she can no longer volunteer in church because of the progression of her disease. The hospice nurse should do which of the following?

a. remind the patient that it is not helpful to dwell on how her disease has limited her life
b. advise placement in an outpatient hospice facility given the progression of the heart disease
c. assist the patient in identifying other ways of staying involved with her church
d. remind the patient that things could be much worse

13. The palliative care advanced practice nurse should be proficient in all of the following EXCEPT

a. providing consultation to other medical professionals in complicated palliative care cases.
b. providing direct education to patients and caregivers.
c. administering medication with the primary purpose of hastening death.
d. maintaining knowledge of current evidence-based evaluation and treatments in palliative care.

14. Typical features of late-stage dementia include all of the following EXCEPT

a. urinary retention.
b. swallowing difficulty.
c. inability to walk.
d. incontinence.

15. A 62-year-old hospice patient with lung cancer develops shortness of breath and facial swelling. The hospice nurse notes distended neck veins. The most likely explanation for these findings is

a. pleural effusion.
b. lymphedema.
c. superior vena cava obstruction.
d. hypercalcemia.

16. Disagreement between family members about the plan of care when a palliative care patient lacks the capacity to make treatment decisions should be managed by

a. pursuing legal action to expedite designation of a single family member as medical decision maker.
b. encouraging the family to consider and discuss what they believe the patient would choose if he or she were able to express his or her wishes.
c. informing the family that palliative care planning is inappropriate unless the family can reach an agreement.
d. encouraging each family member to consider what they would choose for themselves in similar circumstances.

17. A 24-year-old hospice patient with terminal leukemia expresses his preference to avoid artificial hydration once he is no longer able to take fluids by mouth. The hospice nurse should explain that

a. artificial hydration can be withheld in accordance with the patient's wishes.
b. artificial hydration must be provided because it is unethical to deny a patient basic nutrition and hydration.
c. dehydration typically contributes to increased respiratory secretions and vomiting during the dying process.
d. without artificial hydration, the patient will likely experience more pain during the dying process.

18. The hospice nurse notices that a 54-year-old palliative care patient with laryngeal cancer is taking unusually frequent sips of oral fluids throughout the day. When asked about it, the patient reports that he is trying to relieve a feeling of dry mouth. Additional therapy for relief of dry mouth that the nurse may recommend to this patient is

a. a topical anesthetic rinse.
b. supplemental oxygen therapy.
c. mouth breathing.
d. saliva substitutes.

19. A 47-year-old patient with metastatic melanoma receiving opioid analgesic medication informs the hospice nurse that she would "rather just be in pain than feel so sleepy from the pain meds." Given this patient's concerns, the hospice nurse should recommend

a. increased fluid intake and daily stool softeners.
b. the addition of a benzodiazepine to help the patient feel less anxious.
c. administration of naloxone before each dose of pain medication.
d. consideration of a psychostimulant medication.

20. Common barriers to providing optimal palliative care to patients living in poverty include all of the following EXCEPT

a. fragile or nonexistent housing.
b. less stable support systems.
c. undependable transportation to medical visits.
d. less effective coping skills.

21. Patients describing neuropathic pain will most likely characterize their pain as

a. achy, throbbing, and dull.
b. burning, "pins and needles," and shooting.
c. pressure, squeezing, and crampy.
d. diffuse.

22. A 39-year-old patient with testicular cancer has progressive disease despite aggressive cancer treatment. He consents to hospice care and is able to articulate his priorities and goals for treatment but continues to state that he is confident he will survive this illness. The patient's wife asks the hospice nurse how to force the patient to "face the truth." The most appropriate response to the patient's wife is

a. "He will acknowledge the severity of his illness when he is ready."
b. "You should just remind him regularly that he will not survive this illness."
c. "There is always a possibility of a miracle cure."
d. "You should point out to him all of the things he can no longer do because of his illness."

23. All of the following features of delirium would be expected in the patient with dementia EXCEPT

a. disturbed sleep.
b. labile mood.
c. rapid onset.
d. impaired short-term memory.

24. Under the Medicare hospice benefit, respite care for relief of the patient's family caregiver refers to

a. inpatient hospice care for up to 5 consecutive days.
b. home hospice care for up to 5 consecutive days.
c. inpatient hospice care for up to 10 consecutive days.
d. initiation of a "do not resuscitate" order.

25. A 43-year-old palliative care patient with amyotrophic lateral sclerosis (ALS) has progressive weakness of the respiratory muscles and complains of dyspnea. Which of the following statements most accurately describes the use of noninvasive positive airway pressure ventilation (e.g., BiPAP) in patients with ALS?

a. BiPAP is not clinically indicated when respiratory insufficiency is due to muscle weakness
b. BiPAP in the patient with ALS can lead to prolonged survival and improved quality of life
c. patients with ALS using BiPAP must be in an inpatient setting
d. the use of opioid medications for dyspnea is contraindicated in patients using BiPAP

26. The malignancy most commonly associated with upper extremity lymphedema is

a. prostate cancer.
b. melanoma.
c. breast cancer.
d. brain cancer.

27. Fentanyl is administered transdermally (i.e., fentanyl patch) to a home hospice patient for treatment of cancer-related pain. Which of the following statements most accurately describes the use of transdermal fentanyl in the palliative care setting?

a. transdermal fentanyl administration is helpful for treating pain in the palliative care patient who develops dysphagia
b. heat applied directly over the patch will slow the rate of fentanyl absorption
c. steady-state levels of serum fentanyl are reached within 6 hours of patch application
d. transdermal fentanyl administration is helpful for treating breakthrough pain in the palliative care patient

28. If a terminally ill 41-year-old patient is concerned that designating a health care power of attorney (i.e., proxy) in an advance directive will result in loss of control over end-of-life decisions, the hospice nurse should explain that the

a. designated proxy will only dictate end-of-life decision making if the patient is unable to express his or her wishes.
b. patient should only complete an advance directive once he or she is willing to relinquish control of decision making to the designated proxy.
c. advance directive is more important with an elderly palliative care patient.
d. patient should designate his or her primary physician as the health care power of attorney.

29. A 44-year-old hospice patient has a malodorous malignant wound, which is debrided and cleaned regularly. The hospice nurse can recommend which of the following additional therapies to decrease wound odor?

a. topical steroid application
b. topical metronidazole application
c. systemic metronidazole administration
d. calcium alginate dressings

30. Impaired coping by the caregivers of a palliative care patient is most likely expressed as

a. uncertainty and fear.
b. hope for the future.
c. resentment about the large amount of attention being paid to the patient.
d. seeking support resources beyond the palliative care plan.

31. Which of the following would most likely lead to inadequate treatment of pain in the palliative care patient?

a. mutual trust between provider and patient
b. frequent multidimensional pain assessments
c. patient concern for developing an addiction to pain medication
d. availability of a variety of pain assessment tools

32. According to the American Nurses Association's position statement, a patient's request to not receive artificial hydration or nutrition in association with end-of-life care may

a. be inconsistent with the primary ethical and professional expectations of a palliative care nurse.
b. be decided on an individual case basis and may be consistent with appropriate end-of-life care.
c. be considered a form of active euthanasia.
d. cause discomfort for the terminally ill patient.

33. The most effective support system for assisting the hospice nurse in coping with the emotional strain of caring for dying patients and their families is

a. a combination of professional and personal support strategies.
b. a change to a different nursing specialty if the nurse is having difficulty coping.
c. a leave of absence to pursue individual stress management treatment.
d. urging the hospice nurse to deal with his or her grief reactions outside of work.

34. Contributors to constipation in the palliative care patient include all of the following EXCEPT

a. *Clostridioides difficile* infection.
b. decreased fluid intake.
c. opioid medications.
d. hypercalcemia.

35. Tricyclic antidepressants are most likely to be effective in treating which of the following types of pain?

a. ischemic pain
b. cancer-related bone pain
c. visceral pain
d. neuropathic pain

36. Extensive patient and caregiver participation in interdisciplinary team discussions is important so that the

a. patient and caregivers can be informed of the plan of care as formulated by the medical providers.
b. cost of hospice care is reimbursed by the patient's insurance provider.
c. plan of care can be crafted to meet the specific needs and goals of the individual patient and family.
d. patient and caregivers come to terms with a terminal prognosis.

37. Malignant bowel obstruction would most likely develop in a patient with which of the following cancers?

a. lung.
b. breast.
c. leukemia.
d. ovarian.

38. A 51-year-old patient with terminal breast cancer asks the palliative care nurse if she should try acupuncture for intractable vomiting. The nurse's best response to this patient should be,

a. "You will need to stop all of your anti-nausea medications if you choose to pursue acupuncture."
b. "Acupuncture cannot treat vomiting."
c. "Some patients find acupuncture a helpful additional therapy for vomiting."
d. "Alternative medicine is not a proven science."

39. A patient with end-stage chronic obstructive pulmonary disease is dyspneic despite upright positioning and supplemental oxygen administration. The first-line pharmacologic therapy of choice for treating dyspnea in this clinical scenario is

a. benzodiazepines.
b. glycopyrrolate.
c. scopolamine.
d. opioids.

40. A 43-year-old patient with ovarian cancer describes a constant, throbbing pain in her lower abdomen for the last 18 hours, which ranges from an intensity of 4 (on a 10-point scale) at rest to 8 with movement. This information best describes which type of pain assessment?

a. physiologic and sensory pain assessment
b. affective pain assessment
c. comprehensive pain assessment
d. sociocultural pain assessment

41. A 27-year-old patient with metastatic cervical cancer is receiving 10 mg of morphine per dose intravenously (IV) for cancer-related pain. Because of the side effects associated with morphine, the palliative care team decides to change the patient's IV pain medication from morphine to hydromorphone. The approximate hydromorphone analgesic dosage that is equivalent to a morphine 10 mg IV dose is

a. hydromorphone 15 mg IV.
b. hydromorphone 1.5 mg IV.
c. hydromorphone 10 mg IV.
d. hydromorphone 0.15 mg IV.

42. Under the Medicare hospice benefit, general inpatient hospice care would be most appropriate for which of the following patients?

a. a 64-year-old patient with esophageal cancer who is receiving artificial nutrition through a feeding tube
b. a 12-year-old patient with leukemia and intractable pain
c. a 37-year-old patient with AIDS who would like to start a new antiretroviral medication
d. a 59-year-old patient with congestive heart failure who develops dyspnea

43. The palliative care nurse demonstrates turning maneuvers for pressure ulcer prevention to a patient's family member after describing the factors that contribute to ulcer development. After completion of verbal teaching and demonstration by the nurse, the caregiver should be asked to

a. complete a written examination about turning maneuvers.
b. practice turning maneuvers, using the nurse as the "patient."
c. sign a document, relieving the palliative care team of liability if the patient develops pressure ulcers.
d. demonstrate the turning maneuvers with the nurse present.

44. Therapeutic touch is most accurately described as

a. stimulation of reflex points on the hands and feet, corresponding to body parts.
b. the use of touch while directing healing energy to the patient.
c. the use of essential oils for the purpose of treating inflammation and infection.
d. body poses with deep breathing to facilitate relaxation and healing.

45. A hospice patient is taking amitriptyline for neuropathic pain. Which of the following is an adverse effect of amitriptyline?

a. hypersalivation
b. weight loss
c. diarrhea
d. cardiac arrhythmias

46. Diuretic medication (e.g., furosemide) for a palliative care patient with severe heart failure would be most helpful for managing which of the following symptoms?

a. depression
b. chest pain
c. dyspnea
d. constipation

47. All of the following are components of normal grieving EXCEPT

a. fear.
b. a mix of good and bad days.
c. anger.
d. hopelessness.

48. Which of the following medications most commonly causes myoclonus in the palliative care patient?

a. benzodiazepines
b. opioids
c. antispasmodics
d. antibiotics

49. A 34-year-old hospice patient with metastatic melanoma develops loud, moist-sounding breathing also known as a "death rattle." Which of the following statements most accurately describes the "death rattle"?

a. the "death rattle" is usually associated with significant patient anxiety
b. suctioning of oral secretions is the first-line treatment of choice for the "death rattle"
c. family members are not usually distressed by the patient's "death rattle"
d. the "death rattle" usually indicates impending death

50. Bisphosphonates (e.g., pamidronate) are most commonly used in the palliative care patient to treat which of the following conditions?

a. syndrome of inappropriate diuretic hormone secretion
b. hypercalcemia
c. Cushing syndrome
d. hyperglycemia

51. A patient with fourth-stage pancreatic cancer is severely malnourished and barely eating because she has a very bad bitter taste in her mouth all of the time, making food revolting and causing nausea. All of the following strategies may be helpful EXCEPT

a. rinse the mouth with a salt and soda solution before eating.
b. use a straw to drink liquids.
c. eat cold foods and liquids.
d. eat highly spiced foods.

52. A patient taking high doses of opioids has had persistent constipation but complains of a sudden episode of diarrhea and increasing urinary incontinence. The most likely cause is

a. enteritis.
b. fecal impaction.
c. allergic response to medication.
d. malabsorption syndrome.

53. Which type of pain most often requires opioids to control it?

a. visceral
b. neuropathic
c. somatic
d. psychological

54. A daughter caring for her dying mother expresses frustration with the constant demands of care, stating, "It will be a relief when she dies." The best initial response is

a. "I'm sure you don't mean that."
b. "I know your mother appreciates what you are doing for her."
c. "Caregiving is very difficult and exhausting."
d. "Why do you say that?"

55. A patient with end-stage renal disease is too confused to make decisions and is still receiving dialysis. Which is the best approach to use to initiate discussion about discontinuing dialysis with family members?

a. "Do you want to continue dialysis?"
b. "There is nothing more we can do to help your mother."
c. "Do you want to stop dialysis and let your mother die?"
d. "We have exhausted all remedies, and the dialysis is prolonging your mother's suffering."

56. An organ procurement organization is required by federal law to ask family decision makers about organ donation in the absence of an advance directive under what condition?

a. the patient's death is expected
b. the patient dies in the hospital
c. the patient dies at home
d. under all circumstances when a patient dies

57. The cracker test is used to assess for

a. nausea.
b. candida.
c. reflux.
d. xerostomia.

58. A daughter expresses fear about dealing with her father's dying at home. What is the best response?

a. "You can call hospice and a nurse will come to be with you during your father's death."
b. "I'm sure you will be fine."
c. "Let's talk about what to expect and what to do."
d. "You can always transfer your father to the hospital when death is imminent."

59. All of the following medications are usually continued during the final days of life EXCEPT

a. antipyretics.
b. antihypertensives.
c. antiemetics.
d. anticonvulsants.

60. A patient with a glioblastoma nearing death has been receiving oral corticosteroids to control cerebral edema but wishes to discontinue the steroids. What is the best approach?

a. discontinue the medication without tapering
b. discontinue the medication after tapering
c. discontinue the medication after tapering and increase analgesia
d. discontinue the medication after tapering and increase anticonvulsant and analgesia if necessary

61. Which of the following is an indication that death may occur in a few hours for a patient with severe cardiorespiratory disease?

a. heart rate doubles
b. radial pulse is no longer palpable
c. mottling of extremities is evident
d. nail beds are cyanotic

62. Anticholinergic drugs may be indicated in the final days of life for treatment of

a. nausea.
b. Cheyne-Stokes respirations.
c. death rattle
d. agonal respirations.

63. Palliative care should be provided to patients with life-threatening diseases

a. throughout the disease process and continuum of care.
b. concurrently with curative treatments.
c. concurrently with supportive treatment only.
d. when the patient is referred to hospice care.

64. An 80-year-old woman is caring for her elderly husband who wishes to die at home and is under Medicare home health hospice care. The caregiver appears exhausted and weepy. The best initial solution is

a. to place patient in a long-term care facility.
b. to tell caregiver to hire an assistant.
c. to make daily nursing visits.
d. to provide in-patient respite care for 5 days.

65. According to Centers for Medicare & Medicaid Services (CMS) regulations regarding the Medicare Hospice Benefit, an interdisciplinary team must include all of the following EXCEPT a

a. physician.
b. nurse.
c. nutritionist.
d. social worker.

66. According to Byock and Merriman's end-of-life construct, which dimension includes patients' emotions as they near death, including anxiety, fear, readiness, and acceptance?

a. physical
b. transcendent
c. interpersonal
d. well-being

67. One of the developmental landmarks for life completion/closure is accepting the finality of life. One of the tasks associated with this landmark is

a. emotional withdrawal.
b. accepting new personal definition of self.
c. life review.
d. self-forgiveness.

68. From a caregiver's perspective, all of the following indicate that the caregiver has accepted the finality of life EXCEPT

a. expressing anticipatory grief.
b. listening to the patient's life review.
c. telling the patient it is all right to die.
d. discussing personal loss.

69. According to Harper's stages of adaptation for hospice nurses, a nurse who overidentifies with the patient's situation is in which stage of adaptation?

a. Stage I, intellectualism
b. Stage II, emotional survival
c. Stage III, depression
d. Stage IV, emotional arrival

70. A patient recently diagnosed with stage 4 ovarian cancer goes into a rage when having blood drawn, accusing the laboratory technician of purposefully hurting her and demanding that the technician be reprimanded or fired. The best response is

a. "It can be painful when blood is drawn."
b. "It's not the laboratory technician's fault."
c. "I'm so sorry you had to experience discomfort."
d. "You are absolutely right. We will deal with the technician."

71. When differentiating normal grief processes from depression, all of the following are normal responses to grief and terminal disease EXCEPT the

a. patient cries periodically.
b. patient does not cry at all.
c. patient openly expresses anger.
d. patient complains of lack of energy.

72. A caregiver is persistently in denial about her husband's impending death, saying repeatedly, "He just needs to rest, and he'll be ok." What is the best response?

a. "Your husband is going to die soon."
b. "It must be very difficult to believe what is happening to your husband."
c. "What do you think is going to happen?"
d. "Do you really believe that?"

73. In a state that does not allow physician-assisted death, a patient asks the nurse to assist him in committing suicide. The best initial response of the nurse is,

a. "Assisted suicide is illegal."
b. "That would be terrible for your family."
c. "I'm sorry. I can't help you."
d. "Tell me why you feel you want to die now."

74. According to Piaget's theory of cognitive development, at what age is a child likely to believe that he is the reason his parent is dying?

a. age 2-7
b. age 7-11
c. age 11-13
d. age 13-15

75. A family member has called to say that a home hospice patient has died, and to request a nurse come to make the death pronouncement. The first thing the nurse should do when entering the home 20 minutes later is

a. check the patient for heart and breath sounds.
b. introduce herself to the family.
c. look at the patient and confirm death.
d. express condolences.

76. A patient who has gone through months of treatment but suffered a relapse is severely depressed and withdrawn. She states, "There's no point to any of this anymore. I want it to be over." Which is the best response?

a. "Don't give up hope."
b. "I can see you are depressed, and I'm worried about you."
c. "Have you considered clinical trials?"
d. "Have you been thinking of ways of hurting yourself?

77. All of the following are risk factors for complicated bereavement EXCEPT

a. history of substance abuse.
b. recent loss of another family member.
c. strong religious faith.
d. loss of income.

78. A woman in the final weeks of life tells the nurse that she feels she has been a failure as a mother. How can the nurse respond to encourage life review?

a. "What would you do differently?"
b. "What positive memory do you have of raising your children?"
c. "I'm sure you did the best you could?"
d. "That's not important now."

79. All of the following are indications that a patient's drugs are being diverted in the home EXCEPT

a. the caregiver is increasingly isolating the patient and refusing home care.
b. the patient has had an abrupt, marked increase of pain.
c. the patient's pain pills are a different color.
d. the caregiver is unconventional in appearance.

80. Which of the following religions views embalming as desecration of the body?

a. Islam
b. Hinduism
c. Buddhism
d. Shintoism

81. A patient with cancer has poorly controlled pain because she forgets to take her hydrocodone and acetaminophen 5/325 mg tablets on schedule but takes one or two tablets every 3-6 hours depending on how severe her pain is. The best solution is probably to

a. educate the patient about the importance of staying on schedule.
b. switch to fentanyl patch.
c. switch to a higher dose of hydrocodone.
d. set up an alarm system to remind the patient when the medication is due.

82. Which type of pain assessment is most indicated for a patient whose pain medication dosage has been increased to better control pain?

a. comprehensive pain assessment
b. assessment of aggravating factors
c. assessment of location and duration of pain
d. assessment of intensity of pain with 0-10 scale

83. The 5 key elements of pain assessment include words, intensity, location, duration, and

a. aggravating/alleviating factors.
b. affect.
c. behavior.
d. response.

84. Poorly localized pain that is described as cramping, distention, deep, and pressure is most likely

a. visceral.
b. neuropathic.
c. somatic.
d. psychological.

85. A patient tells the nurse and doctor that she is barely having any pain and rarely takes pain medications, but her pain medication record shows she has been averaging about 20-25 mg of hydrocodone daily. This probably indicates

a. the patient is actively lying.
b. the patient is reluctant to admit the degree of pain.
c. the patient is giving the medication to someone else.
d. the patient is confused.

86. An older patient with cancer is in much pain and is willing to take other opioids but refuses to take morphine. The probable reason is that the patient

a. associates morphine with dying.
b. wants stronger medications.
c. is confused.
d. is afraid of becoming addicted.

87. Which pain scale is most appropriate for use with a 5-year-old child?

a. CRIES
b. FACES (Wong-Baker)
c. 0-10 pain intensity scale
d. CHEOPS

88. The most appropriate music therapy to aid in relaxation and pain control is

a. classical music
b. patient's preference
c. jazz
d. New Age

89. Which of the following medications is appropriate for use as terminal/palliative sedation?

a. Haloperidol 0.5-5.0 mg every 4-12 hours
b. Olanzapine 2.5 mg twice daily
c. Lorazepam 0.5-2.0 mg every 1-4 hours
d. Midazolam 0.5-6.0 mg per hour intravenously

90. A patient receiving morphine experiences severe respiratory depression. Which medication is indicated to control symptoms?

a. Flumazenil
b. N-acetylcysteine
c. Neostigmine
d. Naloxone

91. An elderly patient has chemotherapy-induced nausea and vomiting. Which of the following antiemetic agents is most likely to be effective?

a. Haloperidol
b. Scopolamine
c. Ondansetron
d. Dronabinol

92. Which of the following adjuvant analgesics is most indicated to relieve pain associated with spinal cord compression?

a. Pamidronate
b. Clonazepam
c. Nifedipine
d. Prednisone

93. A palliative care patient is receiving chemotherapy through a port in the upper chest but complains that the needle insertion is very painful, so he becomes very anxious before treatment. Which therapy is most indicated?

a. EMLA cream
b. extra pain medication
c. relaxation exercises
d. anti-anxiety medication

94. A patient who is nearing death suffers from refractory pain and is administered ketamine for pain crisis. What other medication adjustments/additions should be made?

a. decrease opioid dose by 25%
b. decrease opioid dose by 25% and administer diazepam or lorazepam
c. decrease opioid dose by 50% and administer diazepam or lorazepam
d. no adjustments/additions are necessary

95. A patient who abruptly stops an opioid after radiotherapy shrinks a tumor and exhibits withdrawal symptoms has probably developed

a. addiction.
b. tolerance.
c. physical dependence.
d. pseudoaddiction.

96. A patient has developed persistent skin irritation from use of fentanyl patches but does not want to change to another medication. What treatment may be used to prevent irritation?

a. spray with steroid used for inhalation therapy.
b. apply steroid cream.
c. apply powder to skin.
d. spray with skin barrier.

97. If a patient receives 1.5 mg of hydromorphone, what is the equianalgesic dose of morphine?

a. 50 mcg
b. 10 mg
c. 7.5 mg
d. 130 mg

98. Which of the following is an example of a complementary therapy?

a. cancer-cure diets
b. oxygen therapy
c. aromatherapy
d. biomagnetic therapy

99. Which complementary therapy is based on the idea that "like cures like?"

a. ayurvedic medicine
b. homeopathy
c. naturopathy
d. traditional Chinese medicine

100. Based on general cultural differences, which ethnic group tends to be the least expressive when in pain?

a. Asians
b. Hispanics
c. Middle Easterners
d. Southern European/Mediterranean

101. A patient is using a 72-hour fentanyl patch to relieve pain and has good pain control for 48 hours but routinely experiences increased pain for the last 24 hours. The best solution is to

a. increase the dosage or change the patch more frequently
b. change to a different drug
c. use complementary therapies, such as acupuncture
d. increase the use of oral opioids for the last 24 hours

102. A patient wants to continue to attend a weekly 1-hour book club meeting, but the meeting is up a flight of stairs and the exertion to climb the stairs results in severe incident pain. What is the best solution?

a. the patient should stop attending the meeting
b. the patient should increase baseline analgesia by 25%
c. the patient should take a rapid-onset, short-acting analgesic before the meeting
d. the patient should take a long-acting analgesic after the meeting

103. A patient with end-stage dementia displays an abrupt, aggressive change in behavior. The nurse's initial intervention should be to

a. place the patient in a quiet environment.
b. evaluate the patient for causes of discomfort.
c. administer analgesia.
d. administer chemical restraint.

104. Which electrolyte imbalance occurs with syndrome of inappropriate antidiuretic hormone secretion (SIADH)?

a. hyponatremia
b. hypernatremia
c. hypocalcemia
d. hypercalcemia

105. If a patient has just died and the nurse is preparing the body for family arrival, which of the following should the nurse do?

a. tie the mouth closed
b. place dentures in the mouth
c. close the eyelids
d. cover the deceased body, including the face, with a sheet

106. When a patient has received bad news about prognosis, what is the best approach to ascertain the patient's needs?

a. "Do you need anything to help you cope with this news?"
b. "I know you have received disappointing news. Can you tell me what I can do to help you?"
c. "Is everything all right? Can I help you?"
d. "I feel terrible for you. What can I do?"

107. All of the following are primary benefits of working with an interdisciplinary team EXCEPT

a. effective problem-solving.
b. pooling of expertise.
c. personal support system.
d. independent decision-making.

108. When using hypodermoclysis to provide fluids for a patient who is dehydrated, what is the usual initial rate of infusion?

a. 50 mL/hr
b. 100 mL/hr
c. 150 mL/hr
d. 200 mL/hr

109. All of the following are effects of dehydration on the pulmonary system at the end of life EXCEPT

a. reduced cough.
b. reduced secretions.
c. decreased dyspnea.
d. increased death rattle.

110. A patient has had a right-hemisphere stroke with left-sided paralysis. Which method of communication is probably indicated?

a. speak very slowly, standing on the patient's right side
b. use visual aids, standing on the patient's left side
c. speak normally, standing on the patient's right side
d. use simple vocabulary and gestures, standing on the patient's left side

111. A patient with Parkinson disease has been evaluated for the ability to swallow, and tests indicate pharyngeal phase dysphagia. Which of the following symptoms should the nurse expect?

a. patient chokes while swallowing and often regurgitates food into the nose
b. patient complains of difficulty swallowing but rarely chokes or coughs
c. patient drools, and food remains in the mouth after a meal
d. patient regurgitates food frequently after eating

112. A patient's records indicate heavy smoking and a history of alcoholism and a diagnosis of variant (Prinzmetal) angina. What type of pain should the nurse anticipate the patient might experience?

a. chest pain occurs when the patient is lying flat at rest
b. chest pain occurs cyclically at the same time each day with the patient at rest
c. chest pain occurs after exertion
d. chest pain occurs with increasing frequency after exertion and at rest

113. Which of the follow triads indicates common risk factors for acute venous thromboembolism?

a. Virchow's triad
b. Beck's triad
c. Cushing's triad
d. Waddell's triad

114. Microvascular changes in chronic diabetes can lead to all of the following consequences EXCEPT

a. blindness.
b. diabetic foot ulcer.
c. chronic renal failure.
d. myocardial infarction.

115. A patient with advanced cirrhosis has marked tense ascites and is experiencing severe dyspnea, pain, and orthopnea. The most appropriate treatment is

a. comfort measures only.
b. IV fluid bolus.
c. sodium and fluid restriction.
d. paracentesis.

116. A patient with dysphagia has an order for a mechanically altered diet because of impaired tongue control and limited chewing ability. Which of the following foods is appropriate?

a. raw fruit
b. baked fish
c. baked vegetables
d. soft scrambled eggs

117. A patient has persistent xerostomia because of post-radiation damage to the salivary glands. Which of the following treatment is appropriate to use to stimulate production of saliva?

a. Bethanechol
b. Pilocarpine
c. Vitamin C
d. artificial saliva

118. A patient with gastric cancer and gastric distention has developed chronic hiccoughs, which result in severe pain. Which initial medication is indicated to control the hiccoughs?

a. Simethicone or metoclopramide
b. Baclofen or midazolam
c. Gabapentin or carbamazepine
d. Haloperidol or chlorpromazine

119. Which type of laxative is usually most effective for opioid-related constipation in the chronically ill patient?

a. saline laxatives
b. osmotic laxatives
c. bulk laxatives
d. stimulant laxatives

120. The opioid medication that is most likely to cause pruritus is

a. oxymorphone.
b. fentanyl.
c. codeine.
d. morphine.

121. Which of the following primary cancers has the highest risk of metastasizing to the bones?

a. breast and prostate
b. lung and thyroid
c. pancreas
d. kidney

122. A patient with an inoperable brain tumor has displacement of cerebral tissue, altered cerebral perfusion, and increased intracranial pressure. What is the best position for the patient?

a. flat in bed with head and neck neutral position
b. head of bed raised 10 degrees with head and neck in neutral position
c. head of the bed raised to 30-45 degrees with head and neck in neutral position
d. Trendelenburg position with head and neck in neutral position

123. Cancer patients who report severe fatigue and general debility should routinely be assessed for all of the following EXCEPT

a. depression.
b. sleep disorders.
c. anemia.
d. family conflict.

124. A patient with ovarian cancer has been losing 2-4 pounds weekly because of anorexia/cachexia. All of the following are good strategies to improve intake EXCEPT

a. small frequent meals.
b. nutritional drinks, such as Ensure.
c. advise patient that she must eat to live.
d. explore dietary preferences with patient.

125. A patient with urge incontinence is taking immediate-release oxybutynin to decrease bladder contractility, but complains that the dry mouth it causes makes her very uncomfortable. Which of the following alternative drugs is likely to cause the least mouth dryness?

a. extended-release tolterodine
b. Propantheline
c. Hyoscyamine oral tablets
d. Flavoxate

126. A patient with stage 4 liver cancer is planning to receive care under the Medicare Hospice Benefit. Which of the following services will be covered by this benefit?

a. extended live-in 24-hour care
b. ambulance service, arranged for by family member
c. antibiotics to treat a urinary infection
d. service at a private, non–Medicare-approved hospice

127. A patient under hospice care lives with her son who works outside of the home, so she spends many hours at home alone with her cat. Which of the following volunteer services may provide the most benefit?

a. transportation services
b. friendly visitors
c. pet walkers
d. hair stylists

128. A hospice patient tells the nurse that she has so many questions to ask her doctor but she gets nervous and flustered and forgets what to ask. What is the best response?

a. "Let's make a list of questions to give to the doctor."
b. "You should make a list of questions."
c. "I'll tell the doctor you have questions."
d. "Perhaps I can answer your questions."

129. A patient has severe lower extremity lymphedema. Which prophylactic treatment is generally recommended?

a. corticosteroids
b. antifungal powders
c. antibiotics
d. oral antifungal agents

130. Which of the following support surfaces for prevention of pressure sores has low moisture retention?

a. static water flotation
b. alternating air
c. high air loss
d. foam

131. A hospice patient resists turning and has developed a coccygeal ulcer that appears as a blistered area with a wound bed that is red/pink with slight exudate but without slough and only partial-thickness skin loss (National Pressure Injury Advisory Panel [NPIAP] stage II). The best dressing choice is

a. semi-permeable film.
b. hydrocolloid.
c. alginate.
d. gauze.

132. A patient has Medicare and supplementary insurance but is concerned about direct nonmedical costs, which include

a. durable medical equipment.
b. physician's visits.
c. lost income from employment.
d. emergency services.

133. A patient with breast cancer has complained of increasing fatigue and dyspnea and has developed a dry, nonproductive cough with dull pain in the left chest. The left lung field is dull to percussion with decreased breath sounds and decreased diaphragmatic excursion. The most likely cause is

a. lung metastasis.
b. pulmonary embolism.
c. pleural effusion.
d. pneumothorax.

134. Which of the following is likely to have the most negative impact on a patient's ability to maintain a feeling of hope at the end of life?

a. pain is poorly controlled
b. patient lives alone
c. patient has no religious faith
d. patient has signed a DNR request

135. The gay partner of a closeted man who is dying is not able to openly grieve or acknowledge his loss. This type of grief is

a. uncomplicated.
b. complicated.
c. disenfranchised.
d. unresolved.

136. A patient in palliative care has a 10-year-old daughter, and the patient is concerned how the child will cope with the patient's eventual death. The best advice for the patient is to

a. shield the child from the reality of the illness as long as possible.
b. ensure that the child not be involved in patient care.
c. send the child to live with another family member.
d. involve the child in patient care to the child's ability.

137. The palliative and hospice care program is developing bereavement and follow-up services for family members after patients' deaths. In order to comply with Clinical Practice Guidelines for Quality Palliative Care (guideline 3.2) of the National Consensus Project, bereavement services must be offered for a minimum period of

a. 30 days.
b. 90 days.
c. 6 months.
d. 12 months.

138. Under Element 4: Performance Improvement Projects (PIPs) of the Quality Assurance and Performance Improvement (QAPI), which entity identifies a problem to focus on?

a. Medicare
b. Medicaid
c. facility
d. state

139. A hospice nurse routinely gives patients and family her personal telephone number and calls and visits them, even on days off, and often brings small gifts and offers to do errands. This is an example of

a. professional excellence.
b. professional boundary violation.
c. professional negligence.
d. professional inexperience.

140. The primary principle of palliative care is to

a. provide compassionate care.
b. relieve suffering.
c. guide the patient to acceptance of death.
d. respect the wishes of the person dying.

141. A nurse monitoring pain control for a palliative care patient with a history of drug abuse is concerned that the patient is exhibiting aberrant drug-taking behavior. Which of the following is of most concern?

a. the nurse finds a rolled and partially burned fentanyl patch beside the patient's bed
b. the patient took one extra dose of oral pain medication
c. the patient changed his fentanyl patch in 2 days instead of 3
d. the patient complains that he needs higher doses of medication

142. The primary difference between physician-assisted suicide and terminal sedation is

a. there is essentially no difference.
b. terminal sedation is legal.
c. terminal sedation is intended to provide comfort and alleviate suffering.
d. terminal sedation does not hasten death.

143. When a patient is undergoing terminal weaning and being removed from ventilation, which medication is most indicated to relieve a sense of breathlessness?

a. benzodiazepine
b. bronchodilator
c. SSRI
d. opioid

144. According to the National Cancer Institute Scale of Severity of Diarrhea, 7-9 stools per day with incontinence and/or severe abdominal cramping is classified as

a. Grade 1.
b. Grade 2.
c. Grade 3.
d. Grade 4.

145. The purpose of teaching "huffing" to a patient with cystic fibrosis is to

a. relieve dyspnea.
b. improve cough effectiveness.
c. distract the mind.
d. relieve cough.

146. A patient with a fungating breast cancer tumor has tumor necrosis and a foul odor. Which treatment is most indicated to control odor?

a. topical metronidazole
b. charcoal dressings
c. topical application of yogurt
d. skin cleansers

147. When reviewing costs in relation to clinical outcomes, which of the following is based on the assumption that that two treatments are equal in effectiveness, so the least expensive option should be utilized?

a. cost effectiveness
b. cost utility
c. cost benefit
d. cost minimization

148. The three primary aspects of evidence-based practice are clinical expertise, best available research, and

a. patient values.
b. economic impact.
c. expected outcomes.
d. decision-making.

149. The primary treatment for tumor-related spinal cord compression is

a. corticosteroids.
b. decompressive therapy
c. fractionated external-beam radiation therapy.
d. analgesia.

150. In the ABCDE method of pain assessment, the E stands for

a. eliminate pain.
b. empower patients and family.
c. expectations.
d. examine patient.

Answer Key and Explanations for Test #1

1. C: The Medicare hospice benefit is a federal program for Medicare-eligible patients with an estimated life expectancy of 6 months or less. Because Medicare is a federally funded program, eligibility requirements and benefits do not vary from state to state. The cost of all supplies and medications being used in relation to the terminal illness are covered under the Medicare hospice benefit. Hospice care may be provided in multiple settings, including home, outpatient, and inpatient settings. A patient does not need a "do not resuscitate" order to qualify for the Medicare hospice benefit. Patients who have activated the Medicare hospice benefit may opt to return to “regular” Medicare (i.e., Medicare Part A) at any time.

2. B: Patients who are taking opiates long term become physically dependent on the medication and will experience symptoms of drug withdrawal if the medication is discontinued suddenly or the dose is dropped dramatically. It is important for the palliative care nurse to understand the differences between physical dependence, tolerance, and addiction to pain medications. Physical dependence occurs when the body adapts to the effects of opiate medications (taken long term) to the degree that rapid discontinuation or rapid dose decreases result in withdrawal symptoms. Tolerance to opiate medications describes the phenomenon of the body adjusting to a stable dose of medication, resulting in a need for increased amounts of the medication to achieve the same effect. Psychological dependence (or addiction) on opiate medications is characterized by a lack of control over use of the medication, compulsive use, and continued use despite harmful effects.

3. A: The essence of palliative care involves the relief of pain and suffering in the terminally ill patient. Palliative (or terminal) sedation describes the use of sedative agents (e.g., benzodiazepines, barbiturates) to treat pain or suffering in the dying patient when other treatment measures are ineffective. Palliative sedation is employed to relieve intractable symptoms in the dying patient, not to expedite the dying process. Palliative sedation is somewhat controversial. Some argue that it is the ethical equivalent to euthanizing a dying patient, given that death may be hastened with the use of sedative medications. Palliative sedation is more often administered for relief of intractable physical symptoms, such as dyspnea, pain, or agitation, than for so-called “psychic” suffering. As with other decisions made in palliative care, honest discussion between providers and the patient and family members about the use of palliative sedation should occur.

4. C: The dying patient becomes progressively less mobile as his or her illness progresses. There are numerous complications associated with immobility, some of which should be prevented when possible to avoid causing discomfort in the dying patient. Complications of immobility include muscle weakness due to atrophy, constipation, joint stiffness and pain, urinary tract infection, increased clotting risk, and pressure ulcers. Pathologic fractures, myoclonus, and pruritus are commonly present in the terminally ill patient but are not increased with immobility. Pressure ulcers can be prevented or minimized with the use of turning and positioning techniques, maintenance of optimal nutritional status (when appropriate), and wound management.

5. C: Spirituality and religion may play a large part in how the terminally ill patient experiences and responds to the dying process. Assessing the role of religious or spiritual beliefs in each patient's life is an important component of a patient's assessment and should, ideally, take place as early as possible in the relationship between patient and palliative care providers. Some patients may have extensive involvement in a religious or spiritual community, while others may have deep personal beliefs, which are not necessarily associated with an official organization or community. Patients who do not identify strongly with spiritual or religious beliefs should not be urged to do so.

Spiritual and religious beliefs may influence a patient's beliefs about why they are ill, which medical interventions they are willing to pursue, rituals they would like around the time of death, and potential sources of comfort during the dying process. Although a patient's religious and spiritual beliefs may differ from the nurse's personal beliefs, the primary purpose is not to seek out differences but to discover what will be most meaningful and helpful to the patient.

6. B: Urinary incontinence is a common symptom in the palliative care patient and may significantly affect a patient's self-esteem, sexual activity, and willingness to venture out in his or her community. There are multiple causes of urinary incontinence, including urinary tract infections; limited mobility, affecting a patient's ability to get to a toilet; constipation; mental status changes; medication effects; weak pelvic floor musculature; neuropathic bladder; fistula; and poor urethral sphincter tone. Management of urinary incontinence varies greatly, depending on the cause. A patient with invasive prostate cancer-causing incontinence needs treatment strategies that differ from those needed by a patient with a urinary tract infection. A thorough history, including a medication history, physical examination, and urinalysis, often reveals likely etiologies of urinary incontinence. Additionally, a bladder log, which details fluid intake, voiding, incontinence episodes, and any associated factors (e.g., coughing, laughing) can be helpful in designing a management plan.

7. C: Palliative patients who have young children are often very concerned about the effect their death will have on their children. Helping a patient and his or her family feel more comfortable with assisting the children through the dying and grieving process can bring a patient a great deal of comfort. A child's understanding of illness and death and the way in which their grief is expressed often varies greatly, depending on their age and development. Many adults mistakenly believe that a young child is either unaware of the parent's illness or is unable to understand the severity of a parent's illness. Many families need and desire specific, concrete strategies for explaining the illness and death of a parent to a child. Maintaining as many of the child's usual routines as possible, answering questions directly, and encouraging the child to express any thoughts or feelings are among the helpful tips that families may need.

8. A: Pain assessment is a crucial part of palliative care nursing, and there are many different assessment tools available to the palliative care nurse for this purpose. Although not universal, pain is an extremely common symptom in the dying patient. Pain is far more than a purely physical experience for the patient, and the most effective assessment tools take into account the multiple factors that influence the individual patient's pain experience. Important factors to assess (and reassess) include specific words describing the pain; intensity (e.g., 1–10 scale); location; duration; quality; associated factors; effect on sleep, appetite, mood, and energy; and the patient's attitudes or beliefs about his or her pain. Using a consistent assessment tool allows the nurse to observe trends in the patient's pain in response to therapy. Although a multifactorial assessment tool may discover adverse medication effects, withdrawal symptoms, or warning signs of psychological dependence on pain medications, most pain assessment tools are not designed for the primary assessment of these issues.

9. C: Acquired immunodeficiency syndrome (AIDS) is caused by human immunodeficiency virus (HIV), a retrovirus that primarily affects the T cells of the human immune system. T cells carry a surface protein called CD4, and the disease severity correlates with falling CD4 levels. Although the discovery and use of antiretroviral medications have markedly changed the life expectancy of most patients with HIV/AIDS, it remains a fatal illness. Because HIV affects the patient's immune system, progression of disease is primarily characterized by opportunistic infections (i.e., infections that would not occur in a patient with healthy T cells). AIDS patients may also develop opportunistic malignancies, such as Kaposi sarcoma and lymphoma, although infection is the primary cause of death in AIDS patients. Examples of opportunistic infections that occur as CD4 levels decrease include *Pneumocystis carinii* pneumonia, tuberculosis, and *Cryptococcus*. Aside from the effects of infections, AIDS patients often require end-of-life care for pain, weight loss, weakness, and mental status changes.

10. B: Although each patient's dying process is individual, the signs and symptoms of impending death are often very similar, even in patients with very different terminal illnesses. The palliative care nurse should be familiar with the common signs and symptoms of impending death so that he or she can educate the patient and caregivers about the dying process and support patients and caregivers through the patient's death. As death nears, the patient has decreasing interest in or awareness of his or her surroundings and a reduced desire or ability to move around. He or she has a marked decrease in food or fluid intake and often develops difficulty with swallowing. The dying patient usually develops noisy and irregular respirations, cool extremities, and possibly fast or irregular pulse. Urine output typically decreases or stops as the patient gets closer to dying.

11. C: Pain can be categorized in a variety of ways, and successful treatment of pain is dependent on a multidimensional and frequent assessment of the palliative care patient's pain. Treating pain well depends in part on assessing what type of pain a patient is experiencing, particularly when considering the onset and duration of action of the many different pain medications available. As the name suggests, spontaneous pain occurs spontaneously, and is not predictably associated with a particular movement or event. Incident pain is pain that occurs predictably in association with a particular event, such as walking, a dressing change, or coughing. Spontaneous pain and incident pain are different types of breakthrough pain. End-of-dose failure is pain that occurs as the time for the next dose of a scheduled pain medication approaches. In other words, the medicine is not lasting long enough. Psychic pain refers to pain that is primarily characterized by its impact on the patient's emotional state (e.g., fear of dying, feeling helpless).

12. C: "Fading away" refers to the process through which patients and their loved ones go when facing a terminal illness, in which they come to terms with the change and loss that accompanies progressive illness and death. Like grief, the process of fading away may be characterized by stops and starts with multiple components of the process occurring simultaneously. "Redefining" involves making adjustments as tasks and routines in which the patient was previously able to engage in are no longer possible because of disease progression. Important nursing interventions for patients working through the redefining process include encouraging patients to express their feelings about what has changed, reminding patients of what remains possible, and assisting patients in finding new ways to engage in those activities that are meaningful to them.

13. C: Advanced practice nurses (e.g., clinical nurse specialist, nurse practitioner) have completed a master's degree in nursing and maintain specialized knowledge and skills in their chosen specialty. Palliative care advanced practice nurses should be up-to-date with the latest literature and evidence-based guidelines of care. They are available both for direct patient care and education of patients, families, and other providers. They are a consultation resource in complicated or difficult cases. Administering medication for the express purpose of hastening death is not considered an appropriate palliative intervention, according to the policies of most palliative care organizations, including the American Nurses Association. This may be an evolving issue in palliative care, particularly with the passage of laws in some states that allow for the prescription of medications with the express purpose of hastening death in terminally ill patients.

14. A: Dementia is a progressive, generally irreversible disease characterized by impaired cognitive functioning, which may be caused by a variety of conditions, including AIDS, Alzheimer disease, trauma, and vascular disease. Dementia is usually a progressive disease, although specific stages of dementia are not clearly delineated. The patient in the late (i.e., terminal or advanced) stage of dementia has severely impaired or complete loss of his or her ability to swallow, communicate, walk, or maintain continence. Palliative care patients with terminal dementia may experience any of the symptoms commonly seen in other terminally ill patients, including pain, infection, dyspnea, and agitation.

15. C: Superior vena cava obstruction in the palliative care patient is most commonly associated with tumors or lung cancer and results from obstruction of blood flow through the superior vena cava (SVC). Obstruction may result from either internal (e.g., local cancer extension) or external (e.g., bulky lymphadenopathy) compression of the SVC or may result from a clot in the SVC. Symptoms of SVC obstruction may present gradually or acutely and are often very distressing to the patient and family. The patient may complain of facial, arm, or neck swelling; shortness of breath; a feeling of fullness in the head; hoarseness; or dysphagia. Distended neck veins may be visible on examination. With rapid or complete obstruction, patients rapidly deteriorate as a result of increased intracranial pressure. Lymphedema typically results in extremity swelling, rather than facial swelling.

16. B: When terminally ill patients lack the mental capacity to make end-of-life treatment decisions, family members usually become the primary medical decision makers in the absence of a predetermined health care power of attorney. Family members may have conflicting values and opinions about end-of-life issues. Convening a family conference with palliative care providers is helpful in cases where there is disagreement among family members regarding the plan of care. Once the family members are updated about the medical status of the patient, a respectful and honest conversation should take place in which each family member's opinions and concerns about what the plan of care should be are elicited. Members of the palliative care team can encourage family members to consider what they believe the patient would have wanted if he or she were able to decide. This may be quite different from what they would choose for themselves in a similar situation.

17. A: Whether to administer artificial hydration to the dying patient should be determined within the context of the patient's symptoms and goals. Artificial (nonoral) hydration is considered a medical intervention in the United States, and its use can, therefore, be refused if the patient or care team feels its burdens outweigh the benefits. Family members and care providers may find it emotionally difficult not to provide artificial hydration to the dying patient. Dehydration that occurs as patients reduce their oral fluid intake may lead to improvement in some end-of-life symptoms, such as edema, vomiting, and respiratory congestion. Dehydration is not typically associated with pain in most patients. In some patients, dehydration may exacerbate distressing end-of-life symptoms, such as delirium from electrolyte abnormalities, or impaired consciousness from poor clearance of sedating medications (e.g., opiates). Patients with decision-making capacity can make informed decisions to accept or refuse artificial hydration.

18. D: The sensation of dry mouth (xerostomia) is a common complaint in the palliative care patient and can lead to discomfort as well as difficulty with chewing, swallowing, speaking, and taste. Xerostomia can result in mouth sores, halitosis, and dental decay. Treatment can prevent complications of xerostomia and provides increased patient comfort. Xerostomia may occur for a variety of reasons, including decreased saliva secretion, damage to the buccal mucosa, dehydration, and psychological factors. Many medications used in palliative care (e.g., anticholinergic medications), oxygen therapy, and mouth breathing also contribute to dry mouth. There are multiple treatment options for xerostomia once underlying conditions have been treated (if possible). Nonpharmacologic therapies include basic mouth care (e.g., lip/mouth swabs, toothbrushing), peppermint water, vitamin C, gum or mints, and acupuncture. Pharmacologic therapies include artificial saliva solutions, pilocarpine, bethanechol, and yohimbine. Although topical anesthetic may be helpful for treating painful mouth sores, it is not a primary treatment for xerostomia.

19. D: Opioid medications are commonly used by terminally ill patients and are highly effective for treatment of pain. Long-term opioid use is often accompanied by unpleasant side effects. The goal should be to find a treatment regimen that treats the patient's pain adequately while minimizing uncomfortable or distressing side effects. Sedation is a common side effect of opiate medications. The somnolence associated with opiate administration often improves or resolves within 1-2 days of starting the medication. If sedation continues, it is important to review other potential causes, including other central nervous system depressant medications (e.g., benzodiazepines). If the patient is without pain, reducing the opiate dose may be effective. If the patient is unable to tolerate a reduced opiate dose, psychostimulant medications (e.g., methylphenidate) can be effective.

20. D: Poverty presents additional challenges to providing optimal palliative care to the terminally ill patient. Often, patients living in poverty have unstable (or nonexistent) housing, making it difficult to provide "home" care consistently. Lack of telephone access and dependable transportation options lead to difficulty with arranging or getting to scheduled or urgent medical visits. Patients may be dealing with the challenges of meeting their most basic needs, such as food and shelter. Patients living in poverty may not have a stable support system, leading to lack of a friend or family member who can function as a caregiver as illness progresses. If the patient is dealing with addiction or psychiatric illness in addition to poverty, the challenges are significantly compounded. Contrary to popular stereotypes, patients living in poverty do not necessarily have less effective coping skills. As with all patients, there is a wide range of psychological reactions to end-of-life issues, and many patients who are homeless or struggling to meet their basic needs on a day-to-day basis are resilient, flexible, and pragmatic when faced with the challenge of terminal illness.

21. B: Pain is a common symptom in terminally ill patients, but there are different types of pain, and different therapies are more effective with certain types of pain than with others. Physiologic or sensory pain is generally classified into three categories. Neuropathic pain is fairly localized (but radiating) pain that arises from nerve infiltration or injury (e.g., tumor infiltration, postherpetic neuralgia) and is often described as shooting, burning, tingling, or shock-like. Somatic pain is well-localized pain that arises from stimulation of skin, bone, or muscle (e.g., bony metastases, cellulitis) and is often described as achy, throbbing, or dull. Visceral pain is poorly localized pain that arises from stimulation of abdominal or thoracic viscera (e.g., ischemic bowel, hepatic capsule distention) and is often described as cramping, squeezing, or pressure.

22. A: Hope is an important component of life, even as people face terminal illness and death, and is an adaptive and healthy response to life's challenges. Assisting patients in maintaining hope in the face of terminal illness and impending death is an important tool of the palliative care provider. "False hope" (or "unrealistic hopefulness" or denial) is somewhat controversial among palliative care providers and family members of terminally ill patients. Some providers feel that any attachment to unrealistic hopes is unhealthy and indicative of impaired coping. As with other assessments in palliative care nursing, one can assess a patient's "unrealistic hopes" to establish whether the patient's beliefs and hopes are causing any actual harm. Gentle intervention may be warranted if the patient's beliefs and hopes are leading to risky behaviors, refusal to seek crucial medical care, or social isolation. In the absence of demonstrated harm to the patient, it should be acknowledged that denial is a legitimate coping mechanism, and patients should not be pushed to accept their impending death until they feel ready to do so.

23. C: Delirium is a complex and common clinical phenomenon in the palliative care patient and is characterized by "acute and fluctuating disturbances in attention, level of consciousness, and basic cognitive functions," according to the *Diagnostic and Statistical Manual of Mental Disorders.* Patients may be disoriented, agitated, and hallucinating. Patients with delirium may have increased psychomotor activity (e.g., sleep disturbance, agitation, loud speech, combative), decreased psychomotor activity (e.g., lethargy, apathy), or a combination of the two. Although there are overlapping features of delirium and dementia (e.g., mood lability, memory disturbances), the time course and fluctuating nature of delirium differentiates it from dementia. Dementia is a slow-onset progressive disease, occurring over months and years, as opposed to hours and days. Palliative care patients are at increased risk for delirium because of their serious medical illness and multiple medications.

24. A: The Medicare hospice benefit is a federal program for Medicare-eligible patients with an estimated life expectancy of 6 months or less. The cost of all supplies and medications being used in relation to the terminal illness is covered. The Medicare hospice benefit covers inpatient respite care for up to 5 consecutive days to provide short-term relief to a hospice patient's primary caregiver. Additionally, the Medicare hospice benefit covers routine home care, inpatient care for medical conditions or complications related to the terminal illness, and continuous home care for medical complications that would otherwise require inpatient hospitalization.

25. B: Noninvasive positive pressure ventilation (e.g., BiPAP) may be utilized in the palliative care setting for relief of dyspnea in some patients or for patients who do not wish to be intubated for respiratory failure but would like more aggressive intervention than supplemental oxygen. As with all interventions in palliative care, the benefits of a particular therapy for meeting the patient's end-of-life goals must be weighed against the burdens of therapy. In patients with ALS whose dyspnea and respiratory failure is due to a primary weakness in the respiratory muscles, BiPAP has been shown to improve quality of life and prolong survival. Of course, many patients with ALS choose not to use BiPAP or choose to discontinue BiPAP if its use is no longer meeting their goals for end-of-life care. The use of BiPAP is not a contraindication for the administration of medications commonly used to relieve dyspnea in the dying patient.

26. C: Lymphedema is a distressing and difficult-to-treat edema secondary to impaired drainage of lymphatic fluid. Lymphedema typically occurs in an extremity and is characterized by swelling, skin tightness, variable discomfort, decreased range of motion, and skin changes, such as weeping or thickening. Breast cancer patients who have undergone surgery with dissection of the axillary lymph nodes or radiation therapy account for the most common source of upper extremity lymphedema, although lymphedema may also be associated with other cancers, infection, trauma, or thrombosis. Treatment is long term and may include manual lymphatic drainage, compression devices, skin care, and treatment of underlying conditions, when possible.

27. A: Fentanyl is a highly potent opioid medication, which can be administered in multiple forms, including intravenously, subcutaneously, and transdermally. Transdermal fentanyl is beneficial in palliative care patients who can no longer take oral medications safely or are experiencing intractable vomiting. The analgesic effects of transdermal fentanyl last about 72 hours, but analgesic effect and steady-state serum levels are delayed until at least 12 hours after the patch is applied. Absorption may be altered by patient factors, such as body habitus or fever. External heat applied over a fentanyl patch may increase the rate of medication absorption. Given the slow onset and offset of transdermally absorbed fentanyl, this route is not appropriate or effective for the treatment of breakthrough pain.

28. A: One of the essential tenets of palliative care is respect for the patient's right to make independent, well-informed choices about his or her life and death. However, one of the most effective tools that a patient has for ensuring that his or her wishes are respected as death approaches, the health care power of attorney or medical advance directive, is underused. There are misconceptions both among health care providers and patients and families that impede the use of these legal avenues for maintaining control over medical decision making. Ideally, discussions with patients about advance directives should occur either before serious illness develops or before the terminal phase of an existing illness. Some providers mistakenly believe that bringing up this topic with patients will scare them, but research demonstrates that most patients prefer to be asked about these issues early on. Some patients mistakenly believe that an advance directive makes it less likely that they will receive advanced medical treatment. Patients need to be assured that they will retain full medical decision-making power unless and until they are no longer able to do so.

29. B: Malodorous malignant wounds create a great deal of distress for patients and families and may result in a patient feeling isolated or ashamed. Suggesting and providing therapeutic options for minimizing wound odor is an important service that the palliative care nurse can provide to assist the patient in maintaining his or her dignity as death approaches. The most common cause of wound odor is colonization with anaerobic bacteria. Treatment and prevention strategies include regular wound cleaning, debridement of necrotic tissue, topical metronidazole application, and charcoal dressings or odor-absorbing charcoal in the patient's room. Topical steroids are not indicated for treatment of wound odor. Calcium alginate dressings are used to control bleeding in wounds. Systemic metronidazole use is not indicated for treatment of local wound colonization.

30. C: Patients and family members can have a wide range of adaptive and healthy coping styles, depending on their personality, past experience, and cultural factors. Caregivers of a terminally ill patient experience a great deal of stress and fatigue as they deal with the physical challenges of a progressively sicker loved one and the emotional strain of the impending death of a family member. It is important for the palliative care nurse to assess and assist the patient's caregivers in the often-monumental tasks that accompany caring for a dying loved one. Signs that may indicate unhealthy or impaired coping of a patient's caregivers include expressing almost exclusively "negative" feelings (e.g., anger), withholding information from other family members, refusing to accept assistance, focusing exclusively on their own needs, or refusing to acknowledge or accommodate differences in opinion among caregivers. The palliative care nurse who has taken the time to become familiar with the strengths and weaknesses of the patient's loved ones can often recognize impaired coping and intervene early with appropriate support and resources.

31. C: Pain is a common symptom in terminally ill patients, and many misconceptions and barriers exist that interfere with both adequate assessment and treatment of a patient's pain. Inadequate or overly narrow pain assessment tools, provider prejudices, mistrust between patient and provider, concerns about addiction to pain medication, and cultural variations in communicating pain are just some of the common barriers to adequate pain treatment. Patients may underreport pain for a variety of reasons, such as attempting to avoid side effects of pain medication, concern about hastening death, or family expectations about stoicism in the face of pain. It is important for providers to review the difference between psychological dependence and physical dependence on pain medications if a patient or family member voices concern about drug addiction in the context of analgesic therapy.

32. B: It is important for the palliative care nurse to be familiar with organizational positions and guidelines surrounding common end-of-life issues. The American Nurses Association (ANA) position on artificial hydration and nutrition in the terminally ill patient states that decisions to forgo artificial hydration or nutrition in association with end-of-life care should be made by the patient and the health care team. Artificial (nonoral) hydration is considered a medical intervention in the United States, and its use can, therefore, be refused if the patient or care team feels its burdens outweigh the benefits. Dehydration is not typically associated with pain or discomfort in the dying patient. The position of the ANA on active euthanasia and assisted suicide states that it is in conflict with the ethical and professional traditions and goals of a nurse to participate in either active euthanasia or assisted suicide. This may evolve as states pass legislation that allows terminally ill patients to pursue medications administered with the express purpose of hastening death.

33. A: Caring for patients with terminal illness and their families through the dying process inevitably elicits strong emotional responses in the palliative care nurse. Palliative care nurses become intimately involved with patients and their families and deal with the loss of patient after patient as his or her professional experience grows. Just as patients and families experience nonlinear progression through the grieving and adaptation process, so do palliative care nurses. One model of hospice nurse adjustment (formulated by Bernice Harper) describes five progressive stages: intellectualization, emotional survival, depression, emotional arrival, and deep compassion. Hospice nurses must have both institutional and individual support systems and strategies in place to engage effectively in self-care and to provide the best care for their patients.

34. A: Constipation is an unpleasant and common symptom in the palliative care patient, and the etiology is often multifactorial. It is important for the palliative care nurse to anticipate and regularly screen for constipation in the terminally ill patient. Constipation can cause abdominal or rectal pain, leakage of liquid stool, urinary retention, and agitation. Common contributing factors to constipation in the hospice patient include medications (especially opiates), reduced mobility, reduced fluid intake, mechanical obstruction because of tumor or spinal cord compression, and metabolic derangements (e.g., hypercalcemia or hypokalemia). *Clostridioides difficile* infection typically causes diarrhea rather than constipation.

35. D: Neuropathic pain is not particularly well understood and is difficult to treat. Neuropathic pain does not respond to nonsteroidal anti-inflammatory drugs or opiate medications as reliably as other types of pain. The drug treatment of choice for neuropathic pain is antidepressant medication, generally tricyclics (e.g., amitriptyline) or selective serotonin reuptake inhibitors (e.g., paroxetine). Onset of analgesic effects with tricyclic antidepressants is generally within 3-4 days of beginning the medication, as opposed to the several weeks it typically takes for depressive symptom relief. Adverse effects frequently occur with use of tricyclic antidepressants. Tricyclic antidepressants are not indicated or effective for non-neuropathic pain (aside from so-called "psychic pain") in the palliative care patient.

36. C: Interdisciplinary palliative care teams ensure that providers from multiple specialties (e.g., physician, social worker, nurse, chaplain) can collaborate with the patient and family to craft a care plan that meets the needs and goals of the patient. Care is directed primarily by the patient. Ideally, the team provides information and elicits patient values, preferences, and goals as they pertain to end-of-life care. Once this is completed, specific challenges can be identified and possible solutions planned. Interventions are then provided for the patient and family in accordance with the formulated plan. Reassessments and changes in the care plan are made as illness progresses or preferences or goals change.

37. D: Bowel obstruction in the hospice patient is most commonly seen in the patient with ovarian or bowel cancer due to primary tumor or peritoneal metastasis. Bowel obstruction typically presents with abdominal pain and vomiting. Treatment may consist primarily of palliative symptom management with antiemetics and pain medications. Antisecretory medications or promotility agents may be helpful for symptom management in some patients. If the patient wishes to pursue more aggressive treatment, it may be appropriate to provide intravenous hydration, nasogastric tube placement, gastrostomy placement, or surgical intervention.

38. C: Many patients with terminal illness explore and pursue complementary and alternative therapies to treat either their primary disease or side effects associated with treatment. Nausea and vomiting are very disruptive and unpleasant for most patients, and may be difficult to manage, particularly when medications being used to treat other symptoms (e.g., pain) contribute to nausea and vomiting. Acupuncture is one of the alternative medicine therapies, in addition to massage, progressive muscle relaxation, and meditation, that has been shown to be effective in managing nausea and vomiting in patients with chronic illnesses. Although some complementary and alternative therapies are not proven to help with symptoms, the only good reason to discourage a palliative care patient from exploring other therapeutic modalities is if the therapy is either unsafe or interacts negatively with other treatment the patient is receiving.

39. D: Dyspnea (shortness of breath) is a common and distressing symptom in terminally ill patients, particularly patients with chronic obstructive pulmonary disease, heart failure, respiratory muscle weakness, or pulmonary pathology from cancer. General supportive measures for treatment of dyspnea include upright positioning, placement near an open window or fan, relaxation techniques, and supplemental oxygen administration. The drug treatment of choice for treating persistent dyspnea is opiates. Depending on the etiology and progression of dyspnea, benzodiazepines, glycopyrrolate, steroids, diuretics, or bronchodilators may also be helpful.

40. A: Pain is a multifactorial sensation, encompassing physiologic and sensory components in addition to psychological, spiritual, and social components. Ideally, the palliative care nurse makes use of a valid and consistent multidimensional pain assessment tool. The factors described by this patient encompass physiologic and sensory components of her pain, such as quality, location, duration, intensity, and alleviating or aggravating factors. A description encompassing psychological or affective aspects of pain may include a report of the patient's emotional experience with regard to the pain, particular ways in which the patient expresses pain, and the impact of the pain on the patient's mood. Sociocultural aspects of pain that may be assessed include impact of the pain on the patient's role in his or her family, job, and cultural community.

41. B: It is critically important for palliative care nurses to be aware of the relative potencies of different opiate medications and to understand how to calculate equianalgesic doses of opioids when changing from one opiate medication to another. There are readily available conversion charts for the palliative care nurse to consult when calculating the appropriate dosage of a new opioid. Administration route also needs to be taken into account when calculating drug dosages. The palliative care nurse may be converting the same medication from one route to another (e.g., parenteral to oral), may be changing the drug without changing the route of administration (e.g., parenteral hydromorphone replacing parenteral morphine), or may be changing both the medication and the route (e.g., parenteral morphine to oral hydrocodone). Hydromorphone is more potent than morphine. A 1.5 mg dose of parenteral hydromorphone is equianalgesic to a 10 mg dose of parenteral morphine.

42. B: The Medicare hospice benefit provides for four different levels of hospice care, depending on the needs of the terminally ill patient. Routine home care (most common) is provided wherever the patient lives (e.g., private home, long-term care facility). Respite care consists of up to 5 consecutive days of inpatient hospice care to provide relief to a family caregiver. General inpatient hospice care is provided for the patient whose home environment is no longer a safe environment or the patient who is having intractable symptoms that are unmanageable in the home setting. Finally, continuous home care is available for patients who would like to remain in their homes but are having symptoms that would otherwise require inpatient hospice care. In this case, inpatient hospice care is essentially brought to the patient in their home setting.

43. D: An important component of palliative nursing, particularly if a patient will remain in a home setting, is education of caregivers. Depending on the clinical situation, caregivers may need to learn when and how to administer medications, wound care, patient movement and positioning techniques, and symptoms that commonly develop as the patient nears death. Although the coping skills and cognitive abilities of patient caregivers vary, a very effective technique for solidifying caregiver learning and allowing the nurse to assess the learning is to have the caregiver demonstrate what they have been taught. With turning and positioning maneuvers taught for pressure ulcer prevention, it is most helpful for the caregiver to demonstrate the learned maneuvers with the actual patient.

44. B: There are many different forms of complementary and alternative medicine that palliative care patients may choose to explore at different stages of their illness. These may include Chinese herbs, homeopathy, hypnosis, specialized diets, biofeedback, massage, guided imagery, naturopathy, vitamin supplements, meditation, art and music therapy, chiropractic manipulation, acupuncture, and energy therapies. Therapeutic touch refers to the use of touch, while healing and positive energy is directed to the patient. Yoga involves body poses and breathing techniques to facilitate relaxation and healing. Reflexology involves stimulation of areas of the hands, feet, and ears, which are believed to correspond to different body parts and organ systems. It is helpful for the palliative care nurses to familiarize themselves with complementary therapies that patients may be interested in using.

45. D: Although tricyclic antidepressants are one of the few therapies that may be effective for treatment of neuropathic pain, they have a high incidence of adverse effects. Anticholinergic effects are common, and include dry mouth, urinary retention, tachycardia, delirium, and constipation. Other adverse effects associated with tricyclic antidepressant use include cardiac arrhythmias, sedation, weight gain, sweating, and sexual dysfunction. Patients may be unwilling to continue taking these medications if adverse effects are more distressing than the symptoms for which they are being used to treat.

46. C: Heart failure results in fluid overload, leading to pulmonary edema, hepatic congestion, and peripheral edema. Dyspnea is a common symptom, primarily from pulmonary edema. Patients with severe heart failure also commonly have pain (i.e., chest, extremity or abdominal pain from ischemia and congestion), dysrhythmias, fatigue, sexual dysfunction, anorexia, and depression. Treatment and palliation for symptoms of heart failure may include oxygen, antiarrhythmics, antidepressants, and analgesic medication. Diuretics are commonly administered to manage symptoms that are caused by fluid overload, including pulmonary edema. Dyspnea often improves when patients with heart failure are treated with diuretics, because pulmonary fluid overload is decreased.

47. D: Feelings of sadness and anxiety are normal and appropriate reactions in response to a grave prognosis. Normal adjustment reactions and grief can be difficult to differentiate from depression and anxiety disorders. In general, normal grieving and depression are differentiated by the severity and duration of symptoms, as well as by the degree to which symptoms are interfering with other aspects of the patient's life or relationships. Features that are expected with normal grief include sadness, anger, worry, fear, and potentially some degree of temporary social withdrawal. Features that would be more concerning for a psychiatric diagnosis, such as depression or anxiety, include hopelessness, suicidal ideation, and poor self-image. The palliative care nurse should continue to support and assess a patient through the grieving process so that the patient can be further evaluated or treated with counseling or psychiatric medication as needed.

48. B: Myoclonic jerks are sudden, brief, and uncontrollable movements. They most commonly occur in an extremity. Myoclonus can be very distressing to the palliative care patient and family members and may be uncomfortable or exhausting. Myoclonus is most commonly caused by opiate medications in the palliative care patient. Generally, myoclonus is considered a sign of opiate toxicity and is an indication for changing to a different opiate medication. Providers may also use opiate antagonists, such as naloxone, for acute treatment of myoclonus. Changing to a different opiate often results in resolution of myoclonus. Benzodiazepines and antispasmodics are used for treatment of myoclonus in some patients.

49. D: Noisy breathing is very common in the dying patient, and generally indicates that death is imminent (within hours). Although most patients who have the "death rattle" have a diminished level of consciousness and are not distressed by the respiratory congestion, it can be quite distressing to loved ones when a patient's respirations are loud and appear labored. The "death rattle" is due to pooling of oral and respiratory secretions in the pharynx and upper airways as the airway protective reflexes diminish. If the patient or family desires treatment, the first-line treatment is anticholinergic medications, such as scopolamine, atropine, and glycopyrrolate. This often diminishes the volume of secretions. Repositioning the patient may also improve symptoms. Suctioning can be uncomfortable and lead to patient agitation and is, therefore, not generally recommended unless the patient is essentially comatose.

50. B: Hypercalcemia is an urgent and serious complication of late-stage malignancy (unrelated to bone metastases) with a significant mortality rate if untreated. Hypercalcemia most commonly occurs in the setting of breast cancer and multiple myeloma but may occur with other malignancies as well. Symptoms of hypercalcemia can be somewhat nonspecific and include gastrointestinal symptoms (e.g., nausea, vomiting, constipation, anorexia), neurologic symptoms (e.g., weakness, mental status changes, fatigue), and cardiac symptoms (e.g., bradycardia, electrocardiogram changes). Treatment, if in keeping with the goals of the palliative care patient, includes intravenous hydration for correction of dehydration, calcitonin (inhibits bone resorption and facilitates calcium excretion), and bisphosphonates. Bisphosphonates are very effective at inhibiting bone resorption and reducing serum calcium levels, but their calcium-lowering effects are delayed until about 48 hours after administration.

51. D: Patients with some types of cancer complain of a very bad taste in the mouth, but some strategies may help increase input:

- Avoid highly spiced foods.
- Avoid hot foods and avoid being in the kitchen when food is prepared if possible.
- Rinse the mouth with a salt and soda mixture before eating.
- Use a straw to drink liquids to minimize contact with taste buds.
- Drink very cold liquids and eat cold or room temperature food instead of hot.

52. B: Fecal impaction occurs when the hard stool moves into the rectum and becomes a large, dense, immovable mass that cannot be evacuated even with straining, usually as a result of chronic constipation. In addition to abdominal cramps and distention, the person may feel intense rectal pressure and pain accompanied by a sense of urgency to defecate. Nausea and vomiting may also occur. Hemorrhoids will often become engorged. Fecal incontinence, with liquid stool leaking around the impaction, is common. An impaction may cause pressure on the bladder neck, obstructing urinary flow, resulting in overflow incontinence.

53. A: Visceral pain frequently requires opioids to control it, although in early stages of disease when pain is less severe, patients may respond to NSAIDs. Neuropathic pain often responds poorly to opioids and is better treated with antidepressants, anticonvulsants, and/or benzodiazepines. Somatic pain may be treated with various drugs, including steroids, NSAIDs, muscle relaxants, and bisphosphonates. Psychological pain is usually treated with psychiatric treatment that may or may not include the use of psychotropic drugs.

54. C: "Caregiving is very difficult and exhausting" reflects back what the daughter is saying about the demands for care without being judgmental and/or making her feel guilty. In fact, caregivers often feel some relief mixed with grief when a family member has died because the constant anxiety of anticipating death and providing care is extremely stressful, and reassuring the daughter that her feelings are normal can help to alleviate any guilt she might feel.

55. A: When initiating a delicate discussion about ending treatment, the best approach is to be direct but avoid trying to influence the decision directly: "Do you want to continue dialysis?" The nurse should avoid statements that suggest there is "nothing more we can do" or "we have exhausted all remedies" but should stress the things that can be done, such as providing adequate medication for pain relief and positioning the patient for comfort. Pointing out that a treatment is "prolonging" suffering may make family members feel guilty and distressed.

56. B: Federal law requires that family decision makers be asked about organ donations when patients die in the hospital if there is no advance directive outlining the patient's wishes. In many cases, patients are provided information about organ donation on admission to the hospital. Staff is not legally required to ask about donations if a patient dies at home because organs are often not viable and the deceased may be taken directly to a funeral home. The spouse is usually the family decision maker; if there is no spouse but multiple children, conflicts can arise.

57. D: Three tests are used to assess for the presence of xerostomia:

- Cracker test: The patient is given a dry cracker to eat. If the patient is unable to chew and swallow the cracker without drinking liquid, then the test is positive.
- Tongue blade test: A tongue blade is placed flat on a patient's tongue. Because xerostomia results in pasty thickened saliva, if the tongue blade sticks to the tongue, the test is positive.
- Measurement of saliva (stimulated or unstimulated): Mouth is swabbed or patient spits repeatedly into a container for a set amount of time.

58. C: The best approach is to prepare the daughter with, "Let's talk about what to expect and what to do," because people are often fearful about death, especially if they are unsure what to expect. Death is not always predictable, so assuring the daughter that the hospice nurse will be with her or that she can transfer her father to the hospital is not truthful. The nurse should avoid platitudes, such as "I'm sure you'll be fine," because that doesn't address the daughter's concerns and is not helpful.

59. B: Antihypertensives and other drugs that do not directly contribute to patient comfort are usually discontinued in the final days. These include diuretics, antibiotics, hormones, antidysrhythmics, hypoglycemic agents, and laxatives. Medications that are usually continued as long as possible include sedatives and analgesics. When indicated to control symptoms, other medications that are continued include antipyretics, antiemetics, anticholinergics, and anticonvulsants. Oral medications can be continued as long as a patient can swallow, often in liquid form rather than pills or capsules. Other medications may be administered parenterally.

60. D: Because the patient remains conscious and adverse effects of abrupt discontinuation of corticosteroids can be severe, the medication should be discontinued after tapering. Corticosteroids are commonly given to patients with brain tumors to reduce cerebral edema and intracranial pressure in order to control pain and seizures; therefore, as the corticosteroid dose is tapered, the dosage of anticonvulsant should be increased as the risk of seizures will increase. Analgesia may also need to be increased because the patient may experience more headaches.

61. B: All of these are indications that the patient is nearing death, but lack of radial pulse indicates that the death is likely to occur within a few hours because the strength of cardiac compressions has lessened considerably. As patients with cardiorespiratory disease near death, the pulse rate often doubles and dysrhythmias occur, as well as decreased strength of compressions. Cyanosis may be evident in nail beds, knees, and tip of nose. Mottling of the extremities usually begins to occur within a few days of death.

62. C: As patients near death, they are unable to cough to clear secretions that begin to pool in the oropharynx and bronchi, resulting in rales, usually referred to as "death rattles." Because the sound is often distressing to family members, an anticholinergic, such as glycopyrrolate or atropine, may be given subcutaneously to relieve respiratory distress. A hyoscine hydrobromide transdermal patch is also available, but action is slower, 12 hours compared with 1 minute for injections. Elevating the head of the bed or turning the patient to the side may also relieve rattling.

63. A: Palliative care should be provided to patients with life-threatening diseases throughout the disease process and continuum of care because patients need support and adequate pain management even in earlier stages of disease. Palliative care can provide emotional and spiritual support to help patients during curative treatments and to prepare the patient and family members for the inevitable decline in health and help them to make decisions and plan for the type of supportive care that best fits their wishes.

64. D: Under the Medicare benefit, caregivers are allowed respite care periodically. Respite care is in-patient care for a period of not more than 5 days, usually in a long-term care facility or hospice facility. In this case, the husband can be provided care to allow his caregiver time to rest and decide on other options, such as hiring an assistant if finances allow. Providing daily nursing visits does little to relieve the time-consuming work of caregiving.

65. C: The CMS regulations regarding the Medicare Hospice Benefit include the requirement that an interdisciplinary team providing hospice care must include at least a physician, nurse, counselor, and social worker, but this does not preclude members from additional medical specialties, such as a nutritionist or occupational therapist. The interdisciplinary team should meet regularly to discuss patient needs and should have easy access to data, such as laboratory studies, to help plan patient care. The use of good communication strategies among team members is critical.

66. D: Byock and Merriman's end-of-life construct includes 6 dimensions, all of which apply to both patient and caregiver:

- Well-being: Subjective feelings about condition and emotions, including anxiety, fear, readiness, and acceptance.
- Physical: Comfort level and physical distress.
- Function: Ability to carry out activities of daily living (ADL).

- Interpersonal: Degree and quality of relationships and changes resulting from caregiving.
- Transcendent: Perception of meaning of life, as well as spiritual and/or religious values.

A change in one dimension will have an effect on the other dimensions, for example, an increase in pain may result in decreased ability to function, increased fear and anxiety, stress on relationships, and spiritual conflict.

67. A: One of the tasks associated with accepting the finality of life is emotional withdrawal (decathexis). Other tasks include accepting the need for dependency and acknowledging and expressing feelings of personal loss and impending death. Another landmark is recognition of a "new" self, which includes accepting a new personal definition of self and recognizing that the new self has value. Finding a sense of personal meaning for life includes completing a life review and sharing stories and information with others. Experiencing personal love of self includes being able to forgive and acknowledge oneself.

68. B: While listening to the patient's life review strengthens the personal relationship between the patient and the caregiver, it does not necessarily imply acceptance of the finality of life. As caregivers begin to accept that death is inevitable and final, they may begin to experience anticipatory grief not only for the loss of the patient but also other losses that may ensue, such as loss of financial support and social relationships. Caregivers may be able to articulate personal loss and still be able to tell the patient that it is all right to let go and die.

69. B: Stage II, emotional survival. Stages of adaptation:

- Stage I, Intellectualism (0-3 months): Focus on intellectualism and may feel anxiety while learning policies and procedures and experience superficial acceptance.
- Stage II, Emotional survival (3-6 months): May overidentify with patient's situation and experience increasing discomfort, guilt, and sadness but have increasing emotional involvement.
- Stage III, Depression (6-9 months): Less intellectualism but more grief, discomfort, and depression, overidentifying with the patient personally.
- Stage IV, Emotional arrival (9-12 months): Interactions with patient/family healthy and productive and effectively coping with loss.
- Stage V, Deep compassion (1-2 years): Acceptance of death/loss and able to express compassion and provide care with respect and dignity.

70. C: "I'm so sorry you had to experience discomfort" acknowledges the patient's concern and expresses empathy and support without making excuses or placing blame on the patient or the technician. Patients who are coming to terms with a life-threatening illness often exhibit emotional lability and may experience profound, undifferentiated anger, lashing out at others. They may take this anger out on family members and care providers, overreacting and sometimes fixating on what they consider ill treatment.

71. B: A normal response to grief is to cry, but crying uncontrollably or not at all is often an indication of depression. With normal grief, people experience loss recurrently and may be preoccupied with loss and experience emotional lability, openly expressing anger. They have difficulty sleeping and have vivid, distressing dreams. They may have a loss of energy and mild, weight loss. Depression tends to persist with people in a constant state of unhappiness. Insomnia or hypersomnia without dreaming is common as are extreme lack of energy and pronounced weight loss. People may isolate themselves and show little emotion.

72. B: "It must be very difficult to believe what is happening to your husband" provides support to the caregiver without directly challenging the person's need to utilize denial to deal with the loss. Denial is very common, both for patients and caregivers. Some patients, for example, resist having laboratory or radiographic studies done because they do not want to know the results. Caregivers may express frustration with patients who aren't "trying" hard enough or may try to force patients to eat or take treatments.

73. D: The best response is, "Tell me why you feel you want to die now," because this encourages the patient to express his feelings without being judgmental or citing legal issues. Many patients who want to die feel that way because of uncontrolled pain or other symptoms or unresolved issues, such as depression. If the nurse can find out what is motivating the patient to consider suicide, then the nurse can often help to find a better solution.

74. A: Children in the preoperational stage (ages 2-7) often develop magical thinking, believing that something they have said or done can cause harm or illness to someone, especially if the children have said "I hate you" or "I wish you were dead," because they believe that their words have power of creation. Young children may fear being abandoned. Adolescents may express anger and become withdrawn and uncooperative. They may have difficulty concentrating, so grades may suffer.

75. B: When making a death pronouncement, the nurse should always first acknowledge the family and introduce himself/herself. The nurse should always check the patient for heart sounds and breath sounds even though the patient may appear deceased. Once the nurse is assured the patient is, in fact, deceased, then the nurse should confirm the death with family members and express condolences. The nurse should ask the next of kin (usually spouse or child) about autopsy and organ donation (if appropriate) and which funeral home to contact. The nurse should notify the physician of the patient's death.

76. D: Patients with advanced disease often become exhausted from treatments, adverse effects, and emotional ups and downs, leading to depression. Patients who are severely depressed should always be assessed for suicidal ideation by directly asking them if they have considered hurting themselves and if they have a plan. While acceptance of inevitable death is a normal progression, wanting to die because of depression is different from acceptance. Depressed patients may need referral for counseling and may benefit from antidepressants.

77. C: A strong religious faith often provides comfort to surviving family members and helps them cope with grief. Risk factors for complicated bereavement include a history of substance abuse or mental illness, recent loss of another family member or close friend or associate, concurrent crisis, severe anxiety or anger, concurrent illnesses, difficult death, absence of religious/spiritual belief, lack of adequate support system, and anticipated problems, such as change in economic status. Age may also be a factor, especially with surviving children.

78. B: "What positive memory do you have of raising your children" encourages the woman to think differently about her experience as a mother and can lead to a discussion of what she felt she had done right and wrong. Later in the discussion, the nurse might ask the patient to imagine what she might have done differently, although this may be a painful question for some. Platitudes, such as "I'm sure you did the best you could," are not helpful. Patient's concerns should never be dismissed with statements like, "That's not important now."

79. D: Nurses should not stereotype people based on appearance. Concerns about diversion should center on the patient. Indications include a sudden change in response to pain medications that had been controlling pain well and a difference in the appearance of pain medications (size, shape, color). Patients may also have a pattern of more analgesia use with some caregivers than others, suggesting that records may be falsified. Caregivers who are diverting drugs often begin to isolate patients, refusing home care and missing doctor's appointments.

80. A: Both Islam and Orthodox Judaism consider embalming a desecration of the body. Hindus and Buddhists are usually cremated and have no need for embalming. There is, in fact, no valid health and safety reason for embalming, and it is rarely practiced outside of the United States and Canada. If burial is to be delayed, then the body must be kept refrigerated if it is not embalmed. No state requires embalming (although 3 states require embalming if bodies are transported across state lines), and funeral directors must advise clients of this.

81. B: Because the patient is taking frequent pain pills and is forgetful, probably the best solution is to switch to a fentanyl patch because it will maintain a stable level of pain control and only needs to be changed every 3 days. However, it may take 2-3 days after initial application of the patch to reach the maximum level of pain control, so the patient may need to supplement with oral tablets. After that, the tablets may be used for breakthrough pain.

82. D: Because the patient's medication dosage has been increased, one can assume a comprehensive pain assessment was done initially, so at this time the only necessary assessment is of the intensity of pain with the 0-10 scale, with 0 indicating no pain and 10 the worst possible pain, in order to evaluate the patient's response to the dosage change. Alternate intensity scales may be used for young children or nonresponsive or confused older children or adults.

83. A: The 5 key elements of pain assessment include the following:

- Words: Used to describe pain, such as burning, stabbing, deep, shooting, and sharp. Some may complain of pressure, squeezing, and discomfort rather than pain.
- Intensity: Use of 0-10 scale or other appropriate scale to quantify the degree of pain.
- Location: Where patient indicates pain.
- Duration: Constant or comes and goes, breakthrough pain.
- Aggravating/Alleviating factors: Those things that increase the intensity of pain and those that relieve the pain.

84. A: Visceral pain may occur with ascites, bowel obstruction, and hepatic cancer, and is often poorly localized and described as cramping, distention ("bloated"), deep, squeezing, and stretching. Neuropathic pain may occur with postherpetic neuralgia and diabetic neuropathy, and is described as burning, shooting, and numb or pins and needles. Somatic pain may occur from bone metastases, fractures, and arthritis, and tends to be localized and described as dull, aching, throbbing, and sore. Psychological pain related to psychological disorders is often described as affecting the entire body.

85. B: Because the patient is able to keep a record of pain medications, the patient is probably not confused or giving the medication to someone else. However, patients are often reluctant to admit the degree of pain and minimize their discomfort when asked about their pain, so it is important to determine how much pain medication the patient is actually taking and to observe the patient's behavior for indications of pain. Some patients may believe that having pain indicates their condition is poor and persist in saying they have little pain despite obvious evidence otherwise.

86. A: When the hospice movement first began, there were fewer choices for analgesia, and the use of morphine or "morphine cocktails" to control pain was common, so older patients often associate morphine with dying and are afraid that taking morphine means they are near death. The best response is to educate the patient about the different medications, but patients should be provided alternative medications if they feel strongly about taking morphine because taking it might increase their stress.

87. D: CHEOPS (Children's Hospital of Eastern Ontario Pain Scale) is used for children 1-7 and based on scores of 6 different characteristics (crying, facial expression, verbalization, torso, upper extremities, lower extremities) with scores of 0-2, except for crying, which is scored 0-3. A score more than 4 indicates pain. FACES (Wong-Baker): Facial expression scale for children older than 7. CRIES: Assesses crying, requirement for O_2 or SaO_2 less than 95%, increased vital signs (blood pressure and heart rate), expression, and sleep to evaluate pain in neonates and infants 6 months and younger. The 0-10 pain intensity scale is used with adolescents and adults.

88. B: While it seems logical that soothing music, such as classical music or New Age music, may be the most calming and relaxing, patient preference is more important because people react very differently to music. Playing a patient's favorite music can be very comforting and may help patients focus attention away from their pain or their situation. Dimming the lights and providing a quiet environment for music therapy help to relax the patient as well.

89. D: Midazolam 0.5-6.0 mg per hour intravenously (IV) is used for terminal/palliative sedation for patients who are highly agitated and in severe, uncontrolled pain. Midazolam is a very short-acting benzodiazepine with action beginning within 5 minutes and peaking at 20-60 minutes. Propofol, another IV agent, is also used, with starting does of 0.25 mg/kg/hr. Terminal sedation is indicated for patients when other medications and therapies have been unable to control their refractory symptoms.

90. D: Naloxone is a reversal agent (opiate antagonist) used for opioid narcotics, such as morphine. Patients must be monitored for hypertension and pulmonary edema after administration, and because the half-life is only approximately 20 minutes, repeat doses may be needed. Flumazenil is a reversal agent for benzodiazepines. N-acetylcysteine is a reversal agent for acetaminophen. Neostigmine is a reversal agent for nondepolarizing muscle relaxants. Reversal agents should always be available when patients are receiving high doses of opioids or benzodiazepines.

91. C: Ondansetron: Indicated for chemotherapy- and abdominal radiation–induced nausea and vomiting. It works well for both geriatric and pediatric patients. Dexamethasone may be given concurrently to potentiate effects. Haloperidol: Indicated for opioid-induced nausea as well as chemical- and mechanical-induced nausea, but can result in dyskinesia, although adverse effects are lessened with low doses. Scopolamine: Indicated for nausea and vomiting associated with intestinal obstruction, peritoneal irritation, and increased intracranial pressure. Dronabinol: Used as a second-line antiemetic, but more effective in young adults.

92. D: Corticosteroids, such as prednisone or dexamethasone, are used as adjuvant analgesics to relieve pain associated with spinal cord compression, cerebral edema, and bone pain, as well as visceral and neuropathic pain. Corticosteroids have anti-inflammatory effects that reduce swelling and inflammation. Prednisone may be given in doses of 15-30 mg three to four times daily. Dexamethasone is less likely to result in Cushing syndrome than prednisone. Dexamethasone may be given orally at 2-20 mg/day or IV (up to 100 mg bolus) for severe pain crisis.

93. A: Eutectic Mixture of Local Anesthetics (EMLA) cream provides good pain control. The skin is first cleansed and then the cream is applied thickly (1/4 inch), extending about 1/2 inch past the port to the peri-port tissue. The cream is then covered with plastic wrap, which is secured and left in place for about 20 minutes. The wrapped time may be extended to 45-60 minutes if necessary to completely numb the tissue. The tissue should remain numb for about 1 hour after the plastic wrap is removed, allowing time for the IV needle to be inserted and treatment begun.

94. C: With administration of ketamine, opioid dosage should be reduced by 50% because ketamine is a very strong analgesic at low doses. However, ketamine often causes hallucinations or nightmares, so lorazepam or diazepam (and sometimes haloperidol) is usually given as well, especially with moribund patients who may not be able to indicate that they are having hallucinations. Some people also have increased secretions and may need to receive an anticholinergic, such as glycopyrrolate or scopolamine, as well.

95. C: Physical dependence: Abrupt cessation of a drug and decrease in blood serum levels leads to withdrawal symptoms, which may vary depending on the type of drug. Addiction is a neurobiological disorder that includes lack of control over drug use, compulsive use of drugs, and continued craving for drugs despite negative effects. Tolerance is an adaptation in which a drug's effect diminishes over time so that an increased dose is needed to achieve the same effect. Pseudoaddiction is the mistaken belief that someone who is seeking drugs for pain is instead suffering from addiction.

96. A: Fentanyl patches may cause skin irritation, so it is important to rotate sites when reapplying the patches. Some patients find that spraying the skin with a steroid used for inhalation therapy prevents the skin reaction. The spray dries and does not leave residue that interferes with adherence or absorption. Powders, creams, ointments, and skin barriers cannot be used under the patches. If irritation persists, then patients may need to change to another form of analgesic.

97. B: Morphine 10 mg is equianalgesic to hydromorphone 1.5 mg. Hydromorphone (Dilaudid) is a hydrogenated ketone derivative of morphine. It is more highly lipid soluble than morphine and crosses the blood-brain barrier more readily, so it is faster acting than morphine and stronger (about 8 times). It has potent antitussive qualities. It produces less histamine release, nausea, and vomiting than morphine, so it is a good alternative if patients have an allergic response to morphine.

98. C: Complementary therapies are used in conjunction with conventional medical treatments, usually to help reduce pain, nausea, and anxiety, and to improve the quality of life. Complementary therapies encompass a wide variety of therapies, including aromatherapy, music therapy, acupuncture, massage, yoga, biofeedback, and hypnosis. Alternative therapies, on the other hand, are used in place of conventional medical treatments, usually to the patient's detriment. Alternative therapies include cancer-cure diets, oxygen therapy, and biomagnetic therapy, none of which have been demonstrated to actually work.

99. B: People who practice homeopathy believe that healing must occur from the inside and that they can use small doses of plants or minerals to promote healing by causing similar symptoms to the ones being treated ("like cures like"). Homeopathy prescribes specific substances for different diseases, depending on the patient's physical and emotional condition. The treatment usually does not include active ingredients found in medications, so the treatments rarely interfere with other medical treatment, although some people choose to use homeopathic treatment rather than traditional medication, and this can put the patient at risk.

100. A: Asian cultures tend to value stoicism, so Asian patients may not express pain with moaning or complaints, so the nurse cannot always use behavior as a guide when assessing a patient's degree of pain. Northern Europeans also tend to be fairly stoic. Hispanic, Middle Eastern, and southern European/Mediterranean cultures tend to be more expressive, meaning that in some instances, their behavior may indicate pain is more severe than it actually is. While generalizations about culture may hold true for a culture as a whole, it is important to remember that they cannot necessarily be applied to a given individual in that culture. The nurse's responsibility is to treat the pain as the patient describes or expresses it.

101. A: This type of breakthrough pain is end-of-dose failure because the medication has peaked and the blood level is decreasing. A pain diary can help to establish the pattern of end-of-dose failure. The best solution is to either increase the dosage, usually by 25% to 50%, or to change the patch more frequently, such as every 48 hours. Increasing the use of oral opioids for the last 24 hours is not a good solution because the patient's pain is not being adequately controlled.

102. C: Incident pain follows a predictable pattern in that it occurs repeatedly with the same activity; therefore, the best solution is for the patient to take a rapid-onset, short-acting analgesic before attending the meeting. The pain medication can be titrated based on the patient's experience until the patient can carry out the activity with relative comfort. Oral transmucosal fentanyl citrate (OTFC) is often used for incident pain because the patient can take the medication easily and it works rapidly.

103. B: An abrupt change in behavior in a patient with end-stage dementia often means the patient is experiencing discomfort of some kind, so the nurse's initial intervention should be to try to determine the cause of discomfort, which may be related to constrictive clothing, pain, constipation, urinary retention, or urinary infection. Chemical restraints should be avoided, but a mild analgesic, such as acetaminophen, may be administered, and patients may benefit from a quiet environment with less stimulation if no cause for discomfort is identified.

104. A: SIADH is related to hypersecretion of the posterior pituitary gland, causing the kidneys to reabsorb fluids, resulting in fluid retention and a decrease in sodium levels (dilutional hyponatremia) but with production of only concentrated urine. SIADH may result from central nervous systems disorders, such as brain trauma, surgery, or tumors, as well as tumors of various organs, pneumothorax, acute pneumonia, other lung disorders, and some medications. Symptoms include the following:

- Anorexia with nausea and vomiting.
- Irritability.
- Stomach cramps.
- Alterations of personality.
- Increasing neurological dysfunction, including stupor and seizures, related to progressive sodium depletion.

105. C: As soon as possible after a patient dies, the nurse should gently apply downward pressure on the eyelids to close them. *Rigor mortis* begins in small muscles, so the eyes may remain open if the eyelids are not closed soon after death. This can be disconcerting to family members. The mouth should not be tied closed, although a rolled towel may be placed under the chin to attempt to close the mouth. Dentures should not be placed in the mouth, as loose dentures can easily be lost. Dentures should be sent to the funeral home with the deceased.

106. B: It is important to ask patients directly about their needs, and patients may be more willing to discuss needs if the nurse acknowledges directly that a patient has received bad news, rather than talking around the subject or asking open-ended questions, such as "Do you need anything?" The nurse should stay focused on the patients and their needs and feelings rather than personal feelings, "I feel terrible for you." The nurse can also offer suggestions, "Some patients have needed..."

107. D: Independent decision-making is not a primary benefit of working with an interdisciplinary team because important decisions should be reached by group consensus, although even in groups, some independent decisions, such as when a patient requires pain medication, are reached by an individual. Working in an interdisciplinary group allows people to learn from each other because members have different expertise, and this aids in problem-solving. Additionally, the group can serve as a support system for the members.

108. B: Most patients are able to easily tolerate infusion of subcutaneous fluids per hypodermoclysis at the rate of 100 mL/hr. If this absorbs readily, then the rate may be increased. Up to about 1500 mL can usually be instilled at one site. Hypodermoclysis is usually administered to tissue of the abdomen or anterior or lateral thighs. Patients should be monitored for pain. Complications can include infection, tissue sloughing with over-infusion, third spacing, and local irritation and bleeding.

109. D: Dehydration at the end of life results in effects on all systems, including the pulmonary system. As airways dry, secretions lessen, and the ability to cough is reduced. The death rattle also begins to lessen. Patients exhibit less wheezing and dyspnea. Rehydration, on the other hand, makes suctioning easier and allows for more productive cough, although as patients weaken, their ability to cough decreases and fluids begin to pool, resulting in the death rattle.

110. C: A right hemisphere stroke usually does not interfere with language skills, so the nurse should speak normally. A right hemisphere stroke results in left paralysis or paresis and a left visual field deficit that may cause spatial and perceptual disturbances, so patients may have difficulty judging distance. Fine motor skills may be impacted, resulting in trouble dressing or handling tools. People may become impulsive and exhibit poor judgment, often denying impairment. Left-sided neglect (lack of perception of things on the left side) may occur. Depression is common as well as short-term memory loss and difficulty following directions.

111. A: Oral phase: Patient has difficulty chewing and swallowing and tends to drool liquids and food and has food remaining in the mouth after finishing the meal. Pharyngeal phase: Patient chokes while swallowing and often regurgitates food into the nose during the meal or immediately afterward. Breath sounds and voice may be gurgling after eating because of incomplete swallowing, and patients may feel as though food is "caught in the throat." Esophageal phase: Patient has reflux and regurgitates food frequently after eating and has difficulty swallowing solid foods. Patient may complain of difficulty swallowing but rarely coughs or chokes, and may feel as though food is caught in the chest.

112. B: Variant angina (also known as Prinzmetal angina) results from spasms of the coronary arteries and can be associated with or without atherosclerotic plaques; it is often related to smoking, alcohol, or illicit stimulants. ST-segment elevation usually occurs with variant angina. Variant angina frequently occurs cyclically at the same time each day and often while the person is at rest. Nitroglycerine or calcium channel blockers are used for treatment, but beta-blockers should be avoided.

113. A: Virchow's triad comprises common risk factors for acute venous thromboembolism: blood stasis, injury to endothelium, and hypercoagulability. Some patients may be initially asymptomatic, but symptoms may include aching or throbbing pain, positive Homan's sign (pain in calf when foot is dorsiflexed), erythema and edema, dilation of vessels, and cyanosis.

114. D: Both type 1 and type 2 diabetes can result in macrovascular (atherosclerotic plaques) and microvascular (capillary) damage:

- Microvascular: Retinopathy can lead to blindness; neuropathy causes nerve damage that can lead to diabetic gastroparesis, bladder dysfunction, diabetic foot ulcers, pain, and loss of sensation. Nephropathy can lead to chronic renal failure and the need for dialysis.
- Macrovascular: Atherosclerosis of the coronary and cerebral arteries and peripheral arteries can result in peripheral vascular disease, stroke, and myocardial infarction.

115. D: Because of the severe discomfort and difficulty breathing associated with tense ascites, paracentesis is frequently used to relieve symptoms. The fluid often recurs after a paracentesis, so it is important to educate the patient and family about the importance of restricting fluids and sodium intake. No more than 6 L of fluid should be removed at one time with paracentesis. Spironolactone is the diuretic of choice, but furosemide may also be used to initiate diuresis. Patients should be advised to suck on hard candy or ice cubes to help alleviate thirst.

116. D: A patient on a mechanically altered diet needs foods that are finely ground or chopped and that require minimal chewing but can easily form an adequate cohesive bolus because the patient has limitations in chewing and poor tongue control. These foods include pasta, cottage cheese, moistened ground meats, and soft scrambled eggs. Fruits should be cooked or canned with seeds and skin removed. Foods to avoid include raw or dried fruits and vegetables, nuts, chips (taco, potato), hard rolls, waffles, and any meat that requires extensive chewing.

117. B: Xerostomia (dry mouth) is a common problem with cancer patients and may result from medications, chemotherapy, radiation, and disease processes. Pilocarpine is a nonselective muscarinic that increases saliva production, but it may result in increased perspiration, nausea, flushing, and cramping. Management includes treating cause (if possible), reviewing medications, stimulating flow of saliva, and using saliva substitutes; however, these remedies may provide only partial relief. Acupuncture treatments have increased saliva production for some patients.

118. A: Most cases of persistent hiccoughs result from gastric distention, as in this case. The initial medication treatment should be to reduce gastric distention with simethicone (15-30 mL by mouth every 4 hours) or metoclopramide (10-20 mg by mouth or intravenously every 4-6 hours). Other nonpharmacologic approaches to relieving gastric distention include fasting or induced vomiting, gastric lavage, and insertion of a nasogastric tube for decompression. Other treatments for hiccoughs include muscle relaxants, corticosteroids, dopamine agonists, anticonvulsants, calcium channel blockers, and SSRIs.

119. D: Stimulant laxatives are recommended for opioid-related constipation in the chronically ill patient. A typical protocol begins with Senokot-S (standardized senna concentrate and docusate sodium) 2 tablets at bedtime with dosage increased if no bowel movement. Bulk laxatives are used for mild constipation and may worsen constipation if fluid intake is inadequate. Osmotic laxatives are also useful for opioid-related constipation, but many patients are unable to tolerate the sweet taste or the resulting gas and distention. Saline laxatives can cause severe cramping and pain and should be used as a last resort for chronically ill patients.

120. D: Most opioids can cause pruritus, but morphine, which causes more histamine release, is more likely to cause pruritus than other opioids such as fentanyl, codeine, and oxymorphone. If itching is mild, an antihistamine given concurrently may control itching, but in some cases discontinuing the morphine and switching to another drug or rotating between morphine and another drug may be necessary. Application of cold may help relieve itching to a localized area, but heat often increases itching. Topical antipruritics, such as hydrocortisone, may relieve itching but are not practical if itching is generalized.

121. A: Of the primary breast and prostate cancers that metastasize, two-thirds metastasize first to bone. About one-third of metastasizing primary lung, thyroid, and kidney cancers metastasize to bone. If the metastasizing cancer activates osteoblasts, lytic lesions (holes) form in the bones, weakening the bones and increasing risk of fracture. If the metastasizing cancer activates osteoblasts, blastic lesions cause sclerosis of the bones, which hardens them, so blastic lesions are not as likely to cause pathological fractures as lytic lesions.

122. C: Because of headaches and altered consciousness associated with increased intracranial pressure, the best position is with the head of the bed raised to 30-45 degrees. The head and neck should be maintained in neutral position with bolsters to facilitate jugular venous return because this may help to decrease the intracranial pressure. The patient should be tilted from side to side, keeping head in neutral position, to prevent pressure sores, and good skin care should be provided.

123. D: Studies show that over a quarter of the patients with cancer experience both fatigue and depression, with each condition exacerbating the other. Other factors that may increase fatigue include anemia, especially common with patients who have received chemotherapy, have experienced bleeding, and have nutritional deficits. Fatigue may also be related to sleep disorders, especially in older adults. Other contributing factors include infection, hormonal imbalances, and electrolyte imbalances. Patients may need to modify their activities and include more rest time.

124. C: There is little that has been able to reverse anorexia/cachexia when people are in advanced stages of disease, and telling a patient she must eat to live will only add to her stress. However, some strategies can help to slow the process. Patients often do better eating small amounts every hour or two and supplementing their diet with nutritional drinks, such as Ensure, to increase calories and nutrients. The nurse should explore dietary preferences with the patient, trying to find foods that the patient feels like eating; however, this can prove challenging and may vary from day to day.

125. A: Extended-release formulas of tolterodine and oxybutynin cause mild to moderate mouth dryness, while older preparations tend to cause moderate to severe mouth dryness. For a patient who is having difficulty eating, changing medications and taking the medication at bedtime rather than in the morning can reduce mouth dryness. The patient should also be taught behavioral remedies, such as urge suppression techniques, and be advised to urinate on a timed schedule because medications alone are not always sufficient.

126. C: While the Medicare Hospice Benefit does not cover curative care for the patient's terminal illness, it does cover curative care for incidental conditions such as an infection or injuries and treatment to control pain and symptoms. Hospice does not cover the costs of extended live-in 24-hour care and requires that hospice services be provided by Medicare-approved hospice providers. The hospice benefit also does not cover ambulance and emergency department services unless arranged for by the hospice provider.

127. B: While individual needs vary, many individuals under hospice care find long periods of time alone difficult, so a friendly visitors program in which the same volunteer comes to the patient's home can be invaluable. Friendly visitors usually make visits on a regular schedule, often weekly, in addition to contacting the patient by telephone and in some cases arranging for outings, such as a taking the patient who is able for a drive. Volunteers in hospice programs should undergo screening and training before visiting patients.

128. A: The best solution is "Let's make a list of questions to give the doctor," because this is a practical solution that responds directly to the patient's concerns. Many hospice patients suffer from fatigue and the thought of writing out a list of questions on their own may seem daunting. In the process of exploring questions, the nurse may find some that he or she can respond to, and this can lead to worthwhile discussions because some questions may not require physician input.

129. B: With lower-extremity lymphedema, there is an increased risk of fungal infection of the toes, so antifungal powder should be applied routinely and the patient advised to wear cotton socks and breathable shoes (such as canvas). Signs of fungal infection include redness, itching, and peeling of skin. Antibiotics are given for infections, which are common complications because of stasis and accumulated debris in tissues. Antibiotics may be given prophylactically if patients have repeated infections. Oral antifungal agents are not generally used prophylactically.

130. C: High-air-loss support surfaces promote the evaporation of moisture by passing air over the skin. High-air-loss (air-fluidized) support surfaces also provide an increased support area and reduced accumulation of heat. They reduce pressure and shear. The typical standard hospital bed mattress has none of these qualities. The common foam support surface provides little more protection than the mattress.

131. B: Hydrocolloids are probably the best choice because they provide absorption for small to medium amounts of exudate and provide a warm, moist environment for healing. They can be left in place for 2-5 days, but they do pose an increased risk of anaerobic infection. Gauze dressings should not be applied directly to an open wound because they will adhere and damage the tissue. Semi-permeable film is appropriate for dry wounds. Alginate dressings are used for wounds with large amounts of dressing because of their absorptive properties.

132. C: Patients may have insurance coverage for direct medical costs, such as medications, treatments, physician's visits, durable medical equipment, and emergency services. Direct nonmedical costs are those that result from the illness, such as lost income from missed employment, transportation costs, and caregiver costs. These direct nonmedical costs are usually not covered by insurance and may pose a severe financial hardship on patients and their families, so these costs need to be considered when people are planning care.

133. C: These symptoms are consistent with pleural effusion, with increasing dyspnea as the most common symptom. As the pleural fluid builds, the pressure may cause the lung to collapse. Patients often exhibit a dry, nonproductive cough and pain and heaviness in the chest. If the pleural effusion is extensive, it may result in a mediastinal shift. Thoracentesis may relieve symptoms, but fluid usually accumulates again within a few days. Other treatment options include sclerotherapy, pleuroperitoneal shunt, pleurectomy, indwelling catheters, and subcutaneous access ports.

134. A: Poorly controlled symptoms, such as pain and nausea, are the most likely to have a negative impact on a patient's ability to maintain a feeling of hope at the end of life, so managing symptoms should be the first priority of care. The nurse should ask patients directly how well they are controlling their symptoms and how this is affecting their sense of hope. The nurse should also ask the patient about who provides support—emotional, physical, and spiritual—and methods they use to handle difficult situations.

135. C: Disenfranchised grief: Grief expressed in secret because it is not socially sanctioned, such as that of a lover, unacknowledged illegitimate child, or mistress. The person may not be able to see the dying person or attend memorial services or funerals. Unresolved grief: Grief that persists because the person is unable to work through the grief to find resolution. Complicated grief: Grief that persists more than 1 year and intrudes on thoughts and abilities to function. Uncomplicated grief: Grief that results in an emotional reaction and then a period of recovery.

136. D: The death of a parent is almost always devastating to a child, and a parent's instinct is often to protect and shield the child from the reality of the illness, but this can result in complicated grief and anger. Children need to be involved in care to the level of their ability. For example, a child can do light tasks, such as bringing water or books to the parent, and provide comfort measures, such as reading or singing to the parent, holding the parent's hand, and even just sitting with the parent. Children are less frightened if people are honest with them and if they feel useful and needed.

137. D: According to the Clinical Practice Guidelines of the National Consensus Project, bereavement and follow-up services must be offered to family members after a patient's death for a minimum of 12 months. Grief and bereavement services should be available and offered by trained staff to both the patient and family members throughout the period of illness. Families should be apprised of services with information that is appropriate for their culture and linguistic abilities.

138. C: Under Quality Assurance and Performance Improvement (QAPI), Element 4, performance improvement projects must be identified within the facility and can apply to one area or department or to the entire facility, depending on the breadth of the project. The goal is a continuing effort to identify problems and improve services. QAPI includes 5 elements:

1. Designs and Scope.
2. Governance and Leadership.
3. Feedback, Data Systems, and Monitoring.
4. Performance Improvement Projects (PIPs).
5. Systematic Analysis and Systemic Action.

139. B: This is clearly a professional boundary violation, even though these actions may appear caring. In fact, since a professional relationship exists between the patient and the nurse, there are liability issues if the nurse is visiting when off-duty, especially if the nurse is providing care and a problem arises. Additionally, the nurse is creating a relationship of dependency on the part of the patient and family, and seeking to fulfill personal needs by being overinvested in patients' lives.

140. B: The primary principle of palliative care is to focus on relieving suffering for the dying person. All aspects of care should be focused on that goal while attending to the medical, social, psychological, and spiritual needs of the patient and family members. The nurse must serve as an advocate for the patient and family to help them gain access to needed services and care settings in order to receive excellent care at the end of life.

141. A: Patients with history of drug abuse are entitled to adequate pain control, but they must be assessed and evaluated carefully. Of special concern are patients who roll and smoke fentanyl patches because this releases a 3-day supply of the drug rapidly and can result in a life-threatening overdose. Patients with a history of drug abuse may have developed a tolerance to drugs, so taking medications before the scheduled time and asking for higher doses is not uncommon; however, some patients react in the opposite way and are fearful of taking pain medications.

142. C: Terminal sedation differs from physician-assisted suicide in that it is primarily intended to provide comfort and alleviate suffering, and the hastening of death that may occur is a secondary effect. The primary purpose of physician-assisted suicide is to bring about a patient's death (even though it is also intended to provide comfort and alleviate suffering). These are legal distinctions. In most states, physician-assisted suicide is illegal, but the US Supreme Court has upheld the rights of individuals to have terminal sedation to alleviate symptoms.

143. D: Patients should be medicated prior to extubation and have additional medications available to control symptoms. The medications that are most indicated to relieve a sense of breathlessness are opioids. Benzodiazepines are also usually administered to relieve anxiety. Oxygen is usually continued at about 21%. If family chooses to stay at the bedside while the patient is dying, the nurse should make sure that they can remain close to the patient and can encourage them to hold the person's hand or touch the patient.

144. C: Grade 3. National Cancer Institute Scale of Severity of Diarrhea:

- Grade 0: Normal stools.
- Grade 1: Two to three stools daily but essentially no other symptoms.
- Grade 2: Four to six stools daily with stools at night and/or moderate abdominal cramping.
- Grade 3: Seven to nine stools daily with fecal incontinence and/or severe abdominal cramping.
- Grade 4: More than 10 stools daily with stools grossly bloody and/or fluid depletion results in need for parenteral support.

145. B: "Huffing" is an airway clearance technique to improve cough effectiveness so patients are better able to expectorate secretions. The patient is instructed to lie on his or her side while holding a pillow against the abdomen for support. The patient takes a deep breath and then "huffs" or breathes out sharply three or four times in bursts with the mouth open. This type of coughing is less tiring than a forceful cough and may help to clear mucus for all patients with cough.

146. A: Because bacterial colonization of the necrotic wound results in a foul odor, the most effective treatment is usually application of a metronidazole topical solution (0.5% to 1%) to the wound surface. It can also be used to irrigate the wound and saturate dressings. Metronidazole topical gel (0.75%) is also available and applied in a thin film to the wound. Yogurt has been applied to necrotic wounds with some success, and skin cleansers and charcoal dressings are also helpful.

147. D: Cost minimization: Based on the assumption that two treatments are equal in effectiveness, so the least expensive option should be utilized. Cost effectiveness: Compares treatments and assigns dollar value to each year of life gained by a treatment. Cost utility: Similar to cost-effectiveness but estimates the value in quality of life. Cost benefit: Evaluates treatments in terms of monetary value of life; assigning a dollar value to life is difficult, so this approach is seldom used.

148. A: The three primary aspects of evidence-based practice are clinical expertise, best available research, and patient values. These three aspects guide decision-making in relation to patient care in order to promote optimal outcomes. Clinical expertise includes both education and experience. The best available research is based on research conducted using scientific methodology and often reported on in juried publications and at conferences. Patient values and wishes are important components of evidence-based practice.

149. C: Fractionated external-beam radiation therapy is the primary treatment for spinal cord compression because it inhibits the growth of tumor and is often able to restore and preserve neurological function. After treatment, most patients will retain the ability to ambulate; of those already paraparetic and unable to walk, over a third will regain this ability, although only about 5% of patients with paraplegia progress to the point that they can walk again. Dexamethasone is the corticosteroid of choice. Decompressive surgery is an option for some patients.

150. B: The Agency for Healthcare Research and Quality recommends use of the ABCDE method for assessing and managing pain:

- **A**sking patient about the extent of pain and assessing systematically.
- **B**elieving that the degree of pain the patient reports is accurate.
- **C**hoosing the appropriate method of pain control for the patient and circumstances.
- **D**elivering pain interventions appropriately and in a timely, logical manner.
- **E**mpowering patients and family by helping them to have control of the course of treatment.

CHPN Practice Test #2

1. If a patient is to receive opioid pain management, what constipation prevention regimen should be included?

a. Stool softener and stimulant laxative (e.g., senna, bisacodyl)
b. Psyllium fiber supplement (e.g., Metamucil)
c. Dietary modifications only (i.e., high fiber, increased fluids)
d. Osmotic laxative (e.g., milk of magnesia)

2. If the nurse must make home visits to patients who have various types and sizes of dogs, the BEST solution is to:

a. Befriend the animals.
b. Carry dog repellent.
c. Require the dogs to be restrained.
d. Carry an ultrasonic dog deterrent device.

3. When providing postmortem care, the nurse should:

a. Place dentures and partial plates in the patient's mouth.
b. Place the deceased in a supine, with the head of bed slightly elevated.
c. Secure the patient's hands together with ties.
d. Secure the patient's eyes in a closed position.

4. If a patient under hospice care at home is receiving care from a hospice aide, how often must the RN visit the home to assess the quality of care provided by the hospice aide?

a. Every 7 days
b. Every 14 days
c. Every 21 days
d. Every 28 days

5. A patient on hospice home care has increasingly severe pain despite changes in opioid medications and dosages. The most appropriate response is likely to:

a. Try inpatient hospice care to achieve pain control.
b. Attempt further changes in opioid medications and/or dosages.
c. Suggest complementary therapy, such as acupuncture.
d. Accept that pain control may not be possible.

6. A cancer patient's condition is stable, but the patient's spouse cries frequently and reports experiencing an overwhelming feeling of dread. This most likely represents:

a. Anticipatory grief
b. Depression
c. Complicated grief
d. Denial

7. If a patient develops refractory ascites and has a peritoneovenous (i.e., Denver) shunt inserted, how many times should the patient and caregiver be advised to pump the shunt to maintain patency?

a. 5 times, hourly
b. 10 times, if the ascites increases
c. 20 times, four times daily
d. 20 times, twice daily

8. If a family member who has not been involved in patient care telephones the nurse and asks for information about a patient's condition, the nurse MUST:

a. Provide the information requested.
b. Ask for identifying information.
c. Obtain permission from the patient to provide the information.
d. Suggest that the family member call the patient directly.

9. The most reliable indicator of the degree of a patient's pain is:

a. Verbal description of pain
b. Nonverbal indicators (e.g., facial expression, body position)
c. Changes in vital signs
d. Moaning, crying

10. If a patient is cared for in the home by a family caregiver, the primary responsibility of the nurse to the caregiver is to:

a. Empower the caregiver.
b. Supervise the patient care.
c. Provide a plan of care.
d. Answer questions about the patient's care.

11. Opioid-induced neurotoxicity is most often characterized by:

a. Myoclonus
b. Seizures
c. Somnolence
d. Headaches

12. A patient's spouse complains that the patient has become quite confused at times since beginning opioid therapy for pain management. How long does it usually take for cognitive impairment associated with opioids to resolve after initiation of the drugs?

a. 24–48 hours
b. 2–3 days
c. 1–2 weeks
d. 2–4 weeks

13. If a patient receiving morphine for pain control complains of itching, the initial intervention should be to:

a. Discontinue the morphine.
b. Lower the morphine dose.
c. Administer a steroid.
d. Administer an antihistamine.

14. If a patient is persistently fatigued and has decreased energy reserves, the BEST approach is to instruct him or her on:

a. Energy conservation methods
b. Improving diet and nutrition
c. Improving sleep habits
d. Avoiding triggering factors

15. A patient has had a PleurX catheter inserted to drain ascites every other day. During drainage, the patient complains of mild discomfort. The nurse should:

a. Use the roller clamp to decrease the rate of flow.
b. Notify the physician that the patient has pain.
c. Provide analgesia to relieve discomfort.
d. Discontinue the drainage and disconnect the drainage bottle.

16. The goals in the hospice and palliative care plan should be primarily based on the patient's:

a. Condition
b. Wishes
c. Diagnosis
d. Life expectancy

17. When developing the care plan, the nurse notes that the patient has the following nursing diagnoses: ineffective health management, ineffective airway clearance, impaired social interactions, and anxiety. According to Maslow's hierarchy of needs, which nursing diagnosis should have priority?

a. Ineffective health management
b. Ineffective airway clearance
c. Impaired social interactions
d. Anxiety

18. A patient's daughter insists that the patient wants to explore all options to prolong her life, but the patient tells the nurse that she wants to stop treatments and have comfort care. The most appropriate response is to:

a. Ignore the daughter.
b. Tell the patient to talk to her daughter about this.
c. Facilitate a discussion between the patient and her daughter.
d. Tell the daughter that the patient wants comfort care only.

19. An essentially bedbound home health patient must be transferred from the bed to a wheelchair, and then from the wheelchair into the bathroom and onto the toilet or a shower chair. The BEST solution is likely:

a. A bedside commode
b. A bedpan and bed baths
c. A rolling toilet/shower chair
d. Safety bars and a raised toilet seat

20. A patient with malignant bowel obstruction experiences severe nausea and vomiting. Which pharmacological intervention is indicated?

a. Prochlorperazine
b. Metoclopramide
c. Octreotide
d. Ondansetron

21. If a patient in palliative care has a chronic infected draining wound that is malodorous, what environmental strategy may help reduce the odor?

a. Spray air freshener around the room.
b. Burn aromatherapy candles in the room.
c. Place a fan near the patient's bed.
d. Place kitty litter and dryer sheets in the room.

22. The drug of choice for the treatment of terminal dyspnea is a(n):

a. Anticonvulsant
b. Benzodiazepine
c. Sedative
d. Opioid

23. If a patient's symptoms of dehydration include thirst, fatigue, muscle weakness, fever, and changes in mental status, and laboratory findings show a sodium level of 150 mEq/L, the type of dehydration is most likely:

a. Hyponatremic
b. Hypernatremic
c. Isotonic
d. Mixed

24. If a palliative care patient has frequent nausea and vomiting, which one of the following is a nonpharmacological intervention that may provide some relief?

a. Sip fluids throughout the meal.
b. Ensure that foods are hot.
c. Sit up for 2 hours after eating.
d. Eat frequent, small meals.

25. During the initial home assessment of a patient, the nurse finds that the home is dirty and unheated and there is little food. The most appropriate intervention is to:

a. Provide a list of necessary remedies for the patient/family.
b. Request that a social worker visit to assess the patient's needs.
c. Request the services of a home aide to help clean the home.
d. Refer the patient to a local Meals-on-Wheels program.

26. When determining whether a patient who is dying should be given artificial hydration, the PRIMARY consideration should be:

a. The family's wishes
b. The patient's wishes
c. Signs of dehydration
d. Policies regarding end-of-life care

27. An older patient takes clopidogrel bisulfate because of a long history of atrial fibrillation. She hits her arm against the bed rails during an episode of confusion, resulting in a Payne-Martin category II skin tear. The most appropriate intervention is to clean the wound and:

a. Apply a transparent film.
b. Apply antibiotic ointment and a gauze dressing.
c. Leave it open to the air.
d. Apply a hydrogel dressing.

28. A hospice physician/nurse practitioner is required to have a face-to-face visit with each hospice patient:

a. Before the second benefit period
b. Before the third benefit period
c. Only before the initial benefit period
d. Before every benefit period

29. The most common cause of hiccups in hospice and palliative care patients is:

a. Muscle spasms
b. Anxiety
c. Gastric distension
d. Inflammation

30. Under the Family and Medical Leave Act, employers with 50 or more employees must provide up to how much unpaid leave and job protection for family and medical reasons each 12-month period?

a. 8 weeks
b. 12 weeks
c. 6 months
d. 12 months

31. A patient with heart disease may qualify for hospice care if he or she meets the New York Heart Association's classification criteria for class:

a. I
b. II
c. III
d. IV

32. If a patient lives in a home environment that is cluttered and poorly lit, thereby increasing the risk of falls, the MOST appropriate intervention is to:

a. Make a referral to an occupational therapist.
b. Make a referral to a physical therapist.
c. Draw up a plan for environmental modifications.
d. Make a referral to a home aide to assist with cleaning.

33. If a patient who has elected Medicare hospice care decides to continue with active treatment and must be discharged for ineligibility, the patient should receive the:

a. Detailed Explanation of Non-Coverage
b. Advance Beneficiary Notice of Non-Coverage
c. Notice of Medicare Non-Coverage
d. Medicare Outpatient Observation Notice

34. Respiratory signs and symptoms of approaching death include:

a. Kussmaul respirations
b. Cheyne-Stokes respirations
c. Biot respirations
d. Apneustic respirations

35. A caregiver frequently searches the internet to find new treatments for a patient and repeatedly asks about unproven treatments found on various websites and chat rooms. The BEST solution is to:

a. Advise the caregiver to stop searching for information.
b. Advise the patient to discuss the treatments with the physician.
c. Teach the caregiver how to recognize credible websites.
d. Remain supportive and noncommittal.

36. Which of the following is consistent with oral-stage (i.e., first-stage) dysphagia/impaired swallowing?

a. Heartburn, hematemesis, hyperextension of the neck
b. Drooling and choking before swallowing
c. Gagging sensation and a gurgling voice
d. Regurgitation and repeated swallowing

37. When educating a caregiver about patient care, the first thing to ascertain is the caregiver's:

a. Style of learning
b. Reason for caregiving
c. Commitment to ongoing caregiving
d. Current base of knowledge

38. A patient nearing death states that her mother (who is long deceased) came to visit her. The most appropriate response is:

a. "Your mother has already died."
b. "Perhaps you were having a dream."
c. "That must have been very comforting for you."
d. "She was very happy to be able to see you."

39. Which one of the following drugs may help to relieve metastatic bone pain?

a. Pamidronate
b. Baclofen
c. Gabapentin
d. Metoclopramide

40. If an experienced nurse is serving as a mentor to a newly hired nurse, the mentor's PRIMARY role is to:

a. Supervise the newly hired nurse.
b. Point out any errors or shortcomings.
c. Guide and support.
d. Assess his or her clinical abilities.

41. A 40-year-old woman is caring for her mother, who has Alzheimer's disease and lives at home. The woman is increasingly frustrated and stressed at her mother's confusion and lack of cooperation. If the nursing diagnosis for the patient and caregiver is "risk of caregiver role strain," a desired outcome may be that the caregiver will:

a. Have realistic expectations regarding the patient.
b. Experience no stress related to caregiving.
c. Understand the need to develop coping skills.
d. Find ways to modify the patient's behavior.

42. Which of the following is recommended as a first-line treatment for the relief of neuropathic pain?

a. Anticonvulsants
b. Tricyclic antidepressants (TCAs)
c. Selective serotonin reuptake inhibitors
d. Opioids

43. An older adult with rheumatoid arthritis has a nursing diagnosis of "Self-care deficit, dressing." The patient often sleeps in her clothing and appears unkempt. On examination, the nurse notes that the patient has hand deformities that make dressing and undressing difficult. The most appropriate response is:

a. Referral to occupational therapy
b. Referral to physical therapy
c. Transfer to inpatient facility
d. Recommending clothing that is easy for her to manage

44. A patient with stage 4 (i.e., end-stage) chronic obstructive pulmonary disease insists on being in a chair day and night. The patient should be taught to shift his or her body weight every:

a. 15 minutes
b. 30 minutes
c. 60 minutes
d. 2 hours

45. If a patient with multiple sclerosis is refusing treatment and increasingly isolating herself, the patient should be assessed for:

a. Disease progression
b. Anxiety
c. Dementia
d. Depression

46. Which of the following is a physical sign that a patient with dementia may be experiencing depression?

a. Loss of interest in activities
b. Cardiac dysrhythmias
c. Appetite loss and weight loss
d. Multiple complaints about health

47. If a patient complains of severe pain, which of the following would be a short-acting opioid of choice?

a. Tramadol
b. Morphine
c. Meperidine
d. Propoxyphene

48. For hospice patients, the individual responsible for coordinating care is the:

a. RN
b. Physician
c. Program director
d. Social worker

49. Under NHPCO's Standards of Practice, hospice services MUST be available:

a. At least 40 hours a week
b. 24 hours a day, 5 days a week
c. 12 hours a day, 7 days a week
d. 24 hours a day, 7 days a week

50. If a patient does not have an advance directive, the nurse should:

a. Provide information and resources regarding advance directives.
b. Accept the patient's choice in not having an advance directive.
c. Advise the patient to complete an advance directive.
d. Ask the family members to encourage the patient to complete an advance directive.

51. If a patient's life expectancy is less than 14 days and he or she is experiencing situational anxiety, the medication of choice is:

a. Bupropion
b. Lorazepam
c. Escitalopram
d. Amitriptyline

52. According to the National Consensus Project, if a patient demands treatment with a medication that is not medically necessary, has been proven to be ineffective, and has numerous adverse effects, the BEST recourse for a health-care organization is likely to:

a. Refuse to provide the treatment.
b. Administer the treatment.
c. Discharge the patient from care.
d. Seek legal counsel.

53. A patient with a terminal illness has eaten poorly for several months. What albumin level is indicative of moderate protein deficiency?

a. 3.7 g/dL
b. 3.2 g/dL
c. 2.7 g/dL
d. 2.4 g/dL

54. If a dying patient has impaired bed mobility and is unable to reposition without assistance, the MOST important intervention is to:

a. Tell the caregivers to reposition the patient frequently.
b. Raise the foot of the bed to prevent shear injuries.
c. Implement thromboembolism prophylaxis.
d. Establish a schedule for repositioning.

55. A patient's nursing diagnosis includes risk for aspiration. Which of the following may be an early indication that the patient is developing pneumonia?

a. Chest pain
b. Change in mental status
c. Signs of dehydration
d. Increased respiratory rate and crackles

56. A patient is losing weight rapidly because of a loss of appetite. When assessing the patient, the nurse notes that the patient says he feels full quickly and usually stops eating after a small green salad. The most appropriate intervention is to:

a. Provide nutritional supplements in place of other foods.
b. Suggest that the patient rest between meal courses.
c. Advise the patient to eat the most nutritious foods first.
d. Educate the patient about a healthy diet.

57. Under Medicare's hospice benefit, the service intensity add-on provides additional reimbursement for services provided during the past:

a. 14 days
b. 10 days
c. 7 days
d. 5 days

58. A patient with HIV/AIDS is considered to be in the terminal stage of the disease when the CD4 count falls to:

a. <100 cells/microliter (μL)
b. <50 cells/μL
c. <25 cells/μL
d. <15 cells/μL

59. If a patient with overactive bladder complains that oxybutynin ER is relieving urinary symptoms but is causing dry mouth, the nurse should suggest:

a. Changing to oxybutynin IR
b. Discontinuing the medication
c. Taking the medication at bedtime
d. Taking the medication first thing in the morning

60. A patient weighs less than 200 pounds and must be moved up in bed, and the patient can only partially assist. According to Occupational Safety and Health Administration (OSHA) guidelines, the correct method is to:

a. Pull the patient under the arms from the head of the bed.
b. Raise the foot of the bed and slide the patient toward the head of the bed.
c. Encourage the patient to scoot toward the head of the bed.
d. Use a friction-reducing device and at least two caregivers.

61. Kennedy terminal ulcers are typically characterized by:

a. Rapid deterioration of skin in the sacral/coccygeal area, sometimes within hours
b. Slow deterioration of skin in the sacral/coccygeal area over weeks
c. Pressure sores on the heels of both feet
d. Mouth sores and cracks in the lips

62. A patient with stage 4 lung cancer and the patient's spouse are discussing hospice care with the nurse. The patient and the spouse both begin to cry. The MOST appropriate response is to:

a. Stop the discussion and leave the room.
b. Stop the discussion and wait quietly while they express their grief.
c. Ask them what you can do to help.
d. Tell them that you understand why they are upset.

63. A patient tells the nurse that he doesn't want to suffer at the end of his life. An appropriate response is:

a. "We will give you medications so you don't suffer."
b. "Can you tell me what kind of suffering you mean?"
c. "You don't have to worry about that."
d. "We will do everything we can so that doesn't happen."

64. If a newly hired hospice and palliative care nurse asks how to handle on-the-job stress, the BEST advice is to:

a. Make a plan in advance.
b. Practice mindfulness.
c. Leave concerns in the workplace.
d. Seek out a mentor.

65. According to the National Coalition for Hospice and Palliative Care's National Consensus Project, because dealing with serious illness can be difficult, staff members should:

a. Receive adequate compensation.
b. Have limited on-call hours.
c. Be assessed for distress and grief.
d. Have limited caseloads.

66. A nurse on the hospice interdisciplinary team shows little emotion when patients die, appears to withdraw emotionally from patients and families, and avoids discussing the death of patients. This suggests:

a. The maintenance of healthy barriers
b. Inadequate processing of grief
c. An underlying personality disorder
d. A lack of compassion

67. According to OSHA requirements, Safety Data Sheets (SDSs) must be available for all:

a. Medications administered
b. Durable medical equipment
c. Hazardous materials
d. Needles and other sharps

68. A patient reports consistent skin irritation from fentanyl patches, which are successfully controlling the patient's pain. The BEST solution is to:

a. Change to a different medication delivery system.
b. Apply steroid cream to the site before applying the patch.
c. Spray an inhaled steroid on the site before applying the patch.
d. Administer diphenhydramine orally when the patch is applied.

69. The hospice infection control program MUST include:

a. A bloodborne pathogen exposure control plan
b. A respiratory protection plan
c. A bloodborne pathogen exposure control plan and a medication safety plan
d. A bloodborne pathogen exposure control plan and a respiratory protection plan

70. A patient with cancer has an abdominal fistula with green output. The most likely source of the fistula is the:

a. Stomach
b. Esophagus
c. Small bowel
d. Colon

71. As part of performance improvement, which one of the following events should trigger a root cause analysis (RCA)?

a. A patient's son overdoses and dies after stealing the patient's opioids.
b. A patient needs an increasing dosage of medication to control his pain.
c. A patient dies because of stage 4 breast cancer.
d. A patient is referred to a therapist because of suicidal ideation.

72. A patient states that, although her pain medication usually controls her pain, sometimes it takes a long time to take effect. When questioned about how she takes her medications, the patient states that she waits as long as possible before taking the pain medication. The nurse should:

a. Educate the patient about pain and pain control.
b. Recommend increasing the dosage of pain medication.
c. Tell the patient to take the pain medication more often.
d. Recommend switching to a different pain medication.

73. A palliative care patient expresses feelings of powerlessness because of the complex treatment regimen she is undergoing. When developing a plan of care for this patient, it is MOST important to:

a. Suggest goals that increase the patient's control.
b. Explain the need for the treatments.
c. Suggest that the patient focus on the future.
d. Encourage the patient to specify her treatment goals.

74. As a patient nears death, she has fluctuating periods of extreme agitation and aggression with hallucinations, indications of hyperactive terminal delirium. Which intervention is MOST indicated?

a. Amitriptyline
b. Nonpharmacological interventions such as acupuncture or massage therapy
c. Haloperidol
d. Lorazepam

75. The hospice interdisciplinary team should review the patient's care plan at least every:

a. 5 days
b. 10 days
c. 15 days
d. 20 days

76. After the death of a patient, which one of the following may be an indication that the spouse is experiencing complicated grief?

a. The spouse reports experiencing waves of grief.
b. The spouse is unkempt, haggard, and thin.
c. The spouse appears stoic and unchanged by the death.
d. The spouse has joined a bereavement support group.

77. A patient who has had a right mastectomy has developed lymphedema of the right arm with 1+ pitting at times, leaving a dent when pressure is applied. The swelling resolves when the patient elevates that arm for a period of time. What stage of lymphedema does this represent?

a. Stage 1
b. Stage 2
c. Stage 3
d. Stage 4

78. The first step in pain management is:

a. Conducting a comprehensive pain assessment
b. Selecting an appropriate analgesic
c. Assessing the patient's psychosocial support
d. Educating the patient about pain management

79. On the Braden scale for predicting the risk of pressure sores, which ranges from 6 to 23, a score of 16 indicates:

a. No risk
b. Breakpoint for risk
c. Low risk
d. High risk

80. If a Muslim patient dies at home, the nurse expects that:

a. A family member will bathe and shroud the deceased.
b. The family will want a postmortem examination.
c. The deceased will be cremated.
d. A wake or viewing will be held prior to the funeral.

81. If a patient experiences dyspnea near the end of his life, the treatment response should be assessed based on:

a. Respiratory rate
b. Pulse oximetry
c. Skin color and signs of cyanosis
d. Symptom relief

82. After a patient dies, the caregiver asks if the patient's medications can be flushed down the toilet. The nurse should recommend:

a. Flushing all of the medications
b. Checking the FDA flush list
c. Throwing the medications in the garbage
d. Returning all of the medications to the originating pharmacy

83. If using a transcutaneous electrical nerve stimulator to relieve pain, avoid placing the electrode pads on the:

a. Front or sides of the neck
b. Upper back
c. Lower back
d. Lower leg

84. A caregiver reports feelings of guilt because of feeling relief when the patient died after a long and difficult illness, stating, "It's like I'm happy he died." The most appropriate response is:

a. "Feeling relief is not the same as being happy."
b. "I'm sure you will feel grief as time passes."
c. "Your feelings are normal."
d. "You have no reason to feel guilty."

85. The caregiver reports that a dying patient's feet and lower extremities feel cold to the touch and appear somewhat dark in color. The nurse should advise the caregiver to:

a. Apply a heating pad.
b. Cover the patient's legs with a warm blanket.
c. Carry out range-of-motion exercises to increase the circulation.
d. Massage the patient's feet and lower legs.

86. What is the threshold score on the Palliative Performance Scale (PPS) that may indicate hospice eligibility for an oncology patient?

a. ≤50%
b. ≤60%
c. ≤70%
d. ≤80%

87. Which of the following factors is the MOST predictive of progression of disease?

a. Recurrent/intractable infection (e.g., sepsis, pneumonia)
b. Decreased KPS or PPS score
c. Increased emergency room visits
d. Dependence on assistance with ADLs

88. A recipe used to increase fiber in the diet and prevent constipation consists of 1 cup applesauce, 1 cup prune juice, and:

a. 1 cup yogurt
b. 1 cup yam
c. 1 cup oatmeal
d. 1 cup oat bran/wheat bran

89. The spouse caregiver of a patient with Alzheimer's disease is increasingly distraught at the changes in the patient and reports feeling isolated and unappreciated. What community resource may prove to be the MOST helpful?

a. Senior citizen center
b. Exercise program
c. Religious or spiritual support
d. Caregiver support group

90. Which type of neurolytic block may relieve the pain associated with pancreatic cancer?

a. Sympathetic plexus neurolysis
b. Intercostal nerve neurolysis
c. Superior hypogastric plexus block
d. Celiac plexus block

91. If a patient has a large pressure ulcer on the coccygeal area with an excessive amount of exudate, which type of dressing is the MOST appropriate?

a. Alginate
b. Hydrocolloids
c. Transparent film
d. Hydrogels

92. If a patient's pain control is through hydromorphone 4 mg PO every 6 hours around the clock, and the conversion factor for hydromorphone is 4, what is the patient's daily morphine milligram equivalent (MME)?

a. 16 mg
b. 24 mg
c. 48 mg
d. 64 mg

93. Under the National Hospice and Palliative Care Organization (NHPCO) Standards of Practice, members of a hospice interdisciplinary team must include a:

a. Physician, registered nurse (RN), social worker, and physical therapist
b. Physician, RN, social worker, and pastoral/spiritual counselor
c. Physician, RN, physical therapist, and pastoral/spiritual counselor
d. RN, social worker, and pastoral/spiritual counselor

94. When teaching a caregiver to apply a fentanyl patch, the nurse explains that the patch should be applied:

a. Over the site of the pain
b. At the same site as previous patches
c. On the upper body
d. Where it receives no pressure

95. The purpose of the NHPCO Self-Determined Life Closure Measure is to:

a. Ensure that the patient is informed about advance directives.
b. Allow the patient to stop all curative treatments.
c. Ensure that the patient receives comfort measures at the end of his or her life.
d. Avoid unwanted hospitalizations and cardiopulmonary resuscitation (CPR) at the end of life.

96. A palliative home care patient has impaired walking and expresses a fear of falling. The nurse notes that the patient sways when standing and has poor balance. The most appropriate intervention is:

a. Assistive devices such as a walker
b. Referral to an occupational therapist
c. Referral to a physical therapist
d. Transfer to a skilled nursing facility

97. Professional licenses for hospice/palliative care staff MUST be verified with the licensing bodies at least:

a. Upon hiring
b. Annually
c. Once every two years
d. Twice a year

98. A patient has developed xerostomia. The FIRST step in its management is to:

a. Assess and treat any underlying infection.
b. Modify the diet.
c. Use a saliva substitute.
d. Review the patient's medications.

99. The adolescent child of a patient with amyotrophic lateral sclerosis pretends that nothing is wrong with the patient and ignores the changes that are occurring. The patient is concerned about how to deal with this. The most appropriate response for the patient is likely to:

a. Continue with the same pattern.
b. Engage the child in a conversation about the disease.
c. Give the child literature about the disease.
d. Ask another family member to discuss the disease with the child.

100. If a patient has experienced breakthrough pain and has received an additional medication that has not yet taken effect, what complementary therapy is MOST likely to help to relieve discomfort or prevent further escalation?

a. Aromatherapy
b. Massage
c. Music therapy
d. Relaxation and guided imagery

101. If a patient with terminal cancer and severe pain has a long history of heroin addiction, this may mean that he or she:

a. Should avoid opioids
b. May not respond to opioids
c. Needs a low dosage of opioids
d. Needs a high dosage of opioids

102. A patient nearing death has become increasingly incontinent of urine, exhibiting almost-constant dribbling. On examination, the nurse notes that the bladder is distended. What intervention should the nurse recommend?

a. Incontinence briefs
b. Intermittent catheterization
c. Indwelling suprapubic catheter
d. Indwelling urethral catheter

103. Which one of the following is the primary barrier to patients with leukemia receiving hospice benefits?

a. Lack of information
b. Younger age
c. Transfusion dependence
d. Unavailability of hospice services

104. If using the faith/belief, importance, community, address during care (FICA) format for a spiritual assessment, under what part of the assessment is it appropriate to ask if the patient's beliefs influence their acceptance of treatments or methods of dealing with illness?

a. F—faith
b. I—importance
c. C—community
d. A—address during care

105. If a patient has a high-output external enterocutaneous fistula draining through an opening in the abdominal wall, the best method of handling the fistula is to use:

a. Alginate dressings
b. A Foley catheter
c. A pouching system
d. Fibrin glue for closure

106. If a patient has dysphagia related to an esophageal stricture, the diet modification should likely be a:

a. Liquid diet
b. Pureed diet
c. Mechanically soft diet
d. Soft, moist diet

107. If a patient with a terminal disease states that she has lost faith in her religion, the BEST response is to:

a. Reassure the patient that her faith will return.
b. Remain supportive and actively listen.
c. Ask if the patient would like to see a spiritual advisor.
d. Tell the patient that religion is not as important as the belief in a higher presence.

108. According to OSHA guidelines for preventing workplace violence, if a patient has a history of severe psychiatric illness, then before a home visit, the health-care organization may:

a. Refuse to accept the patient because of the potential risk.
b. Ask for a consultant to assess the risk for violence.
c. Plan to send two nurses to the home each time.
d. Make an initial visit to determine if further assessment is needed.

109. Which type of complementary therapy is meant to open energy channels via meridians in the body?

a. Reiki
b. Tai chi
c. Acupuncture
d. Chiropractic treatments

110. According to the National Consensus Project, the interdisciplinary team should discuss issues regarding autopsy and tissue and organ donations with the patient or health-care agent:

a. Before the patient's death
b. At the time of admission to services
c. After the patient's death
d. At any convenient time

111. In the Orthodox Jewish community, which one of the following treatments may generally be withheld or discontinued near the end of life?

a. Oxygen
b. Nutrition
c. Fluids
d. Medication that may extend a life of suffering for a brief period

112. Under Medicare hospice reimbursement rules, which one of the following levels of care is paid for at an hourly rate ($60 in 2022)?

a. Routine home care
b. Inpatient respite care
c. General inpatient care
d. Continuous home care

113. A patient without an advance health-care directive is no longer able to express wishes about end-of-life care but has previously stated that he did not want further treatment to prolong his life. However, the patient's daughter, who is now making medical decisions for the patient, has insisted on futile treatments, and the physician is honoring the daughter's wishes. This is an example of:

a. Malpractice
b. Negligence
c. Battery
d. An ethical dilemma

114. Ibuprofen is contraindicated for pain control in patients with:

a. Chronic kidney disease
b. Cancer
c. Multiple sclerosis
d. Rheumatic disease

115. If a patient must undergo multiple painful procedures (e.g., central lines, bone marrow tests, or lumbar punctures) as part of cancer treatment, what pain management is MOST appropriate to reduce discomfort?

a. Acupuncture
b. Opioids
c. Topical anesthetics
d. Nonsteroidal anti-inflammatory drugs (NSAIDs)

116. A patient receives 12-hour extended-release morphine at 8 a.m. and 8 p.m. each day but complains of increased pain approximately 10 hours after administration of the drug. This is likely an indication of:

a. Pseudoaddiction
b. Pseudotolerance
c. End-of-dose pain
d. Tolerance

117. If a home health patient is using fentanyl patches to relieve pain, what should the patient and family be advised about disposing of the patches after use?

a. Place the patch in the trash.
b. Burn the patch.
c. Fold the patch and flush it down the toilet.
d. Cut the patch into multiple pieces and place it in the trash.

118. If a patient receiving oral opioid therapy for severe pain experiences breakthrough pain, the patient should be administered:

a. 5% of the 24-hour dose orally
b. 5–10% of the 24-hour dose orally
c. 10–20% of the 24-hour dose orally
d. 20–30% of the 24-hour dose orally

119. A patient has a high-output external enterocutaneous fistula originating in the small bowel. Which of the following electrolytes are MOST in danger of imbalance and must be monitored carefully?

a. Calcium and phosphate
b. Phosphate and magnesium
c. Sodium and phosphate
d. Sodium and potassium

120. A patient nearing the end of life develops "death rattles" from pooled secretions. The initial response should be to:

a. Reposition the patient.
b. Administer an anticholinergic drug.
c. Suction the patient.
d. Administer oxygen.

121. If methadone is used to control severe, chronic pain, the recommended dosing interval is:

a. Every 4 hours
b. Every 8 hours
c. Every 12 hours
d. Every 24 hours

122. Under Medicare hospice coverage, a patient may receive general inpatient care for:

a. Respite for caregivers
b. Treatment to prolong life
c. Treatment for terminal illness
d. Pain control or management of other symptoms

123. If a patient experiences incident pain, the patient should receive a:

a. Long-acting analgesic 1 hour before an activity
b. Short-acting analgesic 30–60 minutes before an activity
c. Continuous-relief analgesic, such as a fentanyl patch
d. Nonopioid adjuvant 1–2 hours before an activity

124. Hospice bereavement services should begin at the start of care and continue for at least:

a. 3 months following the patient's death
b. 6 months following the patient's death
c. 9 months following the patient's death
d. 13 months following the patient's death

125. Which one of the following drugs is NOT likely to be a cause of opioid-induced neurotoxicity?

a. Hydromorphone
b. Fentanyl
c. Meperidine
d. Oxycodone

126. If a patient who was started on opioid therapy develops confusion, vomiting, respiratory depression, pinpoint pupils, and sedation, the immediate response should be to administer:

a. *N*-acetylcysteine
b. Sodium bicarbonate
c. Naloxone
d. Flumazenil

127. Anorexia/cachexia syndrome is most common in terminal patients with:

a. Cancer
b. COPD
c. Heart failure
d. HIV/AIDS

128. Which one of the following allows government programs, such as Medicare, to recover money paid for fraudulent claims, such as claims for care not rendered?

a. The False Claims Act
b. The Omnibus Budget Reconciliation Act
c. The Health Care Quality Improvement Act
d. The Fair Labor Standards Act

129. Which one of the following pain assessment tools is MOST appropriate to use with an older adult with advanced dementia?

a. FACES
b. Numeric scale (1–10)
c. FLACC
d. PAINAD

130. Which type of pain is characterized as sharp or stabbing and radiates from the neck or spine to the extremities?

a. Radicular pain
b. Somatic pain
c. Neuropathic pain
d. Myofascial pain

131. A dying patient is showing no interest in food or drink and chokes easily. The patient is becoming dehydrated. The MOST appropriate intervention is:

a. Offer food and liquid every 2 hours in small amounts.
b. Insert a feeding tube.
c. Provide IV fluids.
d. Provide comfort care.

132. Which one of the following interventions is MOST likely to provide relief of pain associated with bone metastasis?

a. Opioids
b. Chemotherapy
c. Acupuncture
d. Palliative radiotherapy

133. If a Medicare patient is under palliative care and not hospice care, Medicare will cover:

a. All palliative care
b. All pain medications and treatments
c. Caregiver respite care
d. Medically necessary palliative care

134. Which of the following is an indication that hospice care is appropriate for a patient with advanced Alzheimer's disease?

a. Urinary frequency and urgency
b. Requiring a walker for ambulation
c. A Functional Assessment Staging Tool (FAST) score of 5 or higher
d. Lack of intelligible speech

135. A patient on step 1 of the World Health Organization pain relief ladder is taking acetaminophen to control mild pain. The maximum daily dose for an adult with normal liver function is:

a. 2,000 mg
b. 3,000 mg
c. 4,000 mg
d. 5,000 mg

136. Signs of hospice eligibility for a patient with Parkinson's disease include:

a. Chronic depression and suicidal ideation
b. Compromised breathing and recurring aspiration pneumonia
c. The lack of a caregiver or family members in the home environment
d. Instability and recurrent falls

137. If a patient seems to be having a crisis of faith and the nurse asks a few questions to determine if the patient needs a referral to a chaplain or other spiritual counselor, this is referred to as a spiritual:

a. History
b. Assessment
c. Screening
d. Review

138. An example of a myofascial pain syndrome associated with muscle trigger points is:

a. Fibromyalgia
b. Osteoarthritis
c. Rheumatoid arthritis
d. Gout

139. If a patient nearing death has marked death anxiety, which of the following is an appropriate patient outcome?

a. The patient will express feelings about dying.
b. The patient will die peacefully.
c. The patient will complete a life review.
d. The patient will rely on religious faith.

140. The primary treatments for stages 1 and 2 lymphedema include:

a. Diuretics and antibiotics
b. Liposuction
c. Electrical stimulation
d. Elevation and compression garments

141. Non-English-speaking individuals from communities local to the area receiving hospice and palliative care services are entitled to:

a. Translators only
b. Literature in their language and translators
c. Health-care providers that speak their language
d. No special services

142. An intubated patient with a tracheostomy is nearing death, and terminal weaning is being carried out. Following extubation, the patient exhibits stridor, which is distressing to the family. Which treatment may provide some reduction in stridor?

a. High-flow oxygen by mask
b. Dexamethasone
c. Aerosolized racemic epinephrine
d. Lorazepam

143. After a caregiver cries and complains that the burden of caring for a patient is overwhelming, the nurse goes to the patient's house on a day off to sit with the patient and give the caregiver a break. This is an example of:

a. Boundary violation
b. Compassion
c. Malpractice
d. Professionalism

144. If a patient nearing death has become detached, showing little interest in activities or interacting with family, the MOST appropriate response is to encourage the family to:

a. Try to engage the patient more.
b. Avoid interacting with the patient.
c. Maintain a calm, peaceful environment.
d. Move the patient to an inpatient facility.

145. Quality assessment and performance improvement programs should focus on:

a. Fiscal responsibility
b. Patient satisfaction
c. Improved outcomes
d. Legal compliance

146. A patient complains of persistent constipation. The nurse asks the patient to complete the Constipation Assessment Scale, and the patient scores 12 out of 16, indicating constipation. The nurse notes that #4, oozing liquid stool, is scored as a severe problem (2 points). The nurse should:

a. Advise the patient to increase fiber intake.
b. Examine the patient for a fecal impaction.
c. Ask the physician for an order to treat diarrhea.
d. Suggest that the patient take an over-the-counter laxative.

147. If a patient is identified as being a military veteran, the nurse should:

a. Complete the military history checklist.
b. Assume that the patient is at risk for post-traumatic stress disorder.
c. Question the patient about the impact of his or her military service.
d. Complete the same assessment as for other patients.

148. The most common treatment for complex regional pain syndrome is:

a. Spinal cord stimulation
b. NSAIDs
c. Physical therapy/rehabilitation
d. Psychotherapy

149. If using the PQRST pain assessment tool, what is an appropriate question to ask for the P part of the assessment?

a. "When did the pain begin?"
b. "What brings on the pain?"
c. "Where is the pain located?"
d. "Can you describe the pain?"

150. Which one of the following pharmacological interventions is especially indicated to prevent nausea and vomiting associated with chemotherapy or radiation?

a. Metoclopramide
b. Ondansetron
c. Octreotide
d. Lorazepam

Answer Key and Explanations for Test #2

1. A: The constipation regimen should include a stool softener (e.g., dioctyl sodium sulfosuccinate [DSS]) and a stimulant laxative (e.g., senna, bisacodyl). The constipation regimen should begin at the same time as the opioid therapy, usually with a stool softener, and the laxative is included if there are any signs of constipation (e.g., changes in the usual bowel pattern). If constipation occurs despite preventive measures, then the stool softener dosage may need to be increased.

2. C: The best solution is to require the dogs (and all pets) to be restrained, such as by placing them outside or in a separate room before the nurse enters the home. Even though many pets are not dangerous, they may increase the risk of infection and injury and can interfere with the ability of the nurse to carry out his or her duties. Additionally, they may have fleas and ticks, especially if not adequately cared for. Patients and families should be advised of this policy before a visit is made.

3. B: For postmortem care, the patient should be placed in a supine position with the head slightly elevated to prevent pooling of blood in the head and neck. Dentures should not be placed in the mouth, as they are likely to fall out. The hands should be placed across the abdomen but not secured. The eyes should be gently closed, but they should not be secured with tape or subjected to undue pressure. All visible medical equipment (e.g., catheters, oxygen masks, IVs) should be removed. The patient's body should be gently cleaned unless this is prohibited by his or her religious beliefs.

4. B: The hospice nurse must assess and supervise the hospice aide and document the assessment. The aide may or may not need to be present during the care assessment, depending on state regulations. Any concerns raised by the patient or family should be noted and investigated.

5. A: The most appropriate response is likely inpatient hospice care to achieve pain control. This is a time-limited break from home care in order to better manage symptoms so the patient can return to the home. Inpatient hospice care can be provided in a freestanding hospice facility, a hospice unit inside of a hospital, or a hospice unit inside of a skilled nursing facility.

6. A: With anticipatory grief, a person begins to grieve before the actual loss occurs. Anticipatory grief is an unconscious process that takes place as a preparation for the changes that will come, such as the change from partner to caregiver and the physical decline and loss of the patient.

7. D: The patient and caregiver should be advised to pump the shunt 20 times twice daily (first thing in the morning and last thing at night). If a patient is weak, the patient may not be able to do this independently, so a caregiver should be taught how to do it. The shunt drains fluid from the peritoneal cavity to the superior vena cava, where it returns to the general circulation. The pumping is not necessary to make the pump work, but it is necessary to clear any clots and ensure patency.

8. C: The nurse must obtain permission from the patient to provide information, and should respond by saying, "I cannot give out any information about patients without their permission," without acknowledging that the patient is under hospice care. Providing any information about the patient without permission is a violation of confidentiality under the regulations of the Health Insurance Portability and Accountability Act of 1996 (HIPAA).

9. A: The most reliable indicator of the degree of a patient's pain is his or her verbal description of the pain and personal pain rating. Some people are much more stoic than others and may not openly express pain or cry out even when pain is severe, whereas others may appear to be in severe pain even when their pain is mild. Vital signs may change with pain (e.g., increased pulse and respiration rates) but may also change for other reasons, such as anxiety.

10. A: The nurse provides guidance, education, and support to enable the caregiver to feel confident in providing care and to help ensure the safety of the patient and the caregiver. The nurse can help empower the caregiver by providing strategies for caring and solutions to problems encountered, as well as positive feedback.

11. A: Opioid-induced neurotoxicity is most often characterized by myoclonus (i.e., rapid and involuntary muscle jerks). Some patients may develop allodynia and delirium with hallucinations. Opioid-induced neurotoxicity may occur after a few days of beginning treatment with an opioid or when the dose reaches the point that it builds up in the system. Aggravating factors include renal failure, frailty, older age, fever, dehydration, and infection, as well as the use of additional drugs that result in central nervous system depression.

12. C: Some patients may also exhibit some motor impairment. To ensure patient safety, patients and caregivers should be advised that these adverse effects may occur.

13. D: Itching is a common adverse effect that often subsides with time and is usually relieved with antihistamines. If, however, the itching is severe and does not respond to treatment, then the patient may need to change to a different analgesic. The antihistamine most commonly administered is diphenhydramine, although it may cause drowsiness.

14. A: Although all these are important, the best approach is to instruct the patient on energy conservation methods, including the following:

- Identify a person to assist with activities (e.g., answering the phone, preparing meals).
- Prioritize activities in order to save strength for the most important ones.
- Rest when feeling especially fatigued.
- Enjoy passive activities (e.g., listening to music, reading, or watching TV).
- Eliminate or delay nonessential activities.

15. A: The nurse should reassure the patient that this discomfort is normal and use the roller clamp to decrease the rate of flow, which may relieve the discomfort. No more than 2,000 mL of fluid from the abdomen (or 1,000 mL from the chest) should be removed during one drainage period. Patients usually experience some discomfort at the end of the drainage period as well.

16. B: The nurse should ask what the patient's priorities are. For example, the priority for some patients may be to remain as free of pain as possible, but for others the priority may be to remain awake and alert in order to interact with family, and these patients may be willing to tolerate more pain in order to do so. The family should have input into the plan of care as well, especially if family members are caring for the patient in the home environment.

17. B: According to Maslow's hierarchy of needs, the nursing diagnosis that should have priority is ineffective airway clearance because physiological needs take precedence over other types of needs. Physiological needs include oxygen, food, elimination, temperature control, sex, movement, rest, and comfort. Next are safety and security needs, which would include ineffective health management. Then come love and belonging needs, such as managing anxiety. The fourth level comprises self-esteem needs, such as managing impaired social interactions. Self-actualization needs are the highest-level needs.

18. C: Although the patient can choose a level of care without the daughter's input, an open and honest discussion is important so that the daughter is able to respect the patient's wishes when the patient is no longer able to make decisions.

19. C: A rolling toilet/shower chair can reduce the number of transfers necessary, thereby reducing the risk of injury to the caregiver. Patients under hospice care are eligible for necessary assistive medical devices, including hoists and transfer boards.

20. C: The pharmacological intervention that is indicated is octreotide, an antisecretory drug. Octreotide decreases the production of gastrointestinal (GI) tract hormones, thereby also decreasing the production of secretions in the GI tract. Octreotide slows intestinal motility, which allows for the increased reabsorption of fluids. The drug may allow for removal of the nasogastric tube in some patients, reducing their discomfort and distress.

21. D: The kitty litter and dryer sheets can absorb some of the odor. Other strategies include placing coffee grounds in the room or an open container of vanilla extract. The dressings may need to be changed more frequently. Hydrocolloid dressings should be avoided if possible because they produce odor. Some cleaning agents, such as hypochlorous acid or sodium hypochlorite, may help to reduce the odor.

22. D: The most commonly used drug is morphine, usually at 2.5–5.0 mg PO or parenterally every 4 hours as needed. Another drug used is lorazepam. If dyspnea remains severe, then midazolam (1–2 mg PO/subcutaneously [SC or SQ]) may be combined with morphine for a synergistic effect. Morphine is generally well tolerated and does not result in respiratory deterioration in moderate doses.

23. B: A sodium level of 150 mEq/L (the normal range is 135–145 mEq/L), accompanied by symptoms of dehydration, indicates hypernatremic dehydration. The types of dehydration are as follows:

Type of Dehydration	Characteristics
Hyponatremic	Anorexia, weight loss, nausea and vomiting, sluggish movements, skin turgor, dry mucous membranes, orthostatic hypotension, lethargy, restlessness, delirium, seizures, confusion, coma. Lab work: Hyponatremia (<135 mEq/L), hemoconcentration (hematocrit level >44% in men and >40% in women), blood urea nitrogen level is high compared to creatinine, increased urine osmolality.
Hypernatremic	Thirst, fatigue, muscle weakness, fever, changes in mental status. Lab work: Hypernatremia (>145 mEq/L).
Isotonic	Morose, aggressive, demoralized, apathetic, uncoordinated movements. Lab work: Essentially normal.

24. D: Other interventions include avoiding drinking liquids with meals, lying flat for 2 hours after eating, ensuring foods are bland and cold or at room temperature, having fresh air (e.g., by a fan or an open window) in the environment while eating, and avoiding fatty, salty, spicy, and sweet foods, which may trigger nausea.

25. B: The social worker can determine if the patient is eligible for various services or financial assistance, such as through the Supplemental Security Income program, Medicaid, or other resources, and he or she can make an assessment regarding neglect or abuse.

26. B: The primary consideration should be the patient's wishes. Unfortunately, if a patient has no advance directive or has not stated wishes about his or her end-of-life care, the decision is often left to the family, who may seek advice from the physician or nurses. Families should know that hydration may prolong the dying process and that less invasive procedures, such as moistening the mouth and applying lip balm, may provide comfort.

27. A: The most appropriate intervention is to clean the wound and apply a transparent film. This will allow the wound to be monitored for bleeding or hematoma formation, which can occur due to the patient's higher risk for bleeding secondary to clopidogrel bisulfate use.

Payne-Martin Categories for Skin Tears	
I. Skin tear without tissue loss	Linear: Full-thickness wound that is wrinkled or furrowed with the epidermis and dermis pulled apart (an incisional appearance). Flap: partial-thickness wound with a flap that can cover the wound with ≤1 mm of the dermis exposed.
II. Skin tear with partial tissue loss	Scant tissue loss: Partial-thickness injury and ≤25% of the epidermal flap lost. Moderate to large tissue loss: Partial-thickness injury with >25% of the epidermal flap lost.
III. Skin tear with complete tissue loss	Complete partial-thickness injury with loss of the epidermal flap.

28. B: The visit may occur no more than 30 days before the third benefit period and must occur before each benefit period thereafter. Patients may elect to receive hospice services for an initial 90-day period and a subsequent 90-day period or unlimited 60-day periods. Although hospice care is intended for a 6-month period, some patients receive extended hospice care.

29. C: The most common cause (95%) of hiccups in hospice and palliative care patients is gastric distension, so the initial therapy usually targets this. Nonpharmacological interventions for gastric distension may include fasting, inducing vomiting, gastric lavage, and a nasogastric tube (with abdominal distension). Pharmacological treatments include simethicone and metoclopramide. For other causes, treatment may include muscle relaxants (e.g., baclofen), anticonvulsants (e.g., gabapentin), corticosteroids (e.g., dexamethasone), dopamine agonists (e.g., haloperidol), calcium channel blockers (e.g., nifedipine), and TCAs (e.g., amitriptyline).

30. B: This rule applies only to employees who have worked more than 1,250 hours during the previous year. During leave time, the employer must continue the same benefits and insurance coverage, and must maintain the position or provide another that is approximately equal in salary, benefits, and area of responsibility.

31. D: The New York Heart Association classification of heart failure is based on the patient's functioning, as follows:

- Class I: The patient is essentially asymptomatic during normal activities, with no pulmonary congestion or peripheral hypotension. There is no restriction on activities, and the prognosis is good.
- Class II: Symptoms appear with physical exertion but are usually absent at rest, resulting in some limitations in ADLs. Slight pulmonary edema may be evident by basilar rales. The prognosis is good.
- Class III: The patient experiences obvious limitations in ADLs and discomfort on any exertion. The prognosis is fair.
- Class IV: Symptoms are evident at rest. The prognosis is poor.

32. A: An occupational therapist can carry out an environmental assessment and identify assistive devices that may make life easier for the patient and allow the patient to remain independent for a longer period. The occupational therapist can assist the patient in developing the ability to carry out ADLs.

33. C: The patient should receive the Notice of Medicare Non-Coverage, which informs the patient of discharge from Medicare-covered services. The Advance Beneficiary Notice of Non-Coverage is given to patients when a service they are requesting is likely not covered by Medicare, so that the patient can choose whether to proceed or not.

34. B: Cheyne-Stokes respirations are characterized by a crescendo (fast, shallow) and decrescendo (slow, deep) pattern of breathing followed by a period of apnea. This breathing pattern may be evident for the last few days of life or for only a short period. The episodes of apnea usually increase until breathing stops. Family members should be told about this breathing pattern and should be advised that it is part of the normal process of dying.

35. C: The best solution is to teach the caregiver how to search effectively and how to recognize credible websites, such as the following:

- MedlinePlus
- Cochrane
- Websites with URLs ending in .gov
- The CDC, WHO, and Food and Drug Administration (FDA) websites
- Websites of health organizations such as the National Diabetes Association

36. B: The stages of dysphagia/impaired swallowing are as follows:

- Oral (voluntary stage): Food is taken into the mouth, chewed, and moistened.
  - Impairment: Impaired swallowing, bolus pooling in mouth, weak sucking and chewing, nasal reflux.
- Pharyngeal (involuntary stage): Swallowing reflex is present.
  - Impairment: Choking, coughing, delayed swallowing, fever, gurgling voice, gagging.
- Esophageal (involuntary stage): Moves food down the esophagus.
  - Impairment: Foul breath, bruxism, epigastric pain, heartburn, hyperextension of neck, regurgitation, repeat swallowing.

37. D: The caregiver may have had previous experience with caregiving or may be a complete novice, so the approach to teaching may vary from one caregiver to another. Typical caregiving responsibilities that should be discussed include personal care, food preparation/meal planning, medication management, emotional support, and transportation.

38. C: Sensory changes are very common as people near death, and they are often comforting to the patient. Some may mistake what they are hearing, and others may hear voices or see things or people that are not there. Sensory changes may vary from time to time but often intensify during the night.

39. A: Pamidronate (a bisphosphonate) may help relieve metastatic bone pain. Bisphosphonates are osteoclast inhibitors that slow the progression of skeletal problems. Bone is a common site of metastasis from tumors of the lungs, breasts, and prostate. Other medications to treat metastatic bone pain may include corticosteroids (e.g., prednisone, dexamethasone) and NSAIDs. Patients may also be treated with radiofrequency ablation or radiotherapy to reduce pain.

40. C: Mentorships may be formal or informal. Formal mentoring programs usually establish one-on-one mentoring relationships, as opposed to the more informal mentoring that occurs when one nurse assists another. Mentorship differs from preceptorship, which is often time-limited (e.g., happening just through the orientation period) and may involve more direct supervision.

41. A: A desired outcome may be "The caregiver will have realistic expectations regarding the patient." Another desired outcome may be "The caregiver will exhibit adequate coping skills." It is virtually impossible to eliminate all stress in what is inherently a stressful situation.

42. B: Two commonly used TCAs are imipramine and desipramine. If TCAs are not effective, anticonvulsants, such as gabapentin and pregabalin, may be considered. Nonpharmacological treatments, such as ice or massage, may also provide some relief and are often used along with pharmacological treatments.

43. A: An occupational therapist can assess the type of clothing the patient wears and suggest modifications and assistive devices to make dressing and undressing easier for the patient to manage.

44. A: The patient should be taught to shift his or her body weight every 15 minutes in order to prevent pressure sores. If possible, the patient should be assisted to stand momentarily and then sit again every hour, because sitting causes pressure directly on the ischial tuberosities. Placing the patient's feet on a footstool may help to distribute the pressure and reduce some of the pressure on the ischial tuberosities.

45. D: The rate of depression among patients with multiple sclerosis is double that of the general population. Depression occurs equally among those in early and in later stages, so routine screening should be carried out to assess for signs of depression. Depression may be associated with changes within the brain as well as life changes necessitated by the disease.

46. C: Physical signs that a patient with dementia may be experiencing depression include appetite loss and weight loss. Loss of interest in activities and multiple complaints about health are behavioral indications of depression. To screen patients with dementia for depression, scales that are available include:

- The Cornell Scale for Depression in Dementia: Assesses mood-related signs, behavioral disturbances, physical signs, cyclic functions, and ideational disturbance.
- Montgomery-Asberg Depression Rating Scale: Assesses apparent sadness, reported sadness, inner tension, reduced sleep, reduced appetite, concentration difficulty, lassitude, inability to feel, pessimistic thoughts, and suicidal thoughts.

47. B: Other acceptable drugs include hydromorphone, oxycodone, and fentanyl. The drug should be titrated rapidly to provide relief of pain. Because of possible adverse effects, meperidine and propoxyphene are generally avoided. Tramadol is more appropriate for mild to moderate pain. Severe pain is generally considered pain that rates as a 7 or higher on a scale of 0–10.

48. A: The RN essentially serves as a case manager. The RN ensures that the patient and family receive the services that they need, and that those involved in patient care are kept informed about changes in the patient's condition or needs. The RN coordinates care provided by health-care professionals as well as volunteers.

49. D: Patients are entitled to a timely response, and professional staff, including an interdisciplinary team, must be available at all times to provide assessment, education, necessary interventions, and support. The hospice must have a communication system in place that ensures that staff are updated on their patients' conditions. Patients should receive written information outlining how to access care outside of regular business hours.

50. A: Information should be provided verbally and in written form. Giving information may include providing a sample advance directive form, reviewing it with the patient, and discussing the benefits of outlining what the patient wants rather than leaving it to health-care providers or family members to make decisions. Having an advance directive can help relieve some of the family's burden.

51. B: The usual dosage is 0.5–1.0 mg PO two or three times daily. Escitalopram, bupropion, and amitriptyline can all be used to treat anxiety but may take weeks to be effective, so they are not indicated if the patient's life expectancy is short.

52. D: Discharging the patient rather than otherwise dealing with the issue may be construed as abandonment, and refusal to provide the treatment must be dealt with sensitively and within legal parameters.

53. C: Albumin has a half-life of 18–20 days, so it is sensitive to long-term protein deficiencies more than short-term.

- Normal values: 3.5–5.5 g/dL
- Mild deficiency: 3.0–3.5 g/dL
- Moderate deficiency: 2.5–3.0 g/dL
- Severe deficiency: <2.5 g/dL

Levels of less than 3.2 correlate with increased morbidity and death. Dehydration (e.g., from poor intake, diarrhea, or vomiting) elevates albumin levels.

54. D: The most important intervention is to establish a schedule for repositioning the patient, such as every 2 hours. The nurse must educate caregivers about repositioning the patient and have them demonstrate turning the patient with proper body mechanics in order to prevent injury. The patient's positioning will depend on the underlying diagnosis and symptoms. For example, the head of the bed may need to be elevated if the patient has increased intracranial pressure and headaches.

55. D: The patient's vital signs and temperature should be monitored for any changes, the lungs should be auscultated frequently (especially before and after feedings), and any signs of crackles or wheezing should be noted. The patient's gag reflex should be evaluated before oral feedings, and the patient should be fed slowly while sitting up or having the head elevated to at least 30–45 degrees.

56. C: Green salads are generally low in calories and nutrition. The patient should begin with meat or another source of protein, vegetables, and fruit. Nutritional supplements should be taken with or between meals rather than in place of other foods.

57. C: Under Medicare's hospice benefit, the service intensity add-on provides additional reimbursement for services provided during the past 7 days if certain criteria are met:

- The patient is provided routine home care.
- An RN or licensed social worker provides direct patient care.

Other levels of care include routine home care, continuous home care, inpatient respite care, and general inpatient care. The appropriate level of care is determined by the initial assessment and plan of care.

58. C: A patient with HIV/AIDS is considered to be in the terminal stage of the disease when the CD4 count falls to fewer than 25 cells/μL, or if the patient has a persistent viral load of greater than 100,000/mL. Additionally, the patient should score ≤50% on the Karnofsky Performance Status (KPS) scale or the Palliative Performance Scale (PPS). Additional signs and symptoms that indicate the terminal stage include chronic diarrhea, serum albumin of less than 2.5 g/dL, age >50, drug resistance, substance abuse, and comorbidities such as toxoplasmosis, congestive heart failure, and liver failure.

59. C: Dry mouth tends to be more of a problem with oxybutynin IR, so changing to this medication would not be indicated. Oxybutynin is a urinary antispasmodic that is available as a transdermal patch, topical gel, or tablets. Adverse effects may also include constipation and dry eyes, so patients should be cautioned to drink ample fluids and monitor their bowel status.

60. D: The correct method is to use a friction-reducing device and at least two caregivers—one on each side of the patient. Lifting is a common cause of injury among health-care workers. Although OSHA does not establish a definitive weight limit for lifting because circumstances vary, OSHA does note that experts recommend lifting no more than 35 pounds.

61. A: Kennedy terminal ulcers are typically characterized by rapid deterioration (sometimes within hours) of skin in the sacral/coccygeal area, leaving an abrased area that is red or black and does not respond to treatment. The ulcer occurs because the circulation is impaired, and it is an indication that death is nearing. Although the injury occurs most often in the sacral area with an irregularly shaped or pear-shaped injury, it can occur on the heels, elbows, and posterior lower legs, and the area of ulceration may increase from stage 1 to stage 4 within a matter of hours.

62. B: Discussions about hospice are difficult for the patient and family because they have to accept that the patient is dying, so simply remaining present and supportive is all that is generally necessary unless the patient indicates that the discussion needs to be continued at another time.

63. B: Although many people refer to pain when they think of suffering, for some people a prolonged death or the inability to breathe easily may be equally or more frightening than pain, so it is important to always clarify what the patient is really trying to say rather than making assumptions.

64. A: The best advice is to make a plan in advance because trying to decide how to respond when already feeling stressed is difficult. Plans should include listing current coping strategies that help the person relax, as well as activities that make the person feel good. The plan should include a list of strategies for dealing with stressful situations, such as practicing mindfulness, listening to music, and performing positive self-talk. The plan should also include a list of people with whom to discuss concerns, and a list of people and things (such as drinking to reduce stress) to avoid.

65. C: Emotional support, such as through counseling or time off, should be provided without judgment or stigma, and staff members should be given opportunities to discuss their feelings and the emotional impact of care provision. Workloads should be designed for the benefit of patients, families, and staff members.

66. B: One way of coping with the repeated deaths that occur is to deny the effects that they have, but the stress of doing this can build up over time and lead to burnout. Additionally, this response often leaves the nurse emotionally unable to respond to the needs of patients and their families.

67. C: According to OSHA requirements, Safety Data Sheets (SDSs) must be available for all hazardous materials, such as disinfectants and other chemicals. SDSs outline proper handling and storage of chemicals, procedures for cleanup and dumping of caustic substances, procedures in the event of a chemical spill or injury, and proper locations in the facility for cleanup. The SDS should also contain information indicating which substances may cause allergic effects or asthma from contact or inhalation.

68. C: The best solution is to spray the site with an inhaled steroid (the type used for asthma treatment) and allow it to dry on the skin prior to applying the patch. The inhaled spray does not interfere with adhesion, but the cream does. If this does not prevent irritation, then a different delivery system, such as oral medications, may be necessary.

69. D: The hospice infection control program must include a bloodborne pathogen exposure control plan and a respiratory protection plan, as well as plans to deal with a pandemic, such as COVID-19. For the respiratory protection plan, the hospice must provide fit-tested N95 masks for those providing direct care of patients with airborne disease. Staff must be educated at least annually regarding the bloodborne pathogen control plan.

70. A: An esophageal fistula is likely to have clear or white output. A fistula originating in the small bowel is likely to have tan or light-brown output with a thin, watery consistency, whereas output from the colon tends to have more of a stool appearance and tends to be thick and pasty in consistency.

71. A: This should trigger a root cause analysis (RCA) to determine if this could have been avoided by a more extensive family history or by taking measures to limit access, such as by restricting the number of doses available in the home, or securing them in a locked container or another secure location. The RCA is a retrospective attempt to determine the cause of an event, often a sentinel event such as an unexpected death, or a cluster of events. The focus of the RCA is on systems and processes rather than on individuals.

72. A: The patient needs to learn that it takes longer to control pain if the pain is allowed to become severe before taking the medication. The patient may benefit from regularly scheduled doses.

73. D: It is most important to encourage the patient to specify her treatment goals, especially those that will increase her sense of well-being and control. The nurse should assess factors that may be contributing to the patient's feeling of powerlessness, such as lack of a support system or inadequate knowledge about the treatment and its expected outcomes.

74. C: The intervention that is most indicated is an antipsychotic, such as haloperidol. Although haloperidol is usually the first-line drug, other choices may include chlorpromazine, olanzapine, or risperidone. Nonpharmacological interventions have not been proven successful. If the symptoms are intractable, the patient is suffering, and death is near, terminal sedation may be administered.

75. C: The hospice interdisciplinary team should review the patient's care plan at least every 15 days or with any changes in the patient's status. This review and any revisions should be documented in the patient's health-care record. During the review, the needs of the patient and the patient's family/caregivers must be reassessed, and any findings are communicated to other team members and staff involved in caring for the patient.

76. B: It may be an indication that the spouse is experiencing complicated grief if the spouse is unkempt, haggard, and thin—suggesting that he or she is having difficulty carrying out routine daily activities of living (e.g., dressing, bathing, and eating). It is normal to experience waves of grief, and joining a support group is a sign that the person is trying to come to terms with the loss. Stoicism is not an absolute indication of complicated grief or even that the spouse is not experiencing internal distress. Individuals express grief differently and sometimes in a delayed fashion.

77. B: Stages of lymphedema are as follows:

1	Abnormal flow but no obvious signs or symptoms.
2	Accumulation of fluid with swelling, but the swelling resolves with elevation. Pressing on the area may leave a dent.
3	The swelling is permanent, and limb elevation does not resolve it. The tissue is thickened and scarred, and pressure does not leave a dent.
4	The limb is large and deformed (i.e., elephantiasis), with thickened, scarred skin and wart-like growths.

78. A: A comprehensive pain assessment includes the following:

- Rate the pain on a scale (numerical, pictorial).
- Describe the pain (e.g., aching, burning, shooting, sharp, throbbing, stabbing).
- Identify any exacerbating and ameliorating factors.
- Identify the pain's onset and duration.
- Review previous and current pain relief methods.
- Review previous and current treatments for disease.
- Collect a medical history.
- Collect a history of recreational drug use and/or substance abuse.

79. B: A score of 16 on the Braden scale indicates the breakpoint for risk, with lower scores indicating higher risk.

Sensory perception	(1) Completely limited, (2) very limited, (3) slightly limited, (4) no impairment.
Moisture	(1) Constantly moist, (2) very moist, (3) occasionally moist, (4) rarely moist.
Activity	(1) Bed, (2) chair, (3) occasional walk, (4) frequent walk.
Mobility	(1) Immobile, (2) limited, (3) slightly limited, (4) no limitations.
Usual nutrition pattern	(1) Very poor, (2) inadequate, (3) adequate, (4) excellent.
Friction and shear	(1) Problem (the skin frequently slides down the sheets during moves, and the patient needs help to move), (2) potential problem (the skin slides somewhat during moves, and the patient needs assistance), (3) no apparent problem.

80. A: If a Muslim patient dies at home, the nurse expects that a family member (typically male) will bathe and shroud the deceased. Muslim individuals generally avoid postmortem examinations because many believe that the body should be intact for the resurrection, and they often do not want cremation for the same reason. Muslim individuals often want the deceased to be buried as soon as possible, so they typically do not have wakes or viewings. Caskets are almost always closed. Traditionally, only males attend funerals, although some communities allow females to attend.

81. D: The treatment response should be assessed based on symptom relief, rather than measures such as the rate of respirations or oxygen saturation. Patients may experience shortness of breath even with improvements in objective measures and without evident changes in skin color. The goal of treatment is to provide comfort to the patient, so the patient's perception is paramount.

82. B: The nurse should recommend checking the FDA flush list to determine if a medication can be safely flushed or if it should be otherwise disposed of. The first choice is to take the medications to a drug take-back program, but these programs are not always available. Opioids, in general, can be flushed because their potential for harm if ingested outweighs the risk to the environment from flushing.

83. A: The electrodes may be placed on the back of the neck to relieve neck pain. The electrode pads should not be applied to the chest area if the patient has any type of cardiac disease or dysrhythmia. Other places to avoid include areas that are infected or numb or lack normal sensation, and directly over the spine.

84. A: The nurse should discuss how having the burden of caregiving lifted, or knowing that the patient is no longer suffering, can bring a feeling of relief, but that does not mean that the person's grief at the loss is any less acute or that the person is happy about the death.

85. B: The nurse should advise the caregiver to cover the patient's legs with a warm blanket (it can be warmed briefly in a clothes dryer). These symptoms are a normal finding as a patient nears death. Applying a heating pad or other direct source of heat, such as a hot water bottle, increases the risk of burns. The hands and feet often exhibit decreased circulation.

86. C: The threshold score that may indicate eligibility for an oncology patient is less than or equal to 70%. For most other disorders, the PPS score that indicates eligibility is less than or equal to 50%. The PPS evaluates patients in six areas: ambulation, activity, evidence of disease, self-care, intake, and level of consciousness. The PPS helps guide decisions about when to apply for hospice care.

87. A: Recurrent/intractable infection, such as sepsis or pneumonia, is the most predictive factor of the progression of disease. The next indicators are a decreased Karnofsky Performance Status (KPS) or Palliative Performance Scale (PPS) score and increased emergency room visits. Dependence on assistance with activities of daily living (ADLs) is the least predictive factor of disease progression because this may occur quite early depending on the patient's underlying condition and general health.

88. D: The recipe consists of 1 cup applesauce, 1 cup prune juice, and 1 cup oat bran or unprocessed wheat bran. The patient should begin by taking 1–2 tablespoons of the mixture followed by 6–7 ounces of liquid each evening. If constipation persists after 1–2 weeks, the patient should increase the amount to 2–3 tablespoons of the mixture each day. The mixture may be stored in the refrigerator or the freezer (in individual servings).

89. D: Talking with others who are in the same situation and dealing with the same problems can be cathartic for caregivers, and can help to provide insight into how to better manage patient care as well as self-care.

90. D: A neurolytic block is one that impairs transmission of the impulses to relieve pain. This may be achieved with injection of a chemical irritant (such as alcohol), through radiofrequency ablation, or through cryoablation. The superior hypogastric plexus block is used to relieve pelvic pain. Intercostal nerve neurolysis may relieve post-thoracotomy rib pain or pain from rib fractures or metastasis. Sympathetic plexus neurolysis may relieve neuropathic or visceral pain.

91. A: Alginates are very absorbent, but they are nonadherent and must be covered with a secondary dressing. Alginate dressings are available in different forms—sheets, ribbons, and ropes—so they can be used to pack deep wounds and absorb exudate from surface wounds. One problem with alginate dressings is that they often develop a foul odor, which can be mistaken for a sign of infection.

92. D: Calculation of the MME is as follows:

- 4 mg × 4 doses per day = 16 mg per day
- 16 mg × 4 (conversion factor) = 64 MME

Conversion factors vary according to the strength of the drug. For example, the conversion factor for codeine is 0.14, hydrocodone is 1, oxycodone is 1.4, and oxymorphone is 3. An Opioid Prescribing Guideline mobile app that contains an MME calculator is available as a free download from the Centers for Disease Control and Prevention (CDC).

93. B: The team may also include additional members, such as aides, physical therapists, occupational therapists, speech-language therapists, volunteers, and pharmacists. The nursing staff, in addition to other team members, should be included when the care plans for hospice patients at their facility are reviewed.

94. C: The patch should be applied on the upper body, with the sites rotated so it is not placed on the same site as the previous patch. The patch may be applied to the chest, upper arms, back, or sides of the waist, but it should not be applied below the waist. If patients are confused and remove the patch, then applying it to the back may protect it from removal. The patch should be applied to clean, dry skin.

95. D: This is a one-page form completed on the patient's admission to service. The form asks if the patient/designated health-care agent wants to avoid hospitalization if the patient's condition worsens, and if the patient wants CPR if the patient's heart or lungs stop working. The form also allows for a preference change if at some time later the patient/designated health-care agent wants hospitalization and/or CPR.

96. C: A physical therapist can more thoroughly evaluate the patient's condition and needs and determine whether he or she may benefit from strengthening exercises and balance rehabilitation.

97. B: The verification must be documented in the staff member's personnel record. No licensed personnel may work if their license has expired, or been revoked or suspended, until it is reinstated. The hospice must use appropriate staffing guidelines and follow professional standards.

98. A: The first step is to assess and treat any underlying infections, such as candidiasis. If there is no infection, then the patient's medication should be reviewed, because hundreds of medications may induce oral dryness. Salivary stimulation (e.g., with chewing gum, mints, or pilocarpine) may help, and saliva substitutes may relieve discomfort and improve swallowing. Oral spray preparations that are generally well tolerated are also available.

99. B: Younger adults and adolescents often feel vulnerable and sometimes ashamed at changes brought about with disease. Adolescents, especially, may simply deny what is happening as a way to cope. Engaging the child in a conversation about the disease, and encouraging the child to express his or her feelings, may break down some barriers. If the patient is able to redefine his or her role and face the changes that are occurring, this often makes it easier for a child to do the same.

100. D: Relaxation and guided imagery can help the patient relax and prevent the muscle tightening that often occurs with and exacerbates pain. The patient should be taught how to use these techniques and should practice them before the pain becomes severe, if possible.

101. D: He or she may need a high dosage of opioids because the patient's body has likely built up a tolerance to the drugs. Patients who are addicted are still entitled to pain management, including opioids, but managing their pain may be difficult. In some cases, physicians may be reluctant to order high dosages, and pharmacists may be reluctant to fill the orders. Medications must be monitored carefully in the home because patients may easily overdose if they have free access to the drugs.

102. D: With constant dribbling, the patient may be difficult to manage with incontinence briefs, and this may be resulting from the bladder distension. Incontinence increases the risk of skin irritation and breakdown. Intermittent catheterization may help to relieve the bladder distension but may increase patient discomfort. Indwelling suprapubic catheters are intended for extended use.

103. C: The primary barrier to patients with leukemia receiving hospice benefits is transfusion dependence. Although transfusions may be considered a palliative treatment because they relieve symptoms, the costs associated with transfusions are high, so many hospice facilities do not offer transfusion services for patients. Because of this, leukemia patients in general have a 51% shorter average duration of hospice care than patients with solid tumors. Patients with leukemia who do receive hospice care tend to have lower overall costs to Medicare because of fewer emergency room visits and hospitalizations.

104. B: This question would fall under the importance category of the FICA spiritual assessment tool:

F	Faith	Do you have a faith or belief system that gives your life meaning?
I	Importance	What importance does your faith have in your daily life? Do your beliefs influence your acceptance of treatments or choices dealing with illness?
C	Community	Do you participate in and gain support from a faith community? Are your family and friends supportive?
A	Address during care	What faith issues would you like your health-care providers to address in your care?

105. C: If a patient has a high-output external (i.e., cutaneous exit) enterocutaneous fistula draining through an opening in the abdominal wall, the best method of handling the fistula is to use a pouching system, which can be easily drained to accommodate the high output without necessitating a dressing change, and can also provide protection for the surrounding skin. The output from a high-output enterocutaneous fistula can reach 3,000 mL/24 hours, compared to an output of 500 mL/24 hours for a low-output fistula.

106. B: A pureed diet is also appropriate for patients with reduced tongue function and impaired pharyngeal contractions. For the pureed diet, solid foods may be blended with liquids. Other acceptable foods include yogurt, custards, puddings, applesauce, mashed potatoes, blended cream soups, and cooked cereals (cream of wheat or cream of rice). Oatmeal should be smooth or blended.

107. B: Patients who are undergoing a spiritual crisis or change in their belief system often are not looking for advice but do need to express and explore their feelings. If the patient is distressed about her loss of faith, it is appropriate to ask if there is anyone that the patient would like to talk to about this issue.

108. B: Most patients with psychiatric illness are not violent, so the diagnosis alone should not cause the patient to be rejected. If there is concern that a worker may be in danger from a patient or family, then no home visit should be made.

109. C: Acupuncture, which involves the insertion of very thin needles into the skin, is thought to open energy channels via meridians in the body. Studies have indicated that acupuncture may relieve pain as well as nausea. Tai chi increases muscle strength and improves balance. Reiki, a form of energy healing, uses gentle touch to promote healing. In some cases, Reiki practitioners hold their hands above the skin without touching the patient. Chiropractic treatments involve manipulations of the spine and soft tissue.

110. A: This discussion should be carried out sensitively using age-appropriate, culturally sensitive language. The time following a patient's death can be very emotional, making it a difficult time for people to make decisions, and family members or health-care agents may be unaware of the patient's wishes.

111. D: In the Jewish tradition, every possible effort must generally be made to extend a patient's life. Medicine and those who practice medicine are considered an extension of God's divine power, so the active use of all available means of healing is supported. That said, many in the Orthodox Jewish community believe that, if medications may extend a life of suffering for a brief period but do not offer hope for saving the patient's life, they should generally be discontinued. This may not, however, be allowed in ultraconservative groups. Oxygen, nutrition, and fluids are generally not considered to be medical treatments (however they are provided) and must be continued as needed until the patient's death.

112. D: Continuous home care is provided for a time-limited period during an acute crisis. Routine care is reimbursed at daily rates, with a higher rate for days 1–60 than for subsequent days, whereas inpatient respite care and general inpatient care are reimbursed with set fees. Aggregate hospice payments for each patient are capped each year, and exceeding this limit may affect the subsequent year's cap.

113. D: The daughter has the legal right to make decisions, but she is disregarding the wishes of the patient. This situation places the physician and other health-care workers in a conflicted position.

114. A: Other contraindications include heart failure and peptic ulcer disease. Ibuprofen increases the risk of bleeding and the risk of heart attack or stroke. Ibuprofen should also be avoided in patients with cirrhosis of the liver. Ibuprofen is used to control mild to moderate pain and fever. Ibuprofen may be taken by itself, or it may be combined with acetaminophen or used as an adjuvant to opioid therapy.

115. C: The most appropriate pain management to reduce discomfort is topical anesthetics, such as lidocaine and tetracaine. A eutectic mixture of local anesthetics (EMLA) is an emulsion of 2.5% lidocaine and 2.5% prilocaine cream that is used as a topical anesthetic to provide anesthesia through the skin. It is frequently used to reduce pain associated with venipuncture or IV catheterization.

116. C: This is likely an indication of end-of-dose pain, when the blood level of the drug drops to less than the therapeutic amount. The solution is to increase the medication frequency (such as to every 8 hours) or to increase the dosage by 25–50%.

117. C: The patient and family should be advised to fold the used patch in half (with the sticky sides contacting each other) and flush it down the toilet. The patches should not be disposed of in the trash because someone could retrieve them. Children have died from chewing on the patches. Substance abusers have been known to smoke leftover patches, resulting in a sometimes-fatal dose of the drug.

118. C: The patient should be administered 10–20% of the 24-hour dose orally or 10% of the 24-hour dose intravenously. The pain should be assessed within 60 minutes for oral medication and within 15 minutes for intravenously administered medication. If the pain has decreased to a moderate level, then the same dosage may be repeated. If the pain has increased or has not improved, the dose may be increased by 50–100%.

119. D: The electrolytes that are most in danger of imbalance and must be monitored carefully are sodium and potassium.

- Sodium: Normal value: 135–145 mEq/L.
    - Hyponatremia: <135 mEq/L. Critical value: <120 mEq/L.
    - Hypernatremia: >145 mEq/L. Critical value: >160 mEq/L.
- Potassium: Normal value: 3.5–5 mEq/L.
    - Hypokalemia: <3.5 mEq/L. Critical value: <2.5 mEq/L.
    - Hyperkalemia: >5 mEq/L. Critical value: >6.5 mEq/L.

120. A: The initial response should be to reposition the patient by raising his or her head and turning the patient to one side. This may relieve some of the rattling. An anticholinergic drug, such as glycopyrrolate or atropine, may be administered if the breathing pattern is distressful for the patient's family. The rattling lessens as the patient becomes increasingly dehydrated.

121. B: The recommended dosing interval is every 8 hours, even though methadone has an extended half-life of 24–36 hours. If the patient is transitioning from morphine and the dosage is less than 100 mg, then the patient switches to methadone 5 mg every 8 hours. If the patient is taking more than 100 mg of morphine, then a 3-day rotation period is indicated, with the dose of morphine decreased 30–50% the first day and 35–50% the second day while the dose of methadone is slowly increased.

122. D: Under Medicare hospice coverage, a patient may receive general inpatient care for pain control or management of other symptoms if he or she cannot be managed in other settings, such as the home environment. Respite care is separate, and it allows the patient to receive inpatient care for up to 5 days to give the caregiver a break. Patients must agree to forgo treatment for their terminal condition when they sign on to hospice care.

123. B: If a patient experiences incident pain, which is triggered by an activity such as walking or bathing, he or she should receive a short-acting, rapid-onset analgesic 30–60 minutes before an activity in addition to the routine pain control that the patient already receives. If possible, the patient should use the same drug that is used for routine pain control. Incident pain differs from spontaneous pain in that incident pain is predictable but spontaneous pain is not.

124. D: Hospice bereavement services should begin at the start of care and continue for at least 13 months following the patient's death. The risk assessment should be carried out at the beginning of care, and factors that may lead to complicated grief should be identified. The interdisciplinary team must encourage the patient and family to express their feelings and help prepare them for the patient's death. Family members should be educated about the signs and symptoms associated with the dying process.

125. B: Fentanyl is not a cause of opioid-induced neurotoxicity because it does not contain active metabolites. Methadone also lacks active metabolites. Opioids with active metabolites are implicated in opioid-induced neurotoxicity; these include morphine, codeine, meperidine, oxycodone, and hydromorphone. The most common treatment or preventive is opioid rotation. Some patients may require a reduction in dosage or a switch to fentanyl or methadone.

126. C: The immediate response should be to administer naloxone, a reversal agent for opioids. The patient is exhibiting signs of opioid overdose. Naloxone may be administered by injection or nasal spray and should take effect within 1–2 minutes. *N*-acetylcysteine is the reversal agent for acetaminophen, flumazenil is the reversal agent for benzodiazepines, and sodium bicarbonate is a reversal agent for TCAs.

127. A: Anorexia/cachexia syndrome is most common in terminal patients with cancer, affecting up to 86%, so it is important to be alert to its indications. Anorexia/cachexia syndrome is associated with loss of appetite, fatigue and reduced activities, decreased muscle protein synthesis and immune response, and decreased response to treatments. As anorexia persists, it leads to fatigue, which in turn leads to increased anorexia. Treatment includes identifying underlying causes and providing nutritional support.

128. A: Liability results from knowingly submitting a false claim or making a false record or statement in order to receive payment for a false claim. False claims are those that the entity knows or should know are violations. These claims may include claims for care not rendered, care already billed for, miscoding/upcoding, and services not supported by documentation.

129. D: The most appropriate tool is the Pain Assessment in Advanced Dementia scale (PAINAD). Patients with dementia are typically unable to appropriately respond to verbal questions about pain or to make a decision about where their pain falls on a scale. PAINAD depends on careful observation of nonverbal indicators of pain: respirations, vocalization, facial expression, body language, and consolability.

130. A: Somatic pain may be sharp and localized or dull and aching, and results from damage to muscle, bone, or connective tissue. Neuropathic pain is often described as shocking, shooting, burning, or stabbing. Myofascial pain initially begins as sharp and localized but tends to become dull and aching over time.

131. D: Losing interest in food and drink is a normal progression that occurs as a patient is dying, and forcing food or fluids may result in aspiration. The family or caregivers should be advised to maintain the patient's oral hygiene and to apply lip balm to keep his or her lips from cracking.

132. D: Studies show that many patients receive relief within 10 days of a single palliative radiotherapy treatment. Radiotherapy treatments intended for relief of symptoms rather than treatment of the disease are acceptable while a patient is under hospice care. Radiotherapy may prevent fracture of the affected bone and may relieve spinal cord compression.

133. D: Although Medicare does, in general, cover palliative care separately from hospice benefits, it covers only medically necessary palliative care; therefore, some of the benefits extended to patients receiving palliative care under hospice may not apply. Medically necessary care may include inpatient treatment, skilled nursing facility care, and qualifying home health care. Palliative care is not treated as a separate form of care like hospice care is. Inpatient care is covered by Medicare A or Medicare Advantage (Medicare C) plans. Medicare B covers medically necessary outpatient services, such as home health services, physical therapy, mental health counseling, and durable medical equipment.

134. D: With Alzheimer's disease, multiple factors must be present to qualify for hospice care:

- Lack of intelligible speech or speech limited to six words/phrases or repetitive phrases
- A Functional Assessment Staging Tool (FAST) score of 7 or higher (a score of 1 is normal; scores of 2–5 represent mild to moderate impairment)
- Assistance being required to ambulate, dress, or bathe
- Incontinence of urine and feces

Additionally, one or more of the following should have been present in the previous year: aspiration pneumonia, upper respiratory infection, septicemia, decubiti (stages 3–4), and recurrent infection; and in the previous 6 months: weight loss of 10% or more or a 10% decrease in albumin.

135. C: If patients have reduced liver function, the maximum dose should be reduced by half. Because acetaminophen is metabolized in the liver, if liver function is impaired, the blood level of acetaminophen may reach toxic levels. If a patient is in liver failure, other medications should be used.

136. B: Signs of hospice eligibility for a patient with Parkinson's disease include compromised breathing and recurring aspiration pneumonia because these are life-threatening symptoms. Other indications of eligibility include increased dyspnea that is unrelieved with oxygen, frequent choking resulting in the need for a pureed diet, persistent weight loss, and an inability to manage ADLs.

137. C: This is referred to as a spiritual screening because it is short and not in depth. A spiritual history is more comprehensive and usually involves the use of a standard set of questions. A spiritual assessment is typically conducted by a chaplain and depends more on actively listening to the patient rather than obtaining answers to specific questions.

138. A: Fibromyalgia is a complex syndrome with symptoms that include fatigue, chronic generalized muscle pain, and focal areas of tenderness persisting for at least 3 months. Symptoms may also include irritable bowel syndrome; sleep disorders; mood disorders; sensitivities to odor, noises, and lights; and paresthesia in the hands and feet. Treatment may include analgesia, antidepressants, physical therapy, and pregabalin (Lyrica).

139. A: An appropriate patient outcome is that the patient will express feelings about dying or seek help to deal with concerns. Sometimes, assisting a patient with a life review can help the patient come to terms with dying. Indications of death anxiety include sadness, fear of dying, fear of pain associated with dying, fear of the unknown, concerns about leaving family members, and the family's ability to cope.

140. D: During stage 1 lymphedema, elevation above the heart is often adequate on its own to control swelling, but as lymphedema progresses, compression garments can provide better control. A variety of compression garments and devices are available. Decongestive therapy for stages 1 and 2 lymphedema also includes exercise, use of an arm pump, and infection prevention strategies.

141. B: These individuals are entitled to literature in their language (such as hospice pamphlets and guidelines) and translators that are available 24 hours a day, 7 days a week. Although patients are not entitled to health-care workers who speak their language, staff members should make an effort to learn at least a few words in languages that are commonly encountered locally in order to improve communication and establish rapport.

142. C: Aerosolized racemic epinephrine is administered by a nebulizer, with a response occurring within 10 minutes and a duration of effect of 60-90 minutes. The dose may be repeated in 1 hour. If family members are prepared in advance for the possibility of stridor, it may be less distressing. Dexamethasone may be administered 12 hours prior to extubation if airway edema is anticipated.

143. A: A more appropriate response would be to arrange for respite care, refer the caregiver to an online or in-person support group, or arrange for homemaker assistance to give the caregiver a break.

144. C: A period of detachment before death is common. The family may play soft music, dim the lights, talk softly, and gently touch the patient. The family should be advised that patients can often hear what is said even if they are not responding.

145. C: Although fiscal responsibility, patient satisfaction, and legal compliance are important components of a quality assessment and performance improvement program, the focus should be on improved outcomes. These may apply not only to patient outcomes but also to other factors, such as staff retention, financial stability, service delivery, and accreditation. Staff members at all levels of the organization should work to identify areas for potential improvement.

146. B: The following items are scored with 0 (no problem), 1 (some problem), or 2 (severe problem):

1. Abdominal distension/bloating	5. Rectal fullness/pressure
2. Change in the amount of gas passed (rectally)	6. Rectal pain with bowel movement
3. Less-frequent bowel movements	7. Small stool size
4. Oozing liquid stool	8. Inability to pass stool despite urges

147. A: If a patient is identified as being a military veteran, the nurse should complete the military history checklist, which is a one-page form used to elicit information about the patient's service experience, branch and duration of service, and possible VA benefits. In addition, the form asks how the patient views his or her military experience and whether the patient has service-connected conditions (such as injuries, disabilities, or post-traumatic stress disorder), and asks for contact information for the patient's VA physician or primary care provider.

148. C: Physical therapy improves circulation and maintains mobility and muscle strength. Other treatments include psychotherapy (depression is common), medications (e.g., TCAs, anticonvulsants), spinal cord/neural stimulation, drug pumps, medical marijuana, acupuncture, sympathetic nerve blocks, and surgical sympathectomy.

149. B: The PQRST pain assessment tool is explained as follows:

- P—Provoking factors/palliative: What brings on the pain? Makes it better? Worse? What medications are you using? How often? Are they effective? Any side effects? Are there any other medications?
- Q—Quality/quantity: Can you describe the pain?
- R—Region/radiation: Where do you feel the pain? Does it spread to other areas? S—Severity: How severe is the pain? Now? At its worst? At its best? Does it affect your ability to perform ADLs?
- T—Timing/treatment: When did the pain start? Is it constant or intermittent? What is its duration and frequency?

150. B: The usual dose is 4–8 mg PO or parenterally every 8 hours on the day of treatment, with an initial dose 30 minutes before treatment. Alternate dosing includes 16–24 mg in one dose orally or 8–16 mg IV in one dose. Ondansetron is an antiemetic and a selective serotonin receptor antagonist.

How to Overcome Test Anxiety

Just the thought of taking a test is enough to make most people a little nervous. A test is an important event that can have a long-term impact on your future, so it's important to take it seriously and it's natural to feel anxious about performing well. But just because anxiety is normal, that doesn't mean that it's helpful in test taking, or that you should simply accept it as part of your life. Anxiety can have a variety of effects. These effects can be mild, like making you feel slightly nervous, or severe, like blocking your ability to focus or remember even a simple detail.

If you experience test anxiety—whether severe or mild—it's important to know how to beat it. To discover this, first you need to understand what causes test anxiety.

Causes of Test Anxiety

While we often think of anxiety as an uncontrollable emotional state, it can actually be caused by simple, practical things. One of the most common causes of test anxiety is that a person does not feel adequately prepared for their test. This feeling can be the result of many different issues such as poor study habits or lack of organization, but the most common culprit is time management. Starting to study too late, failing to organize your study time to cover all of the material, or being distracted while you study will mean that you're not well prepared for the test. This may lead to cramming the night before, which will cause you to be physically and mentally exhausted for the test. Poor time management also contributes to feelings of stress, fear, and hopelessness as you realize you are not well prepared but don't know what to do about it.

Other times, test anxiety is not related to your preparation for the test but comes from unresolved fear. This may be a past failure on a test, or poor performance on tests in general. It may come from comparing yourself to others who seem to be performing better or from the stress of living up to expectations. Anxiety may be driven by fears of the future—how failure on this test would affect your educational and career goals. These fears are often completely irrational, but they can still negatively impact your test performance.

Elements of Test Anxiety

As mentioned earlier, test anxiety is considered to be an emotional state, but it has physical and mental components as well. Sometimes you may not even realize that you are suffering from test anxiety until you notice the physical symptoms. These can include trembling hands, rapid heartbeat, sweating, nausea, and tense muscles. Extreme anxiety may lead to fainting or vomiting. Obviously, any of these symptoms can have a negative impact on testing. It is important to recognize them as soon as they begin to occur so that you can address the problem before it damages your performance.

The mental components of test anxiety include trouble focusing and inability to remember learned information. During a test, your mind is on high alert, which can help you recall information and stay focused for an extended period of time. However, anxiety interferes with your mind's natural processes, causing you to blank out, even on the questions you know well. The strain of testing during anxiety makes it difficult to stay focused, especially on a test that may take several hours. Extreme anxiety can take a huge mental toll, making it difficult not only to recall test information but even to understand the test questions or pull your thoughts together.

Effects of Test Anxiety

Test anxiety is like a disease—if left untreated, it will get progressively worse. Anxiety leads to poor performance, and this reinforces the feelings of fear and failure, which in turn lead to poor performances on subsequent tests. It can grow from a mild nervousness to a crippling condition. If allowed to progress, test anxiety can have a big impact on your schooling, and consequently on your future.

Test anxiety can spread to other parts of your life. Anxiety on tests can become anxiety in any stressful situation, and blanking on a test can turn into panicking in a job situation. But fortunately, you don't have to let anxiety rule your testing and determine your grades. There are a number of relatively simple steps you can take to move past anxiety and function normally on a test and in the rest of life.

Physical Steps for Beating Test Anxiety

While test anxiety is a serious problem, the good news is that it can be overcome. It doesn't have to control your ability to think and remember information. While it may take time, you can begin taking steps today to beat anxiety.

Just as your first hint that you may be struggling with anxiety comes from the physical symptoms, the first step to treating it is also physical. Rest is crucial for having a clear, strong mind. If you are tired, it is much easier to give in to anxiety. But if you establish good sleep habits, your body and mind will be ready to perform optimally, without the strain of exhaustion. Additionally, sleeping well helps you to retain information better, so you're more likely to recall the answers when you see the test questions.

Getting good sleep means more than going to bed on time. It's important to allow your brain time to relax. Take study breaks from time to time so it doesn't get overworked, and don't study right before bed. Take time to rest your mind before trying to rest your body, or you may find it difficult to fall asleep.

Along with sleep, other aspects of physical health are important in preparing for a test. Good nutrition is vital for good brain function. Sugary foods and drinks may give a burst of energy but this burst is followed by a crash, both physically and emotionally. Instead, fuel your body with protein and vitamin-rich foods.

Also, drink plenty of water. Dehydration can lead to headaches and exhaustion, especially if your brain is already under stress from the rigors of the test. Particularly if your test is a long one, drink water during the breaks. And if possible, take an energy-boosting snack to eat between sections.

Along with sleep and diet, a third important part of physical health is exercise. Maintaining a steady workout schedule is helpful, but even taking 5-minute study breaks to walk can help get your blood pumping faster and clear your head. Exercise also releases endorphins, which contribute to a positive feeling and can help combat test anxiety.

When you nurture your physical health, you are also contributing to your mental health. If your body is healthy, your mind is much more likely to be healthy as well. So take time to rest, nourish your body with healthy food and water, and get moving as much as possible. Taking these physical steps will make you stronger and more able to take the mental steps necessary to overcome test anxiety.

Mental Steps for Beating Test Anxiety

Working on the mental side of test anxiety can be more challenging, but as with the physical side, there are clear steps you can take to overcome it. As mentioned earlier, test anxiety often stems from lack of preparation, so the obvious solution is to prepare for the test. Effective studying may be the most important weapon you have for beating test anxiety, but you can and should employ several other mental tools to combat fear.

First, boost your confidence by reminding yourself of past success—tests or projects that you aced. If you're putting as much effort into preparing for this test as you did for those, there's no reason you should expect to fail here. Work hard to prepare; then trust your preparation.

Second, surround yourself with encouraging people. It can be helpful to find a study group, but be sure that the people you're around will encourage a positive attitude. If you spend time with others who are anxious or cynical, this will only contribute to your own anxiety. Look for others who are motivated to study hard from a desire to succeed, not from a fear of failure.

Third, reward yourself. A test is physically and mentally tiring, even without anxiety, and it can be helpful to have something to look forward to. Plan an activity following the test, regardless of the outcome, such as going to a movie or getting ice cream.

When you are taking the test, if you find yourself beginning to feel anxious, remind yourself that you know the material. Visualize successfully completing the test. Then take a few deep, relaxing breaths and return to it. Work through the questions carefully but with confidence, knowing that you are capable of succeeding.

Developing a healthy mental approach to test taking will also aid in other areas of life. Test anxiety affects more than just the actual test—it can be damaging to your mental health and even contribute to depression. It's important to beat test anxiety before it becomes a problem for more than testing.

Study Strategy

Being prepared for the test is necessary to combat anxiety, but what does being prepared look like? You may study for hours on end and still not feel prepared. What you need is a strategy for test prep. The next few pages outline our recommended steps to help you plan out and conquer the challenge of preparation.

Step 1: Scope Out the Test

Learn everything you can about the format (multiple choice, essay, etc.) and what will be on the test. Gather any study materials, course outlines, or sample exams that may be available. Not only will this help you to prepare, but knowing what to expect can help to alleviate test anxiety.

Step 2: Map Out the Material

Look through the textbook or study guide and make note of how many chapters or sections it has. Then divide these over the time you have. For example, if a book has 15 chapters and you have five days to study, you need to cover three chapters each day. Even better, if you have the time, leave an extra day at the end for overall review after you have gone through the material in depth.

If time is limited, you may need to prioritize the material. Look through it and make note of which sections you think you already have a good grasp on, and which need review. While you are studying, skim quickly through the familiar sections and take more time on the challenging parts.

Write out your plan so you don't get lost as you go. Having a written plan also helps you feel more in control of the study, so anxiety is less likely to arise from feeling overwhelmed at the amount to cover.

Step 3: Gather Your Tools

Decide what study method works best for you. Do you prefer to highlight in the book as you study and then go back over the highlighted portions? Or do you type out notes of the important information? Or is it helpful to make flashcards that you can carry with you? Assemble the pens, index cards, highlighters, post-it notes, and any other materials you may need so you won't be distracted by getting up to find things while you study.

If you're having a hard time retaining the information or organizing your notes, experiment with different methods. For example, try color-coding by subject with colored pens, highlighters, or post-it notes. If you learn better by hearing, try recording yourself reading your notes so you can listen while in the car, working out, or simply sitting at your desk. Ask a friend to quiz you from your flashcards, or try teaching someone the material to solidify it in your mind.

Step 4: Create Your Environment

It's important to avoid distractions while you study. This includes both the obvious distractions like visitors and the subtle distractions like an uncomfortable chair (or a too-comfortable couch that makes you want to fall asleep). Set up the best study environment possible: good lighting and a comfortable work area. If background music helps you focus, you may want to turn it on, but otherwise keep the room quiet. If you are using a computer to take notes, be sure you don't have any other windows open, especially applications like social media, games, or anything else that could distract you. Silence your phone and turn off notifications. Be sure to keep water close by so you stay hydrated while you study (but avoid unhealthy drinks and snacks).

Also, take into account the best time of day to study. Are you freshest first thing in the morning? Try to set aside some time then to work through the material. Is your mind clearer in the afternoon or evening? Schedule your study session then. Another method is to study at the same time of day that you will take the test, so that your brain gets used to working on the material at that time and will be ready to focus at test time.

Step 5: Study!

Once you have done all the study preparation, it's time to settle into the actual studying. Sit down, take a few moments to settle your mind so you can focus, and begin to follow your study plan. Don't give in to distractions or let yourself procrastinate. This is your time to prepare so you'll be ready to fearlessly approach the test. Make the most of the time and stay focused.

Of course, you don't want to burn out. If you study too long you may find that you're not retaining the information very well. Take regular study breaks. For example, taking five minutes out of every hour to walk briskly, breathing deeply and swinging your arms, can help your mind stay fresh.

As you get to the end of each chapter or section, it's a good idea to do a quick review. Remind yourself of what you learned and work on any difficult parts. When you feel that you've mastered the material, move on to the next part. At the end of your study session, briefly skim through your notes again.

But while review is helpful, cramming last minute is NOT. If at all possible, work ahead so that you won't need to fit all your study into the last day. Cramming overloads your brain with more information than it can process and retain, and your tired mind may struggle to recall even previously learned information when it is overwhelmed with last-minute study. Also, the urgent nature of cramming and the stress placed on your brain contribute to anxiety. You'll be more likely to go to the test feeling unprepared and having trouble thinking clearly.

So don't cram, and don't stay up late before the test, even just to review your notes at a leisurely pace. Your brain needs rest more than it needs to go over the information again. In fact, plan to finish your studies by noon or early afternoon the day before the test. Give your brain the rest of the day to relax or focus on other things, and get a good night's sleep. Then you will be fresh for the test and better able to recall what you've studied.

Step 6: Take a Practice Test

Many courses offer sample tests, either online or in the study materials. This is an excellent resource to check whether you have mastered the material, as well as to prepare for the test format and environment.

Check the test format ahead of time: the number of questions, the type (multiple choice, free response, etc.), and the time limit. Then create a plan for working through them. For example, if you have 30 minutes to take a 60-question test, your limit is 30 seconds per question. Spend less time on the questions you know well so that you can take more time on the difficult ones.

If you have time to take several practice tests, take the first one open book, with no time limit. Work through the questions at your own pace and make sure you fully understand them. Gradually work up to taking a test under test conditions: sit at a desk with all study materials put away and set a timer. Pace yourself to make sure you finish the test with time to spare and go back to check your answers if you have time.

After each test, check your answers. On the questions you missed, be sure you understand why you missed them. Did you misread the question (tests can use tricky wording)? Did you forget the information? Or was it something you hadn't learned? Go back and study any shaky areas that the practice tests reveal.

Taking these tests not only helps with your grade, but also aids in combating test anxiety. If you're already used to the test conditions, you're less likely to worry about it, and working through tests until you're scoring well gives you a confidence boost. Go through the practice tests until you feel comfortable, and then you can go into the test knowing that you're ready for it.

Test Tips

On test day, you should be confident, knowing that you've prepared well and are ready to answer the questions. But aside from preparation, there are several test day strategies you can employ to maximize your performance.

First, as stated before, get a good night's sleep the night before the test (and for several nights before that, if possible). Go into the test with a fresh, alert mind rather than staying up late to study.

Try not to change too much about your normal routine on the day of the test. It's important to eat a nutritious breakfast, but if you normally don't eat breakfast at all, consider eating just a protein bar. If you're a coffee drinker, go ahead and have your normal coffee. Just make sure you time it so that the caffeine doesn't wear off right in the middle of your test. Avoid sugary beverages, and drink enough water to stay hydrated but not so much that you need a restroom break 10 minutes into the test. If your test isn't first thing in the morning, consider going for a walk or doing a light workout before the test to get your blood flowing.

Allow yourself enough time to get ready, and leave for the test with plenty of time to spare so you won't have the anxiety of scrambling to arrive in time. Another reason to be early is to select a good seat. It's helpful to sit away from doors and windows, which can be distracting. Find a good seat, get out your supplies, and settle your mind before the test begins.

When the test begins, start by going over the instructions carefully, even if you already know what to expect. Make sure you avoid any careless mistakes by following the directions.

Then begin working through the questions, pacing yourself as you've practiced. If you're not sure on an answer, don't spend too much time on it, and don't let it shake your confidence. Either skip it and come back later, or eliminate as many wrong answers as possible and guess among the remaining ones. Don't dwell on these questions as you continue—put them out of your mind and focus on what lies ahead.

Be sure to read all of the answer choices, even if you're sure the first one is the right answer. Sometimes you'll find a better one if you keep reading. But don't second-guess yourself if you do immediately know the answer. Your gut instinct is usually right. Don't let test anxiety rob you of the information you know.

If you have time at the end of the test (and if the test format allows), go back and review your answers. Be cautious about changing any, since your first instinct tends to be correct, but make sure you didn't misread any of the questions or accidentally mark the wrong answer choice. Look over any you skipped and make an educated guess.

At the end, leave the test feeling confident. You've done your best, so don't waste time worrying about your performance or wishing you could change anything. Instead, celebrate the successful completion of this test. And finally, use this test to learn how to deal with anxiety even better next time.

Review Video: Test Anxiety
Visit mometrix.com/academy and enter code: 100340

Important Qualification

Not all anxiety is created equal. If your test anxiety is causing major issues in your life beyond the classroom or testing center, or if you are experiencing troubling physical symptoms related to your anxiety, it may be a sign of a serious physiological or psychological condition. If this sounds like your situation, we strongly encourage you to seek professional help.

Online Resources

Due to our efforts to try to keep this book to a manageable length, we've created a link that will give you access to all of your online resources:

mometrix.com/resources719/chpn-19006

It's Your Moment, Let's Celebrate It!

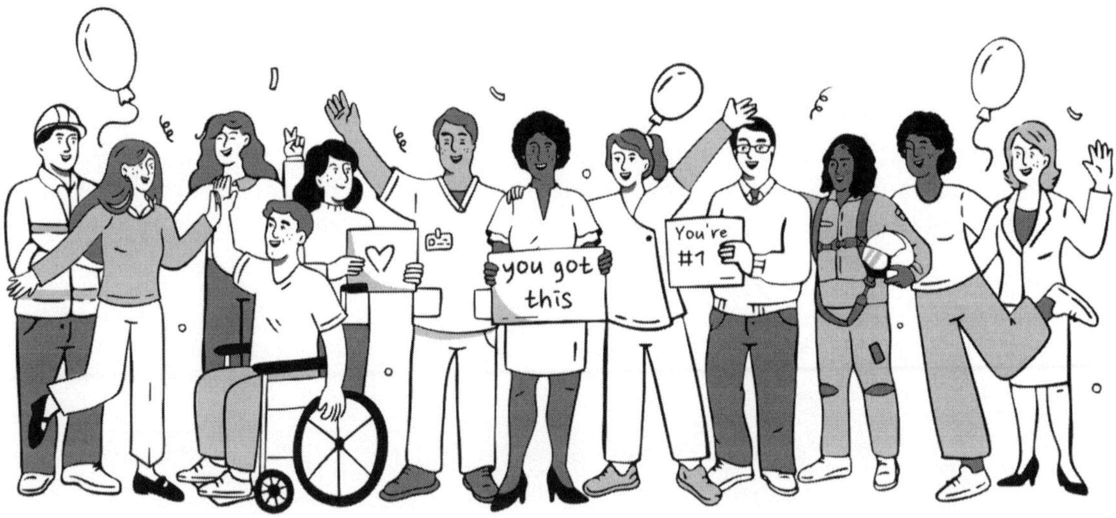

Share your story @mometrixtestpreparation